KEY TOPICS IN

SPORTS MEDICINE

Key Topics books contain the information you need for:

- Clinical guidance – rapid access to concise details and facts
- Postgraduate exams – an essential revision guide

Clear and comprehensive, *Key Topics in Sports Medicine* is a single quick reference source for sports and exercise medicine. It presents the essential information from across relevant topic areas, and includes both the core and emerging issues in this rapidly developing field. It covers:

- Sports injuries, rehabilitation and injury prevention
- Exercise physiology, fitness testing and training
- Drugs in sport
- Exercise and health promotion
- Sport and exercise for special and clinical populations
- The psychology of performance and injury.

Based on graduate programme teaching practice and with an international team of contributors, this is a valuable and practical resource for all those interested in sports and exercise medicine, including sports clinicians, general practitioners, team doctors, orthopaedic surgeons, accident and emergency doctors and physiotherapists.

Amir Ali Narvani is Specialist Registrar in Orthopaedics and Trauma, North West Thames Rotation. **Panagiotis Thomas** is co-director of the MSc School of Human Health and Performance at University College London and Consultant Orthopaedic Surgeon at the Whittington Hospital NHS Trust, London. **Bruce Lynn** is Professor of Physiology and co-director of the MSc School of Human Health and Performance at University College London.

The KEY TOPICS Series

Accident and Emergency Medicine, Second Edition
Anaesthesia, Third Edition
Cardiac Surgery
Cardiovascular Medicine
Clinical Research
Critical Care, Second Edition
Evidence-Based Medicine
Gastroenterology
General Surgery, Second Edition
Human Diseases for Dental Students
Neonatology, Second Edition
Neurology
Obstetrics and Gynaecology, Second Edition
Oncology
Ophthalmology, Second Edition
Oral and Maxillofacial Surgery
Orthopaedic Surgery
Orthopaedic Trauma Surgery
Otolaryngology, Second Edition
Paediatrics, Second Edition
Pain Management, Third Edition
Plastic and Reconstructive Surgery
Psychiatry
Renal Medicine
Respiratory Medicine
Sexual Health
Thoracic Surgery
Trauma
Urology

KEY TOPICS IN

SPORTS MEDICINE

Edited by

A A Narvani, P Thomas and B Lynn

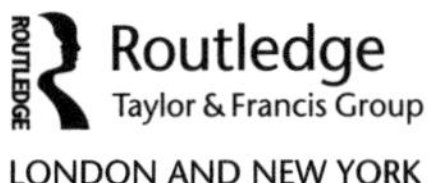

LONDON AND NEW YORK

First published in the United Kingdom in 2006
by Routledge
2 Park Square, Milton Park, Abingdon, Oxon OX14 4RN

Simultaneously published in the USA and Canada
by Routledge
270 Madison Ave, New York, NY 10016

Routledge is an imprint of the Taylor & Francis Group, an informa business

Typeset in Times by Wearset Ltd, Boldon, Tyne and Wear
Printed and bound in Great Britain by TJ International Ltd, Padstow, Cornwall

Although every effort has been made to ensure that drug doses and other information are presented accurately in this publication, the ultimate responsibility rests with the prescribing physician. Neither the publishers nor the authors can be held responsible for errors or for any consequences arising from the use of information contained herein. For detailed prescribing information or instructions on the use of any product or procedure discussed herein, please consult the prescribing information or instructional material issued by the manufacturer.

British Library Cataloguing in Publication Data
A catalogue record for this book is available from the British Library

Library of Congress Cataloging in Publication Data
Narvani, A. A. (Amir Ali), 1971–
Key topics in sports medicine / A.A. Narvani, P. Thomas, and B. Lynn.
p. ; cm. — (Key topics series)
Includes bibliographical references and index.
1. Sports medicine—Handbooks, manuals, etc. I. Thomas, P. (Panagiotis), 1960– II. Lynn, Bruce, 1943– III. Title. IV. Title: Sports medicine. V. Series.
[DNLM: 1. Athletic Injuries—Handbooks. 2. Sports Medicine—Handbooks. QT 261 N238k 2006]
RC1211.N37 2006
617.1′027—dc22

2006008644

ISBN10: 0-415-41122-X (hbk)
ISBN10: 1-841-84441-1 (pbk)
ISBN10: 0-203-48015-5 (ebk)

ISBN13: 978-0-415-41122-6 (hbk)
ISBN13: 978-1-84184-441-1 (pbk)
ISBN13: 978-0-203-48015-1 (ebk)

To my father, who taught me how a father could also be his son's best friend, defined kindness and generosity for me and introduced me to the wonderful world of sport.

To my mother, who is the main reason for every success that I have ever had and whose sacrifices I truly appreciate.

To my wife without whose support and patience this book would not have been possible.

I would also like to thank my co-editors, all of the contributing authors and the publishing company Routledge.

A A Narvani

To my parents, my wife Jennie and my two daughters Bethany and Jessica Thomas.

P Thomas

To my long-suffering family.

B Lynn

Contents

List of contributors

T Betts BSc(Hons), Grad Dip Phys, Grad Dip Sports, MSCP, SRP
Chartered Physiotherapist – Sports Medicine
Royal National Orthopaedic Hospital

O Haddo BSc, MBBS, MRCS
Specialist Registrar in Trauma & Orthopaedics
North East Thames Rotation

A Kamvari MBBS
United Medical School of Guy's & St Thomas' Hospitals

MF Khan MS, MD, MRCP
Cardiology Research Fellow
Harvard Medical School & Department of Clinical Biometrics
Brigham and Women's Hospital
Boston, USA

JL Livingstone BSc, D.Pod.M, M.Ch.S, S.R.Ch
Consultant Podiatrist
Barnet General Hospital

B Lynn BSc PhD
Professor of Physiology
Director, MSc School of Human Health and Performance
University College London

B Modarai BSc MB BS MRCS (Eng & Ed)
Specialist Registrar in General Surgery, St Thomas' Hospital, London
South East Thames Rotation

F Monibi BDS, MFDSRCS, MRDRCS(Eng), MRDRCPS(Glas), Master of Clinical Dentistry
Specialist Prosthodontist

N Munir MBBCH, MRCS(Eng), DO-HNS
Registrar in Otorhinolaryngology and Head and Neck Surgery, Queen's Medical Centre, Nottingham

AA Narvani BSc, MBBS(Hons), MRCS(Eng), MSc(Sport Med.)(Hons)
Specialist Registrar in Trauma & Orthopaedics, Chelsea and Westminster Hospital, London
North West Thames Rotation

S Parnia MBBS, PhD, MRCP
Fellow in Pulmonary & Critical Care Medicine,
Weill Cornell Medical Center, New York, USA
Honorary Senior Research Fellow
School of Medicine, University of Southampton, UK

M Ramachandran BSc(Hons), MBBS(Hons), MRCS(Eng), FRCS(Tr & Orth)
Paediatric and Young Adult Orthopaedic Fellow, Children's Hospital Los Angeles and Westmead Hospital, Sydney
Base rotation: Royal National Orthopaedic Hospital, Stanmore, Middlesex

R Sreekumar FRCS, M.Ch(Orth)
Lower Limb Fellow
Wrightington Hospital, Wigan

P Thomas MD, CCST(Orth), FRCS
Director of MSc in Sports and Exercise Medicine, Hon. Senior Lecturer University College London
Consultant Orthopaedic Surgeon at the Whittington Hospital NHS Trust

EE Tsiridis MD, MSc(Orth), PhD, FRCS
Consultant Orthopaedics and Trauma Surgeon
St James' University Hospital, Leeds Teaching Hospitals

Preface

The principal aim of this book is to provide a quick reference source for sport and exercise medicine. We have been influenced by our experience teaching (and in one case studying on) graduate level courses in this area. The key notes style is ideal for this purpose. We have deliberately kept anatomical illustrations to a minimum to reduce cost. Most readers will have favourite anatomy texts, and these days good anatomical diagrams are easy to find on the web.

The core of the book is a thorough coverage of sports injuries and the related areas of rehabilitation and of injury prevention. Modern sports medicine, however, needs to deal with many other issues such as sports psychology, exercise in extreme environments, or drugs in sport. The widening participation in sport by all sectors of the population means that there needs to be an awareness of the special issues related to women, to older people, and to those with disabilities. Finally, coverage of key topics on the exercise aspect of sports and exercise medicine is crucial. In the developed world, exercise and health are high on the political agenda and those involved in sports and exercise medicine are well placed to contribute to the development of effective public health programmes related to exercise and health.

AA Narvani
P Thomas
B Lynn

Abdominal injuries in sport

B Modarai

Aetiology

Sporting accidents can cause serious abdominal injuries that need prompt attention to avoid catastrophic consequences. The abdomen is largely unprotected and may be damaged in blunt impacts and rapid decelerations in sports that include rugby, football, ice hockey and downhill skiing. Penetrating injuries are associated with cycling, motor cycling, fencing and shooting.

Blunt trauma can damage solid organs including the spleen, the liver and retroperitoneal organs. Penetrating trauma frequently involves the small bowel, colon, diaphragm and liver. It is more important to recognise the need for urgent laparotomy in the unstable patient than to waste time determining the specific injury.

Sports-related abdominal trauma may cause non-specific symptoms and signs and can pose a diagnostic challenge to the unsuspecting clinician. A high index of suspicion is, therefore, required to avoid pitfalls. Athletes have a substantial cardiovascular reserve which may mask the effects of ongoing intra-abdominal haemorrhage. A large volume of blood has usually been lost by the time a drop in systolic blood pressure is evident and this will worsen the prognosis.

Clinical features

Specific symptoms and signs are initially absent in as many as 20% of athletes with a serious abdominal injury, therefore, serial examinations are essential. The abdomen should be inspected for abrasions and bruising, especially to the right and left upper quadrants and flanks. Ecchymosis involving the flanks (Grey Turner sign) or the umbilicus (Cullen sign) indicates retroperitoneal haemorrhage. Localised swelling, fullness in the flanks and generalised abdominal distension may be present. Tenderness, guarding and rebound indicate peritoneal irritation by blood or visceral contents. Localised tenderness may arise from the musculature of the abdominal wall or from damaged internal organs.

Penetrating wounds can be gently explored under aseptic conditions to ascertain depth of the wound and to determine whether the peritoneal cavity has been breached. Examination of the external genitalia and a digital rectal examination is mandatory.

Investigations

Useful blood tests include a full blood count, group and save and a blood cross match if the patient is haemodynamically unstable. Deranged liver function tests are associated with liver injury. A sample of urine should be tested for blood and βHCG in females.

An erect chest X-ray may show free air under the diaphragm or a ruptured hemidiaphragm. The presence of lower rib fractures should raise the suspicion of damage to the spleen or liver.

Displacement of the gastric air bubble and loss of the psoas shadow on an abdominal X-ray are associated with, respectively, splenic rupture and free intra-peritoneal fluid.

An ultrasound scan, carried out by an experienced sonographer, can identify free intra-peritoneal fluid.

A contrast-enhanced abdominal CT scan is the investigation of choice in the haemodynamically stable patient and can demonstrate a pneumoperitoneum, free intra-peritoneal fluid or specific signs of organ damage. This investigation is particularly useful for imaging the pancreas, duodenum and genitourinary system.

Management

The immediate priority in any patient with a suspected abdominal injury is to assess the airway, breathing and circulation. Two large-bore peripheral intravenous lines should be sited and used to administer 2 litres of intravenous fluid. The haemodynamically unstable patient who does not respond to fluid resuscitation requires an urgent laparotomy provided all other sources of haemorrhage have been excluded.

Some of the indications for urgent laparotomy are:

- Blunt abdominal trauma with persistent hypotension despite resuscitation
- Hypotension associated with a penetrating abdominal wound
- Peritonitis
- Evisceration
- Free air seen on erect chest X-ray.

Diagnostic imaging in the haemodynamically stable patient can demonstrate injuries that are amenable to non-operative treatment. Splenic, liver and kidney injuries are increasingly being treated conservatively.

Specific injuries

The abdominal wall

Contusions of the abdominal wall musculature are common in athletes and must be remembered as a cause of pain. It is important to distinguish simple contusions from rectus sheath haematomas, which develop after bleeding from the inferior or superior epigastric arteries. A rectus sheath haematoma may be palpable as a tender mass above or below the arcuate line and may represent a significant blood loss. Contraction of the abdominal muscles increases the pain associated with injuries to the abdominal wall (Fothergill's sign) whereas it improves the pain related to deeper visceral injury.

Both ultrasound and CT scanning will demonstrate a suspected rectus sheath haematoma but the latter is the investigation of choice. Most non-expanding haematomas can be managed conservatively with rest and analgesia. The condition usually improves within 3–5 days but complete resolution, depending on the size of the haematoma, will usually take 1–4 months.

Abdominal wall hernias, commonly inguinal and femoral, can develop or worsen after heavy lifting or following a sudden increase in intra-abdominal pressure. The "sports hernia", first described by Gilmore, refers to a subtle disruption of the inguinal canal that occurs with repeated twisting and turning in activities such as ice hockey. A torn external oblique aponeurosis causing dilatation of the superficial inguinal ring, a torn conjoint tendon and a dehiscence between the torn conjoint tendon and the inguinal ligament are most often described as the causes of Gilmore's hernia. Non-operative management is rarely successful. The operations carried out are variations on the standard technique employed for inguinal hernia repair. Return to sporting activity is usually allowed 6–8 weeks after surgery.

Liver and spleen

The spleen is the most frequently injured abdominal organ. Bruising in the left hypochondrium, lower rib fractures, left upper quadrant tenderness, left shoulder tip pain (Kehr's sign), tachycardia and hypotension should alert the clinician to a splenic injury. Liver injuries present with similar, but right-sided symptoms and signs. The liver may be lacerated by blunt or penetrating trauma. The haemodynamically unstable patient who does not respond to resuscitation needs an urgent laparotomy. A contrast-enhanced CT scan in the haemodynamically stable patient will show the severity of organ injury and has increased non-operative management of both splenic and hepatic injuries.

Small bowel

The entire small bowel is at risk in penetrating trauma. A sudden deceleration can cause tearing at a point where the bowel is fixed (e.g. the duodeno–jejunal flexure) and direct blows to the abdomen can lead to bowel rupture. Rupture of the duodenum and jejunum has been reported in football, ice hockey, biking and motorcycling accidents.

The patient may have minimal symptoms and signs immediately after the injury and may only start to deteriorate after 2–3 days. A bloody aspirate from a nasogastric tube, chest X-ray showing air under the diaphragm or retroperitoneal air on abdominal X-ray should raise suspicion. An urgent laparotomy is required.

Blunt abdominal injury may also cause mural haematomas of the duodenum and jejunum and the thickening of the bowel can lead to obstruction. Small bowel obstruction presents with vomiting, abdominal distension and constipation, sometimes days after the initial injury. Stable patients can be managed conservatively with nasogastric suction and intravenous fluid resuscitation.

Stomach

Gastric rupture can occur with both penetrating and blunt trauma. It has also been reported after swift ascents from deep scuba dives where rapid expansion of air trapped within the organ causes rupture. Presentation can be insidious with diffuse abdominal pain developing into perotinism.

Pancreas

A direct blow to the abdomen can crush the pancreas against the vertebral column and cause pancreatitis. Diagnosis of this condition is notoriously difficult and delayed recognition often worsens the prognosis. Symptoms include vague upper abdominal pain radiating to the back, accompanied by nausea and vomiting. A normal serum amylase does not exclude pancreatic injury. A contrast-enhanced CT is the most useful investigation. Treatment is usually non-operative but this depends on the severity of injury.

Return to sport

Most abdominal injuries necessitating a laparotomy will require 7–10 days in hospital and return to competitive sport may take 4 months or longer. The decision to allow athletes with a single kidney or testicle to participate in contact sports is controversial. The possible mechanisms of injury and the risk of further trauma must be considered on an individual basis before making a decision. The young athlete with a single testicle should be counselled about storing a sample of semen before resuming participation in contact sports.

Further reading

Ryan JM. Abdominal injuries and sport. *Br J Sports Med* 1999; **33**: 155–60.
Cramer FS, Heimbach RD. Stomach rupture as a result of gastrointestinal barotrauma in a SCUBA diver. *J Trauma* 1982; **22**: 238–40.

Achilles tendon rupture

AA Narvani

The Achilles tendon is formed by the merging of the tendinous portions of the gastrocnemius and soleus muscles. The incidence of Achilles tendon rupture in the general population is estimated to be around 18 per 100,000 and appears to be increasing. Between 40 to 80% of the ruptures occur when patients are participating in sports (most common in racquet sports especially badminton). Athletes who start training after a period of inactivity are at a higher risk of rupturing their Achilles tendon. It is more common in males and the mean age of presentation is 40 years. There may be an association between the incidence of Achilles tendon rupture and blood group O.

Aetiology

Aetiology of Achilles tendon rupture is poorly understood, however several pathological processes have been suggested to contribute. Histologically, many of the ruptured Achilles tendons exhibit degenerative changes. This degenerative process may also be related to decreased blood supply to the tendon with increasing age. Mechanical factors such as overpronation of the foot, training errors and poor sports equipment may also play a part on increasing the stress imposed on the tendon. There is also an association with previous history of Achilles tendon tendinopathy and corticosteroid injections. Fluroquinolone antibiotics have also been implicated in the aetiology of the Achilles tendon rupture.

Clinical features

Typically the patient presents with sudden pain, reporting that at the time of injury they thought that they had been struck behind the ankle. Some also report an audible snap. There are mainly two mechanisms of injury. In over 50% of the patients the rupture occurs while pushing off with the weight-bearing forefoot while extending the knee joint. Sudden and violent dorsiflexion of the ankle is reported by approximately 30% of the patients.

On examination there is a palpable defect in the tendon, however the bruising and the swelling might mask the gap. There may be some weakness of plantar flexion but some active plantar flexion may be possible due to plantaris, flexor hallucis longus and tibialis posterior function. Simmond's test (lack of full plantar flexion in response to calf squeeze with patient prone) is positive.

Investigations

Achilles tendon rupture is a clinical diagnosis, however ultrasound and MRI are the studies of choice if diagnosis is in question.

Treatment

Achilles tendon rupture can be managed non-operatively or surgically. The choice remains controversial as there are very few well-controlled prospective randomised trials conducted.

Non-operative treatment

This involves reapposing the tendon ends by plantar flexing the ankle (with an equinus cast), and then gradually bringing the foot to neutral position over 2 months before removing the cast. A below-knee cast is acceptable and protected weight bearing is allowed after 6 weeks and usually continued for 4 or more weeks after cast removal.

Surgical treatment

This involves repair of the Achilles tendon. There are various techniques, including open and percutaneous methods, which range from simple end to end suturing to more complex repairs using fascial reinforcement or tendon grafts. Traditionally, a similar regime of cast treatment to conservative management is required with weight bearing at 4 weeks; however, there has been a trend over recent years towards a more aggressive mobilisation post surgery.

Non-operative versus surgical treatment

There appears to be a higher re-rupture rate in patients treated non-operatively compared to patients managed surgically. It has also been argued that with conservative management there is a higher degree of tendon lengthening and muscle weakness, which can lead to loss of strength. With surgical repair, there is always a risk of wound complications, infection, skin necrosis and fistulas. Athletes are candidates for surgery whereas sedentary, elderly or those with chronic illness could be offered the non-operative management.

Return to sport

Return to play is permitted once the athlete is pain free, able to achieve a full range of movement and has regained enough strength to perform their sport-specific activities. With surgery this may take 4 months.

Further reading

Maffulli N, Wong J. Rupture of the Achilles and patellar tendons. *Clin Sports Med* 2003; **22**(4): 761–76.

Movin T, Ryberg A, McBride DJ, Maffulli N. Acute rupture of the Achilles tendon. *Foot Ankle Clin* 2005; **10**(2): 331–56.

Ageing and sport

AA Narvani

The numerous benefits of regular exercise are well established. These effects can even become more pronounced as we become older. These health benefits include:

Cardiovascular

- Reduction in risk of, and premature mortality from:
  —ischaemic heart disease
  —cerebral vascular disease
  —hypertension
  —thrombo/embolic disease
- Decreased morbidity caused by conditions such as:
  —congestive heart failure
  —peripheral vascular disease
- Improved cardiac function

Endocrine and metabolic

- Reduction in risk, morbidity and mortality of diabetes (see chapter on Diabetes and exercise)
  —better glycaemic control
  —enhanced insulin sensitivity
- Improvement in lipid profile
- Reduced risk of obesity

Musculo-skeletal

- Decreased risk and morbidity of osteoporosis
  —reduction in rate of bone density loss in post-menopausal females
  —reduction in rate of osteoporotic fractures
- Decrease in morbidity of osteoarthritis

Respiratory (see chapter on Pulmonary disorders and exercise)
- Decreased morbidity caused by asthma and chronic obstructive pulmonary disease

Psychology and psychiatry
- Better self-motivation
- Feeling of well-being and self-importance
- Improved sleep
- Reduction in rate and morbidity of depression
- Improvement in memory
- Self-independence
- Social integration

Cancers
- Potential reduction in rate of some type of malignancies

In the view of the above benefits, our more senior citizens should be encouraged to participate in some form of regular exercise. It is, however, important to have an understanding of physiological changes accompanying ageing that can limit the "exercise capacity".

Cardiovascular alterations
It can be difficult to differentiate those changes that occur as a consequence of ageing from those due to inactivity; however, the following alterations are thought to occur:

Decrease in
- VO_2max.
- maximum cardiac output
- maximum heart rate
- myocardial contractibility
- stroke volume
- vascular compliance
- sensitivity of myocardial to catecholamines
- systemic blood pressure regulation function
- vessel wall extensibility
- microcirculation to muscle and major organs

Increase in
- circumference of all cardiac valves
- lipid, calcium and collagen deposition on the valves
- rate of atherosclerosis
- calcium deposition in the elastin of the vessel walls

Respiratory alterations
Ageing is generally believed to be associated with progressive deterioration of respiratory function resulting in shortness of breath with lighter exercise than that experienced in youth. This is thought partly to be due to:

Reduction in
- total lung capacity
- vital capacity

- tidal volume
- inspiratory capacity
- inspiratory airflow
- forced expiratory volume
- efficiency of alveolar gas exchange
- elasticity (diminished elastic recoil in expiration)
- lung compliance

Increased

- chest wall rigidity
- airway resistance
- residual lung volume caused by loss of structural support for pulmonary tissue leading to earlier airway closure

Skeletal muscle alterations

Like cardiovascular changes, these have been challenging to investigate as it is difficult to isolate those due to ageing from those due to inability. The following transformations are thought to occur:

- loss of muscle tissue
- relative increase in type I muscle fibres
- loss of muscle strength
- decrease in maximal velocity of muscle contraction leading to reduced power
- increased collagen content in muscle leading to stiffness and higher risk of injury

Ligament and tendon alterations

Ageing is associated with

- decrease in compliance
- reduced micro-circulation
- decrease in collagen fibre thickness
- reduced water content
- decrease in glycoaminoglycan content
- increased risk of injury
- impaired healing once injury occurs

Bone and joint alterations

- The progressive reduction of bone density associated with ageing is more pronounced in post-menopausal females
- Decrease in articular cartilage water content leading to reduced tissue compliance, making it more brittle and therefore an increased risk of damage with stress as well as reducing its capacity to act as a shock absorber.

Neurological alterations

These include:

- a decrease in number of neurones
- an increase in ventricular sizes
- reduced CSF turnover

- decreased nerve conduction speed
- slower processing of information

The above changes contribute to impaired

- hearing
- vision
- sensation
- proprioception
- coordination
- speed and reaction time
- motor skill
- concentration
- balance

Renal function alterations

Renal function becomes less efficient. Contributing factors include decline in the number of glomeruli, reduced renal blood flow and glomerular filtration rate.

Adequate exercise?

It is important to appreciate that as well as reducing the risk of many diseases, in addition to their morbidity as mortality, adequate exercise can reduce the rate of physiological decline that occurs in many organs as mentioned above. It is suggested that as little as 30 to 50 minutes of aerobic exercise of moderate intensity (60–90% of the maximum heart rate), three to five days a week, can result in significant health benefits and a decrease in physiological decline. The type of exercise that should be recommended is dependent on a number of factors including individual's

- preference
- existing physical limitations
- existing medical conditions
- specific health needs and goals

Any recommended exercise programme should, however, for optimal gains, consist of a mixture of exercises involving rhythmic contraction of large muscle groups over a period of time, and resistance exercises in order to improve cardiorespiratory fitness, strength, coordination, balance and flexibility. It is also important at this stage to mention that, although few, there are a number of contraindications to exercise training as suggested by the American College of Sports Medicine (see Further reading). These are thought to include:

- recent myocardial infarction
- ischaemic ECG changes
- unstable angina
- acute heart failure
- uncontrolled arrhythmias
- third degree heart block
- uncontrolled hypertension (relative contraindication)

- valvular heart disease (relative contraindication)
- cardiomyopathies (relative contraindication)
- complex ventricular ectopy (relative contraindication)
- uncontrolled metabolic disease (relative contraindication)

Injuries in ageing athletes

The majority of injuries in senior citizens are chronic and overuse injuries. Acute injuries occur less frequently than in young athletes, which is partly due to the fact that ageing athletes tend to participate in lower intensity exercises and less aggressive sports.

Chronic and overuse injuries

Age-related changes that occur in muscle, tendons, ligament and cartilage, increase the vulnerability of older athletes to chronic and overuse injuries. The combination of degeneration and repetitive injury result in significant damage to various soft tissue structures. Common examples of these injuries include:

- tendinopathies and tears
  —tendo-achilles
  —rotator cuff
  —tibialis posterior and other foot/ankle tendons
  —wrist tendons
- epicondylitis
  —lateral
  —medial
- osteoarthritis
  —Although this may not be thought as a chronic or overuse injury, coupled with age-related cartilage changes, repetitive torsional loading can result in cartilage damage (see the chapter on Osteoarthritis and sport).

Acute injuries

Acute injuries sustained by older athletes include:

- acute muscular strain
  —stiffer and less efficient muscle function are believed to be contributing factors.
  —tend to occur at the muscular-tendinous junction as terminal sarcomeres are thought not to be as extensible as middle sarcomeres
- tendo-Achilles rupture
- quadriceps tendon rupture
- acute fractures

Further reading

American College of Sports Medicine position stand: Exercise and physical activity for older adults. *Med Sci Sports Exerc* 1998; **30**: 992–1008.

Chen AL, Mears SC, Hawkins RJ. Orthopaedic care of the aging athlete. *Journal of American Academy of Orthopaedics Surgery* 2005; **13**: 407–16.

Galloway MT, Jokl P. Aging successfully: the importance of physical activity in maintaining health and function. *Journal of American Academy of Orthopaedics Surgery* 2000; **8**: 37–44.
Menard D. The ageing athlete. In: M Harries, C Williams, WD Stanish, LJ Micheli (Eds) *Oxford Textbook of Sports Medicine*, 2nd edn. Oxford University Press, 1998: 787–814.
Young A, Dinan S. Active in later life. In: M Harries, J King, C Williams (Eds) *ABC of Sports Medicine*, 2nd edn. BMJ Books, 2000: 51–6.

Ankle – acute sprains

AA Narvani

Ankle sprains represent 15–20% of all sporting injuries. They are in fact the most common injury sustained by athletes; furthermore, up to 40% of the patients with acute ankle sprains may develop some type of chronic problem such as instability, chronic pain and recurrent swelling, particularly in those who are inadequately treated. Ankle sprains are more common in the younger age group as they participate more often in sports. They are more common in sports that require rapid changes of direction.

Pathology

Sprains of the lateral ligament complex represent 85% of all the ankle sprains. The lateral ligament complex consists of the anterior talofibular ligament (ATFL), the calcaneofibular ligament (CFL), and the posterior talofibular ligament (PTFL). The ATFL has a flat band appearance and passes from the tip of the fibula anteriorly to the lateral talar neck. The CFL fans out from the tip of the lateral malleolus to the lateral side of the calcaneum. The PTFL is the strongest of the three and runs posteriorly from the fibula to the talus.

Damage to this ligament complex occurs as a result of supination and inversion of the foot. As the foot twists medially in relation to the lower leg, the ATFL is the first ligament damaged followed by the CFL and finally the PTFL.

Traditionally these injuries are divided into three grades. Grade I injuries result in tearing of some fibres with minimal haemorrhage. In Grade II injuries there is an incomplete tear of the ligament and moderate haemorrhage. Grade III injuries are characterised by complete disruption of the ligament.

Clinical features

There is a history of twisting injury to the ankle. Patients may recall hearing a pop at the time of the injury. There is usually a combination of pain, swelling, weakness and instability, the degree of which is dependent on the severity and the grade of the injury as demonstrated in Table 1.

Table 1 Classification of acute ankle sprains.

Grade	Severity	Clinical features
I	Mild	Pain, but able to carry on with activity Able to bear weight Mild or minimal swelling Pain reproduced by stressing the ligaments but there is no laxity No functional and strength loss
II	Moderate	Pain severe enough to stop the patient from carrying on with activity Able to bear weight Moderate swelling Pain on stressing the ligament with some degree of laxity, but a firm end point Slight reduction in function with possible decrease in strength
III	Severe	Pain and inability to bear weight Severe swelling Gross laxity without an endpoint Potentially a complete loss of function, strength and proprioception

Investigations

Plain X-rays are important in ruling out malleolar, talus, calcaneum, base of fifth metatarsal fractures, and osteochondral injuries (however, osteochondral injuries may not be apparent on the initial X-ray).

Magnetic Resonance Imaging (MRI) can be a very valuable tool for the assessment of lateral ligament complex damage as well as in excluding other injuries, including osteochondral lesions.

Differential diagnosis

Fractures

- Malleolar
- Talus
- Base of 5th metatarsal
- Calcaneum
- Tibial platfond
- Stress fractures

Osteochondral injuries
Syndesmosis injuries
Tendon rupture

- Tibialis posterior
- Peroneal tendons
- Achilles tendon

Peroneal tendon dislocation
Tendinopathies
Other ligament injuries
- Medial ligaments
- ATFL sprain

Treatment

This can be divided into three phases irrespective of how severe the injury is; however, rate of progression from one phase to another is dependent on the grade of the injury.

Phase I – ***Control of pain and inflammation***
This phase starts immediately after injury and is achieved by protection, rest, ice, compression and elevation.

Phase II – ***Restoration of full range of movement and muscle strength***
There is a progression from no weight bearing to partial weight bearing to full weight bearing. Mobilisation of the ankle, subtalar and the midtarsal joints are commenced. Muscle strengthening involves progression from active exercises to resistive exercises.

Phase III – ***Restoration of proprioception function, functional exercises, restoration of general fitness and return to sport, prevention of future injuries***
Patients need to be weight bearing before this phase starts. Proprioception exercises include use of rockerboards. Functional exercises involve jumping, hopping, twisting and figure of eight running. When these exercises can be performed without pain, return to sport is permitted. Taping or bracing may offer protection and prevention of further injury once the athlete returns to sport.

Surgery
Surgery is mainly indicated in those patients with severe/Grade III injuries who, despite six weeks of conservative treatment, still have instability symptoms. In these patients surgical reconstruction of the lateral ligaments is recommended.

Return to sport

As with other sports injuries, return to play is permitted once the athlete is pain free, able to achieve a full range of movement and has regained enough strength to perform their sport-specific activities. Exactly when this occurs is dependent on the severity of the problem, the type of management chosen and whether this management plan has been successful or not. If the non-operative regime is successful, athletes are usually able to return to play within 3 months. With surgical intervention, return to play may take 3 to 6 months following surgery.

Further reading

Di Giovanni BF, Partal G, Baumhauer JF. Acute ankle injury and chronic lateral instability in the athlete. *Clinics in Sports Medicine* 2004; **23**: 1–19.

Ankle – persistent problems following sprains: overview

AA Narvani

Ankle sprains are thought to account for approximately 20% of all sports injuries. Some studies suggest that up to 40% of those athletes with acute ankle sprains suffer from recurrent sprains or have residual symptoms 6 to 18 months after surgery. This can result in performance impairment in a very significant portion of these athletes.

Persistent problems following ankle sprains may be due to:

(i) inadequate rehabilitation
(ii) lateral instability
(iii) incorrect diagnosis/failure to diagnose associated injuries or the presence of conditions such as inflammatory disorders, neoplasm or congenital abnormalities.

Inadequate rehabilitation

This is thought to be the most common cause of persistent ankle pain following sprain.

Pathology

Several mechanisms have been proposed to explain how inadequate rehabilitation following sprains may lead to pain. These include:

(i) Inadequate muscle power, control and coordination leading to instability and failure to prevent the ankle from further injury.
(ii) Persistent capsular adhesions and intra-articular adhesions causing pain and reduced range of movement.
(iii) Inadequate proprioception.
(iv) Without adequate rehabilitation, chronic inflammation may result in excessive scar tissue formation. This may, in turn, lead to synovitis and irritation.
(v) Inadequate rehabilitation may result in an abnormal sympathetic response.

Clinical features

- Pain and tenderness
- Weakness and instability
- Stiffness and decreased range of movement

Investigation

Various imaging modalities may be used to exclude other conditions (see below).

Treatment

A full, adequate, appropriate rehabilitation programme must be restated (see the previous chapter).

Further reading

Bassewitz HL, Shapiro MS. Persistent pain after ankle sprain: targeting the causes. *The Physician and Sportsmedicine* 1997; **25**(12).

Ankle – persistent problems following sprains: lateral ankle instability

AA Narvani

This is thought to occur in up to 20% of athletes who have had sprains. Chronic ankle instability may be functional or mechanical. Functional instability refers to an athlete's subjective feeling of giving way in the ankle, usually due to neuromuscular deficits. Mechanical instability is increased mobility of the talus in the ankle joint, beyond the physiological range caused by structural damage.

Pathology

The following processes have been proposed to contribute to the pathology of lateral ankle instability following sprains:

- Healing of the ligaments in a lengthened position.
- Persistent peroneal weakness.
- Heredity hypermobility of the ankle joint.
- Impaired proprioception/neuromuscular deficits (see above).
- Impingement of soft tissue in the joint.

Clinical features

- History of initial ankle sprain
- Recurrent ankle sprains
- Feeling of ankle giving way
- Pain
- Suboptimal performance
- Localised tenderness
- Muscle weakness
- Positive anterior draw test (in mechanical instability)
- Positive varus stress test (in mechanical instability)

Investigations

Plain radiographs

- Anterior–posterior and lateral will aid in excluding other pathologies.

- Stress views are helpful, however without anaesthesia they may not be very accurate.

Arthrography
- Not used as much as previously because of emergence of magnetic resonance imaging.
- Can diagnose ligament and capsular rupture.

Ultrasound
- This may be used to assess the integrity of the lateral ligament complex.

Magnetic Resonance Imaging
- As well as demonstrating lateral complex ligament damage, MRI will also help to exclude other pathologies (see below).

Examination under anaesthesia and arthroscopy
- Stress testing under anaesthesia would allow a more accurate assessment of mechanical instability.
- Although an invasive procedure, arthroscopy will enable the clinician to detect the presence of other pathologies, such as osteochondral defects, loose bodies and impingement lesions (see below).

Treatment

Before deciding on the treatment options, the clinician must be able to answer the following questions:

(i) Are there any other associated pathologies?
(ii) Is the athlete's main problem pain or instability?
(iii) Is the instability mechanical or functional?

Treatment may be non-operative or by operative means.

Non-operative
- This involves a complete and adequate rehabilitation programme, which should consist of:
  —Muscle strengthening (especially peroneal muscles)
  —Proprioception exercises
  —Coordination exercises
- Functional ankle bracing, preventing inversion of the subtalar joint, may be used during this rehabilitation period.
- Some athletes may also benefit from lateral heal wedge.

Operative
- Surgery is indicated for athletes with mechanical instability who are symptomatic despite having been through a complete and comprehensive rehabilitation programme. It is important to emphasise that those who suffer mainly from pain rather than instability may not benefit from surgery.
- Surgical options for chronic mechanical lateral instability include:

Anatomical repairs

- Brostrom procedure:
  This involves identification of the ligament ends which are then sutured or plicated.
- Gould's modification of Brostrom procedure:
  This involves shortening of the anterior talofibular ligament (and calcaneofibular ligament in some) followed by reinforcement of the ligaments with extensor retinaculum.

Non-anatomical repairs

- These include a number of procedures that use peroneal, plantaris or free grafts to reconstruct the lateral ligament complex.

Return to sport

As with other sports injuries, return to play is permitted once the athlete is pain free, able to achieve a full range of movement and has regained enough strength to perform their sport-specific activities. Exactly when this occurs is dependent on the severity of the problem, the type of management chosen and whether this management plan has been successful or not. If the non-operative regime is successful, usually athletes are able to return to play within 3 months. With operative intervention, return to play may take 3 to 6 months following surgery.

Further reading

Baker JM, Ouzounian TJ. Complex ankle instability. *Foot Ankle Clin* 2000; **5**(4): 887–96.

DiGiovanni BF, Partal G, Baumhauer JF. Acute ankle injury and chronic lateral instability in the athlete. *Clin Sports Med* 2004; **23**(1): 1–19.

Hertel J. Functional instability following lateral ankle sprain. *Sports Med* 2000; **29**(5): 361–71.

Ankle – persistent problems following sprains: other injuries

AA Narvani

Persistent pain following sprain may be due to other missed or associated pathologies. A practical way of classifying these other pathologies is by the exact site of the pain as described below. It is important to emphasise that persistent pain following sprains may also be due to missed fractures, stress fractures and referred pain from other sites. These are not covered in this chapter.

Anterior

- Impingement syndrome
- Syndesmosis injury

- Tibialis anterior tendinopathy
- Nerve injury

Lateral
- Sinus tarsi syndrome
- Impingement syndrome (antero-lateral)
- Peroneal tendon pathology

Posterior/postero-medial
- Tibialis posterior tendinopathy
- Flexor hallucis longus tendinopathy
- Achilles tendon tendinopathy
- Os trigonum syndrome
- Posterior impingement
- Tarsal tunnel syndrome and other nerve entrapments

Ankle impingement syndrome

Anterior impingement may occur secondary to either an osseous or soft tissue lesion. Osseous impingement, also referred to as "footballer's ankle", is due to osteophyte formation in the talus or anterior tibia. As well as being common in kicking sports, this condition is also seen in ballet dancers as it occurs in activities that involve forced dorsiflexion of the ankle joint. Soft tissue impingement is due to fibrous connective tissue formation and impingement in the antero-lateral or antero-medial ankle following a sprain. This dense fibrous connective tissue formation occurs either as a result of torn ligament ends of anterior talo-fibular ligament impingement in the ankle joint or synovial hypertrophy. This dense fibrous connective tissue's arthroscopic appearance is not dissimilar to that of knee meniscus, therefore it is also referred to as a "meniscoid lesion".

Clinical features
- History of initial ankle sprain
- Anterior or antero-lateral ankle pain
- Pain worse on dorsiflexion
- Stiffness
- Suboptimal performance
- Anterior/lateral ankle joint tenderness
- Positive anterior impingement (pain when athlete moves forward while the heel remains on the floor)
- Decreased range of movement

Investigations
Plain radiographs
- With osseous impingement, osteophytes may be detected.
- Will aid in excluding other pathologies.

Magnetic Resonance Imaging
- MRI may reveal the impingement lesion as well as helping to exclude other pathologies.

Arthroscopy

- Will show the impinging lesion (meniscoid lesion in case of soft tissue impingement, see above).

Treatment

Non-operative

- NSAIDs
- Physical therapy
- Bracing
- Shoe modification (heel lift)

Operative

- Either arthroscopic or open osseous/soft tissue debridement.

Posterior impingement syndrome is common among those athletes whose sport involves maximum plantar flexion of the ankle. These athletes include ballet dancers and gymnasts. Causes include os trigonum (see below), posterior talar tubercle, flexor hallucis longus pathologies, impingement by other soft tissues. Athletes present with posterior ankle pain and reduced range of movement. Pain is worse with passive plantar flexion. Athletes are first managed with NSAIDs, physical therapy, injection and bracing. Surgery could be considered for those who do not respond to non-operative measures.

Syndesmosis injury

The anterior and posterior inferior tibio-fibular ligaments, the transverse tibio-fibular ligament and the interosseous membrane make up the ankle syndesmosis complex. This ligament complex, together with the deltoid ligament on the medial side, provides important resistance to external rotation forces. Damage to the structures of this complex occurs most frequently in collision sports. It is thought that between 1 to 10% of the ankle sprains may be associated with syndesmosis injuries. The actual damage to the individual ligament ranges from stretch to partial tear to complete tear.

Clinical features

- History of initial ankle sprain (usually forced external rotation)
- Pain
- Swelling
- Instability
- Suboptimal performance
- Tenderness
- (+) squeeze test (compression of the tibia and fibula together above the level of injury produces pain at antero-lateral aspect of the ankle)
- (+) external rotation test (application of external rotation force to the ankle in neutral position produces pain in the syndesmotic area)
- (+) shunk test (application of medial and lateral force to the talus causes pain in the syndesmosis area or a feeling of looseness)

Investigations

Plain radiographs

- In severe injuries, weight-bearing views may demonstrate medial space widening and talar lateral subluxation. This subluxation becomes more apparent with external rotation stress radiographs.

CT scan

- This may also illustrate the medial joint space widening.

Bone scan

- This is a quite sensitive diagnostic tool for acute syndesmosis injuries.

Magnetic Resonance Imaging

- MRI is becoming a popular choice as it is sensitive yet non-invasive and does not expose the athlete to ionising radiation.

Treatment

- Treatment is dependent on the severity of the injury.
- Stretch or partial tear injuries, which are not associated with bony fractures, may be treated non-operatively. This involves:
  —RICE
  —Once swelling and pain are decreased, athlete may bear weight, start range of motion, strength and coordination exercises.
- Complete rupture injuries, which have normal appearance on unstressed radiographs, may also be treated non-operatively. However, the period for non-weight bearing should be 8 to 10 weeks.
- Complete rupture injuries with which there is syndesmosis opening on unstressed radiographs may be treated surgically with open reduction internal fixation.
- More recent techniques involving syndesmosis fixation using "TightRope", without screw insertion, are gaining popularity.

Sinus tarsi syndrome

This is thought to occur due to residual synovitis from injury to interosseous talocalcaneal ligament. The sinus tarsi itself is a small osseous canal which forms part of the subtalar joint. Its contents include fat, connective tissue, blood vessels and ligaments.

Clinical features

- There may be a history of initial ankle sprain
- Pain
- Stiffness
- Suboptimal performance
- Tenderness just anterior to the lateral malloelus
- Reduced subtalar joint range of movement
- Inversion and eversion of the subtalar joint will reproduce the pain
- Injection of local anaesthetic into the sinus tarsi will provide pain relief (this can be a valuable diagnostic test)

Investigations

MRIs

- This condition may be diagnosed clinically and with injection in the sinus tarsi, however MRI can confirm the diagnosis and aid to exclude other pathologies.

Treatment

- For the vast majority of athletes, treatment is non-operative with injection of local anaesthetic and corticosteroids in the sinus tarsi followed by physical therapy.
- Those very few who do not respond to non-operative measures may benefit from surgical excision of the contents of the sinus.

Tibialis anterior tendinopathy

This could be a cause of chronic anterior ankle pain. This is usually an overuse injury resulting from repetitive ankle dorsiflexion. Athletes will have pain and tenderness which is made worse by resisted dorsiflexion and inversion. Management is mainly non-operatively with NSAIDs and physical therapy.

Flexor hallucis tendinopathy

See the chapter on Heel pain.

Peroneal tendon pathology

Possible pathologies with the peroneal tendons include:

- Peroneal tendinopathy
- Tears and rupture
- Peroneal tendon instability (subluxation/dislocation)

Peroneal tendinopathy

This is not an uncommon cause of chronic lateral ankle pain. It is an overuse injury seen in sports such as dancing and basketball and is associated with excessive pronation. It may also occur secondary to peroneal instability.

Clinical features

- Pain and tenderness over the peroneal muscles, which are made worse by resisted eversion and plantar flexion.
- Passive inversion may also reproduce the pain.
- Any predisposing factors, such as excessive pronation, must also be looked for during assessment.

Investigations

- MRI will demonstrate features of peroneal tendinopathy as well as helping to exclude other pathologies.

Treatment

- Treatment in the vast majority of athletes with peroneal tendinopathy is non-operative including:
  —RICE
  —NSAIDs
  —Physical therapy
  —Correction of any predisposing conditions.
- In those very few athletes who do not respond to a comprehensive non-operative regime, surgical debridement of the peroneal tendons may be required.

Peroneal tendon tear and rupture

Although peroneal ruptures occur more frequently with longus than brevis, they are still relatively uncommon. They usually occur in tendons with macroscopic and microscopic features of tendinopathy, even though the athlete may have been asymptomatic with these features, prior to rupture.

Clinical features

- There may be a previous history of lateral ankle pain (tendinopathy) or chronic ankle instability.
- In acute ruptures, athletes usually complain of acute pain accompanied by a popping noise.
- Swelling.
- Tenderness posterior to distal fibula or between the tip of the fibula and the base of the fifth metatarsal.
- Weak ankle eversion.
- Resisted ankle eversion is painful.

Investigations

Plain radiograph

- May reveal a fracture or change of position of os perineum (both indicative of peroneus longus rupture).

MRI

- This is the investigation of choice as it will demonstrate the tear or rupture.

Treatment

Peroneus longus

- Treated surgically in most athletes with either a direct repair or tenodesis to brevis.

Peroneus brevis

- These are usually chronic and longitudinal
- May be treated both non-operatively or operatively
- Non-operative management includes:
  —NSAIDs
  —Immobilisation
  —Shoe modification
- Operative treatment would involve debridement of the tear followed by repair of the tendon.

Peroneal tendon instability

This includes peroneal tendon subluxation or dislocation, which can occur as a result of sudden forceful passive dorsiflexion of the inverted foot. The superior peroneal retinaculum, which normally maintains the peroneal tendons behind lateral malleolus in the peroneal groove, is disrupted. As a result, the peroneal tendons can slip out of the groove (either one or both of them). Once dislocated or subluxed, the tendons either relocate back or remain dislocated. If they relocate back, they can become unstable, resulting in recurrent dislocation. Peroneal tendon instability can lead to peroneal tendinopathy and/or tears.

Clinical features

- With acute subluxation/dislocation there is usually a history of initial injury.
- Athlete may recall a snapping noise at time of the injury.
- Pain and tenderness over the course of the peroneal tendons.
- Recurrent episodes.
- Athlete may be able to demonstrate the tendons dislocating to the clinician, or the clinician may be able to dislocate the tendon him/herself.

Investigations

Plain radiograph

- This may show a small avulsion fracture of the posterolateral margin of the fibula (superior peroneal retinaculum attachment).

MRI

- This will demonstrate any peroneal tendon lesion as well as any disruption of the superior peroneal retinaculum.

Treatment

- First acute dislocation can be treated non-operatively with immobilisation using a modified below-knee cast. Those athletes with chronic dislocation are candidates for surgical repair and reconstruction of the superior peroneal retinaculum.

Os trigonum syndrome

Present in up to 10% of normal feet, os trigonum is an accessory centre of ossification of the posterior talus, just lateral to the groove for the flexor hallucis longus. It may be symptomatic in athletes pursuing activities that involve repetitive forced plantar flexion (causing it to impinge against the posterior tibia) such as ballerinas, basketball and volleyball players. Occasionally it may result in secondary flexor hallucis tendinopathy.

Clinical features

- Insidious onset of posterior ankle pain
- Pain is made worse with plantar flexion of the ankle
- Tenderness over posterior talus
- Reduced subtalar joint range of movement

Investigations

Plain radiograph

- This will show the os trigonum.
- Posterior impingement may be illustrated with lateral radiographs taken with ankle in plantar flexion.

CT

- Will provide a more comprehensive view of the os trigonum.

Bone scan

- May demonstrate increased uptake of the os trigonum in symptomatic athletes.

MRI

- Again in symptomatic athletes, MRI may illustrate os trigonum bone oedema in addition to the presence of surrounding fluid.

Treatment

- Non-operative management, including immobilisation and NSAIDs, should be tried first.
- Those who do not respond to the non-operative regime are candidates for surgical excision of the os trigonum.

Osteochondral lesions of the talar dome

These are common sporting injuries. They may occur in up to 6.5% of all ankle sprains. Furthermore, they are associated with premature ankle arthritis. They occur as a result of shearing/compression impaction force between the tibial plafond and the talar dome. Various classification systems have been developed, but one of the common classifications used is Berndt and Harty's classification – see Table 1.

Clinical features

- Progressive pain
- Usually a history of injury
- Swelling and stiffness
- Clicking/locking
- Sub-optimal performance
- Tenderness over talus
- Reduced range of movement

Table 1 Berndt and Harty's classification for talar osteochondral defects.

Stage	Lesion
I	Compression fracture
II	Partial undisplaced fracture
III	Complete but still undisplaced fracture
IV	Displaced fragment present

Investigations

Plain radiograph

- May show the lesion or loose body.

CT and MRI

- Both very useful in demonstrating the lesion.

Treatment

- Stage I and II lesions can be treated non-operatively.
- Stage III lesions are less likely to heal and, in many athletes, require surgery (in children a trial of non-operative treatment may be appropriate).
- Stage IV usually requires surgery.
- Operative procedures may be open or arthroscopic (see the chapter on Osteoarthritis – treatment) and include:
  —Excision of lesion
  —Curettage
  —Internal fixation of the lesion
  —Cancellous bone grafting
  —Microfracture
  —Drilling
  —Mosaicplasty
  —Autologous chondrocyte implantation

Further reading

Brown TD, Micheli LJ. Foot and ankle injuries in dance. *Am J Orthop* 2004; **33**(6): 303–9.

Maquirrian J. Posterior ankle impingement syndrome. *J Am Acad Orthop Surg* 2005; **13**(6): 365–71.

Mizel MS, Hecht PJ, Marymont JV, Temple HT. Evaluation and treatment of chronic ankle pain. *Instr Course Lect* 2004; **53**: 311–21.

Patterson MJ, Coz WK. Peroneus longus tendon rupture as a cause of chronic lateral ankle pain. *Clin Orthop Relat Res* 1999; **(365)**: 163–6.

Back pain – overview

AA Narvani

Eighty percent of the general population are thought to suffer from back pain at some stage during their life. It is also common among athletes, in particular in those competing in sports such as wrestling, gymnastics and weight lifting. The forces imposed on the athlete's back are often much greater than those of non-athletes. Furthermore, these larger forces are often sustained for longer duration. Back pain in athletes occurs either as the result of an acute traumatic event or a repetitive activity that causes fatigue injuries.

Aetiology

Back pain is not a diagnosis, but a symptom, which could occur as a result of a number of conditions. Some of the causes are listed in Table 1.

Management

In 90% of low back pain sufferers, symptoms resolve within 6 weeks regardless of treatment. Unfortunately, in a small percentage of patients this pain can become chronic and in all those who have become disabled for more than 1 year, up to 90% will never work again without aggressive intervention. Furthermore, in a small number of patients, back pain may be the presenting symptom of serious diseases such as cancer. Therefore it is important that clinicians who assess athletes with back pain recognise the "red flag" signs of serious diseases. These are listed in Table 2.

Table 1 Differential diagnosis for low back pain.

Spinal pathology
Strain/sprain
Discogenic
  Annular tears
  Degenerative disc disease
  Disc herniation
Spondylolysis
Spondylolisthesis
Facet joint OA
Fractures
  Acute lumbar vertebra fracture
  Stress fractures
    Sacral stress fractures
    Facet stress fractures
Infection
  Discitis
  Osteomyelitis
Malignancy
  Primary
  Metastatic
Metabolic
  Osteoporosis

Sacroiliac joint pathology
Hip and groin pathology
Gynaecological
Urological
Rheumatological
Gastrointestinal
Vascular
Soft tissue tumours

Table 2 Red flag signs.

Red flags for cancer
Age >50
Cancer history
Night pain
Gradual onset
Constitutional symptoms, i.e. fever, weight loss
Red flags for infection
Constitutional symptoms
Gradual onset
Night pain
Immune suppression
History of other infections
IV drug abuse
Previous surgery

Athletes with any of the red flag features require imaging. Imaging is also indicated in all those patients with radicular symptoms or neurological features, in those who have sustained significant trauma, and in all those who remain symptomatic despite a trial of conservative treatment. This may be in the form of plain radiographs, MRI, CT scan, bone scan or single photon emission computed tomography (SPECT), depending on the particular case.

Further reading

Bono C. Low-back pain in athletes. *J Bone & Joint Surgery (Am)* 2004; **86**(2): 382–96.

Wilk V. Acute low back pain: assessment and management. *Aust Fam Physician* 2004; **33**(6): 403–7.

Back pain – lumbar strains and sprains

AA Narvani

Disruptions of muscle fibres are referred to as strains whereas tears in the ligament fibres are known as sprains.

Epidemiology

These are the most common cause of low back pain in athletes as well as the general population. Seventy percent of the cases of all low back pain are thought to be due to lumbar strain and sprains.

Aetiology

This is not completely understood. Acute trauma or prolonged mechanical stress can cause ligamentous and/or muscular damage and this damage will cause pain. As a consequence of this pain, there is a decrease in muscular activation and patient activity. This may lead to further damage to the ligaments and the muscles as a result of decreased stability of the back. Therefore, a vicious cycle may be established.

Clinical features

Athletes usually recall a recent history of a specific injury that led to the pain. Pain may start immediately after injury, however it will progressively get worse as a result of localised oedema and reflex muscle contraction (pain and stiffness is usually worse the day after the incident). This pain is made worse by activity. With only strain/sprain, there should not be any radicular or abnormal neurological features.

Investigations

Imaging is not indicated unless there are any red flag signs (see the previous chapter: Back pain – overview), any radicular or abnormal neurological clinical features, or if the symptoms have persisted for more than a month. In these cases, it is important to exclude other differential diagnoses.

Treatment

In order to prevent the vicious cycle (see above) becoming established, treatment is aimed at controlling the pain so athletes can regain their range of motion. This is achieved by a period of limited rest (not more than 1 to 2 days) combined with NSAIDs and physical therapy modalities such as ice and heat. Once pain control is established, various exercising programmes may be initiated (see the following chapter: Back pain – discogenic).

Return to sport

There is usually complete resolution of symptoms in 90% of the patients within 2 months; however, it must be ensured that the athlete can achieve sufficient range of motion to prevent subsequent injury before return to full play is permitted.

Further reading

Bono C. Low-back pain in athletes. *J Bone & Joint Surgery (Am)* 2004; **86**(2): 382–96.

Eck JC, Riley LH. Return to play after lumbar spine conditions and surgeries. *Clinics in Sports Medicine* 2004; **23**: 367–79.

Back pain – discogenic

AA Narvani

This refers to low back pain, which occurs as a result of disc pathology. These disc pathologies include annular fibrosis tear, degeneration and herniation. Disc herniation is covered in detail elsewhere (see the chapter on Lumber intervertebral disc herniation), but annular tear and disc degeneration are discussed here.

Annular fibrosis tear and disc degeneration

Epidemiology

These conditions appear to be more common in patients who participate in sports, particularly sports such as weight lifting, gymnastics, golf, ballet and cricket (bowling). It must be mentioned, however, that there are many athletes with degenerative discs who do not have any symptoms at all.

Pathology

During various sporting manoeuvres, large forces are produced within the disc. Prolonged compressive loads lead to a decrease in the water content of the nucleus (this also occurs with ageing). As a result, the ability of the disc to spread the force equally is decreased. This would mean that the annulus is less able to tolerate the compressive load, therefore more likely to deform. It is thought that this deformation with time can lead to fissure formation and disc degeneration.

Excessive stress on the disc can directly lead to annular tears. Initially these tears are circumferential, but with continued stress these can progress to radial tears. This further weakens the disc and a vicious circle is initiated which leads to disc degeneration.

Clinical features

There may be a history of an initial injury. The back pain is usually greater than the leg pain. It is made worse on flexion of the spine. Sitting is particularly painful. Coughing, sneezing and straining worsen the pain through increasing the intra-discal pressure. There are usually no neurological symptoms and signs.

Investigations

Plain radiography may show disc space narrowing. MRI demonstrates decreased signal intensity on the T2 images (disc dehydration) with a degenerate disc and it might reveal a high-intensity zone (T2 images again) in the annulus with an annular tear). Both disc degeneration and annular tears are demonstrated more clearly with discography. Furthermore, discography may be useful in clarifying whether the disc is the source of the pain or not.

Treatment

Management of discogenic low back pain can be non-operative, minimal invasive and/or in the form of surgery.

Non-operative measures include NSAIDs and physical therapy. In the initial stage, various therapeutic modalities such as NSAIDs, heat or ice therapy follows a brief period of rest. Early exercise to restore the range of movement is started once pain control is established. This is then followed by isometric exercises for the abdominal and lumbar extensor muscles in order to stabilise the injured motion segment. The next task is exercises to strengthen all the lumbar muscles. Once this is achieved then the athlete can progress to sports-specific exercises and finally return to the sport itself.

Minimal invasive treatments include epidural injections and intradiscal electrothermal therapy (IDET). IDET is a new procedure, which involves heating the disc to a high temperature. It is very controversial and its efficacy remains to be proven. Surgery involves various forms of fusion. It is reserved for patients who continue to have symptoms despite 6 months of conservative measures and also have a positive MRI and discogram.

Return to sport

With non-operative treatment, return to play is a gradual process. Return to light play is permitted as soon as pain allows, however there must be a complete resolution of pain together with restoration of sufficient range of movement and strength before the athlete returns to full play. Most athletes are able to return to sport within a few weeks; however, some remain symptomatic despite months of non-operative treatment.

Those who undergo fusion should not return to sport before there is radiological evidence of solid fusion as well as restoration of the standard parameters used for non-operative measurement. Usually, return to play is about 1 year for non-contact sports.

Further reading

Bono C. Low-back pain in athletes. *J Bone & Joint Surgery (Am)* 2004; **86**(2): 382–96.

Eck JC, Riley LH. Return to play after lumbar spine conditions and surgeries. *Clinics in Sports Medicine* 2004; **23**: 367–79.

Back pain – spondylolysis

AA Narvani

Spondylolysis is derived from the Greek word "spondylos" which means spine, and "lysis" which means to dissolve. It refers to a condition caused by a defect within the bone of the posterior part of the neural arch. This defect is usually in the pars interarticularis.

Epidemiology

Its prevalence in the general population is reported to be between 3 to 6%. It occurs more commonly in divers, gymnasts, weight lifters, wrestlers, rowers, fast bowlers in cricket, ballerinas and throwing athletes than the general population. It appears to be slightly more common in males than females although high grade slippage is more frequent in girls than boys. The mean age of diagnosis in athletes is about 16 years. Its incidence is particularly high in Alaskan Eskimos (26%). There also seems to be a hereditary predisposition.

Aetiology

The main aetiological factors appear to be a weakened or defective pars interarticularis that is further injured with repetitive hyperextension loading, which is thought to cause stress fractures (therefore it is common in sports that require repetitive hyperextension of the spine). Skeletally immature athletes are particularly at risk because the risk of injury to the spine is greater during times of rapid skeletal growth especially with improper techniques, sudden increases in training frequency, unsuitable equipment, improper footwear choices, different playing surfaces and musculoskeletal weakness and inflexibility.

Pathology

In 85% of the cases, the spondylolysis occurs at the L5 level. It may be unilateral or bilateral. In 25% of symptomatic patients with spondylolysis, there is also slipping of the concerned vertebrae (spondylolisthesis).

Clinical features

Ninety per cent of the patients with spondylolysis are asymptomatic. Those patients who have symptoms typically present with low back pain that is made worse by activity, in particular those which involve hyperextension of the spine. There are usually no radicular symptoms, however there may be some referred pain to the buttocks or the back of the thigh. In general there are no neurological symptoms. Examination may reveal an increased lumbar lordosis due either to greater sacral inclination, which is seen in some patients with spondylolysis, or to an associated spondylolisthesis. On palpation there may be a midline point tenderness with spondylolysis and a step-off with an associated spondylolisthesis. The "one leg hyperextension" test may be positive. (This test involves extending the low back while standing on a single leg. It is positive for the ispsilateral spondylolytic lesion, when there is pain on the side of the standing leg.)

Investigations

A plain X-ray should include an oblique view which demonstrates the "Scotty dog" lesions in the pars interarticularis. The 30 degrees cranially angulated AP view and coned lateral view are thought to demonstrate about 85% of the spondylolytic lesions. A lateral view will also reveal the presence of an associated spondylolisthesis. Those patients who are symptomatic despite a normal plain radiograph require further investigation in the form of a bone scan, single photon emission computed tomography (SPECT) scan or magnetic resonance imaging. A bone scan may be normal with chronic lesions. A SPECT scan can identify acute stress reaction (impending stress fractures) of the pars prior to its radiological manifestation. In addition, it may not detect chronic spondylolytic lesions. Although CT is very good in demonstrating the anatomical features of the lesion, it will not detect impending stress fractures. MRI can reveal stress reactions (bone oedema), however false negatives may occur as a result of facet joint osteophytes obscuring the pars defects.

Treatment

Non-operative management is shown to have a good outcome in the majority of the athletes with spondylolysis and spondylolisthesis with less than 50% slip. This involves a period of analgesia and activity restriction followed by physical rehabilitation. Bracing is controversial but many athletes are generally advised to wear a brace until they are pain free, at which time they start weaning off it.

Surgery is indicated in athletes

(1) who continue to have pain despite 6 to 12 months of non-operative measures.
(2) with spondylolisthesis who also have associated neurological deficits.
(3) with progressive spondylolisthesis.
(4) with more than 50% slip (Grade III spondylolisthesis).

Surgery is in the form of either fusion (with or without decompression) or direct repair of the defect. Techniques used for fusion include posterolateral fusion with or without instrumentation, and interbody fusion. Direct par repair may be performed by wiring, interfragmentary screws, pedicle screw-rod constructs, or pedicle screw-rod-hood constructs.

Return to sport

With non-operative treatment, athletes may return to sport when they are pain free even if there is no radiological evidence of par healing. Stable bony union may not be achieved and despite a fibrous non-union many athletes are able to return to play. This may take in excess of 6–8 weeks.

With operative management, in addition to being pain free, there must be radiological evidence of solid fusion or bone healing in those who undergo pars repair. This delays return to non-contact sports to about 1 year.

Further reading

Bono C. Low-back pain in athletes. *J Bone & Joint Surgery (Am)* 2004; **86**(2): 382–96.

Eck JC, Riley LH. Return to play after lumbar spine conditions and surgeries. *Clinics in Sports Medicine* 2004; **23**: 367–79.

Wiberely RL, Lauerman WC. Spondylolisthesis in the athlete. *Clinics in Sports Medicine* 2002; **21**(1): 133–45.

Biomechanics

B Lynn

Biomechanical analysis has a long history in sports science, where increasingly sophisticated methods are used in the quest for better performance. Biomechanics is also being increasingly used in sports medicine to find ways to prevent injury and to monitor rehabilitation post injury. As the technology becomes more user-friendly one can expect this trend to continue. In addition, there are major applications where bioengineering and biomechanics combine to develop aids for those disabled people who wish to take part in sports activities.

Kinematics

Kinematics is concerned with describing and analysing posture and movement. The methods include goniometry, video and specialised opto-electronic systems (e.g. CODA). Kinematic analysis is widely used in sports medicine. A good example is the use of video analysis to sort out gait problems. A typical situation may be recurring Achilles tendon or related injuries that can be traced to excessive foot pronation during running. Video analysis allows the nature of the problem to be quantified. It can then be used to look critically at treatment options, for example looking at the effect of special orthotic running shoes on ankle alignment during running.

Kinetics

Kinetics deals with forces and moments. In other words, not just observing patterns of motion, but analysing in detail the ways in which those movements are brought about. The necessary equipment comprises dynamometers for measuring forces in any direction or around any joint and force plates, usually used for measuring ground reaction forces. In kinetics, life becomes seriously complicated, but the basis is still just Newton's three laws:

(1) A body will remain at rest unless acted upon by a net force. Many forces may be acting but they all cancel out.
(2) A body (its centre of mass) accelerates at a rate proportional to the net force acting and in the direction of the force. The acceleration is inversely proportional to the mass. $P = m \times a$ where P = force in Newtons, m = mass in kg and a = acceleration in $m\,s^2$.
(3) Action and reaction are equal and opposite. When we measure a force such as the *action* exerted by a subject, an equal and opposite force, the *reaction*, acts upon the subject.

Electromyography (EMG) and anatomy

Detailed analysis of sports movements and how they may cause injury depends firstly on knowing the anatomy. For example, we are going to be in big trouble in trying to understand shoulder overuse problems if we have not come to terms with the complex anatomy. However, it is EMG analysis that often leads to the fullest understanding of what has gone wrong in a repeat injury scenario. It is our muscles that drive all movements, but it is not always clear whether a particular pattern on movement reflects equal activity in all the synergists, or whether a change reflects overactivity in a particular prime mover or under-activity in a stabilising antagonist.

Gait analysis

The analysis of gait illustrates how all the methods of biomechanics can combine to give a very complete picture. The subject is monitored kinematically, either using video or optoelectronically (CODA). Usually the side view is enough, but front, or even top, views can also be analysed if necessary. Whilst being viewed kinematically, the subject steps on a force plate whose signals are synchronised with those from the kinematics. The force plate tells us about forces in three planes:

- the vertical forces associated with supporting the body and accelerating and decelerating it in the up–down direction;
- the anterior posterior directed forces involved in forward locomotion;
- the lateral forces, which for straight motion should be small and symmetrical.

Finally, information about the activity of selected muscles can be obtained, again synchronously, with all the other signals.

With all this going on, there is a serious issue with data overload! Condensing the information to just about lower limb biomechanics can involve three force channels, looking at angular motion around three major joints in each leg, and monitoring EMG from at least four muscles on each side. So 17 channels of continuous data. It is really a case of knowing what you are looking for, plus having a database of normal responses for comparison.

Properties of biomaterials

An important area of biomechanics is the analysis of strength and stiffness of biomaterials, particularly bone, tendons and ligaments. When a force is applied to a structure it will deform, and the extent of deformation will increase as force increases. We normally need to know the material properties of a tissue, i.e. how the material responds whatever the exact shape or size of the specimen. For uniform materials (only a rough approximation for bones, tendons, etc., but we have to start somewhere!) we can define stress as the force per unit cross-sectional area. So a thick tendon can support a greater load than a thin one, but the mechanical properties of the collagen matrix may be the same. If this is the case, then a tendon one-tenth the cross-sectional area of another should stretch by ten times more under the same load. Stretch or compression also need to be normalised to allow for differences in length of the specimen. So *strain* is defined as the percentage change in length. Therefore a tendon 5 mm long will stretch only half as much as an otherwise similar tendon that is 10 mm – but the strain in each will be the same.

The ratio of stress to strain is the elastic modulus of a material. Stiffness of tendons is approximately 600 MN/m^2 (MN = mega Newtons), for bone it is 15 GN/m^2, 25 times higher. Note, however, that the strength of bone and tendon (the maximum stress that can be tolerated) is pretty much the same; it is just that tendon stretches much more before it breaks. Stress–strain relations are also important as they allow the calculation of the energy storage during, for example, tendon stretch.

For acute injuries, immediate breaking strain is important. For overuse injuries the response to repeated stresses is also important. One factor here is the viscoelastic nature of all biomaterials. They do not show simply elastic responses where it does not matter at what speed the stress is applied. Biomaterials characteristically deform further to slowly-applied stresses, and show "creep", continued slow deformation, in the face of prolonged steady stresses. With repeated brief stresses, there can be accumulation of microdamage and this can build up until failure occurs. This is, of course, not just a property of biomaterials and has been much studied by mechanical engineers. Unfortunately we still do not have a very good understanding of these phenomena in biomaterials.

Further reading

Brukner P, Khan K, Agosta T. Biomechanics of common sporting injuries. In: P Brukner, K Khan (Eds) *Clinical Sports Medicine*, 2nd edn. Sydney: McGraw Hill, 2001: 43–81.

Nigg BM. Biomechanics as applied to sports. *Oxford Textbook of Sports Medicine*, 2nd edn. Oxford University Press, 1998: 153–70.

Structure and function of ligaments and tendons. Published on the Internet. Online. Available http://www.engin.umich.edu/class/bme456/ligten/ligten.htm.

Calf pain

P Thomas

Calf muscle injury

The calf muscles comprise the gastrocnemius and the soleus muscles. The plantaris passes obliquely from the lateral to the medial side between the gastrocnemius and soleus muscles. All three of them form the Achilles tendon distally.

The gastrocnemius crosses both the knee and ankle joint and is prone to injury. The soleus is rarely injured. Most calf strains occur at the mid-belly of the medial head of the gastrocnemius. They present with acute pain, swelling, tenderness and in a few days the appearance of bruising.

Treatment will consist of rest, ice, compression and elevation, and anti-inflammatories. This should be followed by physiotherapy including stretching and strengthening exercises, as a second stage after the acute painful episode has settled. Recovery can take between 2–6 weeks.

Achilles tendon injuries

The Achilles tendon twists as it descends, rotating laterally, raising stresses at about 2–5 cm before its insertion, where the rotation is more pronounced. This area has also less blood supply compared to the rest of the tendon. At insertion there are two bursae, one subcutaneous and the other retrocalcanear between the tendon and the calcaneum bone. The tendon is surrounded by the paratenon which is not a synovial sheath.

Factors contributing to injury include inappropriate footwear, excessive training loads, biomechanical factors of the leg and foot such as overpronation, rear foot varus or valgus and tight gastrocnemius and soleus muscles.

Assessment by an ultrasound scan will confirm the presence of swelling, degenerative cysts, calcification and bursitis on the tendon. HLA-B27 and serum uric acid measurements will exclude the presence of a seronegative rheumatology condition or gout.

Nodular thickening from a degenerative cyst, which moves with dorsiflexion or plantar flexion, suggests a tendon pathology. If the nodule does not move with ankle movements then the pathology lies on the paratenon and not at the Achilles tendon itself. Treatment includes ice application, anti-inflammatories, use of a heel raise orthotics, physiotherapy modalities, other orthotics where necessary and stretching programmes of the gastrocnemius and soleus muscles. When the pain settles then eccentric stretching and loading will improve elasticity and return of function and, eventually, a return to sport activities.

Injections of the tendon with corticosteroids should be avoided due to their softening effect and risk of tendon rupture. New techniques using dry needling under ultrasound guidance and autotransfusion of blood are considered to promote recovery and enhance healing.

Surgery in chronic Achilles tendinopathy addresses adhesive-thickened paratenon and excision of degenerative cysts and repair of partial ruptures.

Tendon rupture

See the chapter on Achilles tendon rupture.

Further reading

Brown PE. Ankle and leg injuries. *Team Phys Handbook*. Philadelphia: Hanley and Belfus, 1997.

Garrett WE. Muscle strain injuries: clinical and basic aspects. *Med Sci Sports Exercise* 1990; **22**(4): 436–43.

Cervical spine injuries – overview

AA Narvani

Sporting activities are among the commonest cause of cervical spine injuries with 5 to 10% of all cervical injuries occurring as a result of sports. Although most cervical spine injuries are minor, a small percentage of these could be catastrophic and pose actual or potential damage to the spinal cord. Around 8% of all spinal cord injuries are due to sporting accidents. Appreciation of a potentially catastrophic cervical spine injury, and appropriate management from the first moments, is of vital importance in order to reduce the risks of extensive morbidity and even mortality.

Cervical spine injuries are common in contact sports including American football, rugby, ice hockey and wrestling. They are also seen in some non-contact sports such as equestrian events, diving, skiing and surfing.

Management

Principles of management of cervical spine injuries are:

(i) ATLS management with attention to *airway*, *breathing*, *circulation* and *disability*.
(ii) At the same time, just as important is *prevention of further damage to spinal cord* by:
  (a) Awareness of potential of cervical spine injury.
  (b) Appropriate on-field management, which includes immobilisation.
  (c) Detection of any neurological deficits.
  (d) Detection of "unstable" injuries. (Instability as defined by White and Panjabi is "loss of ability of the spine under physiological loads to maintain relationships in such a way that there is neither damage nor subsequent irritation to the spinal cord or nerve roots and, in addition, there is no development of incapacitating deformity and pain".)

A thorough assessment of the athlete, which includes history, examination and various diagnostic imaging investigations, would allow the physician to make one of the following diagnoses:

(i) Cervical ligament/muscle injuries:
  - Sprains
  - Strains
  - Contusions
(ii) Cervical disc injuries including herniation
(iii) Nerve root/brachial plexus injuries
  - Stingers
(iv) Cervical fracture/dislocations
  - May be stable/unstable
  - May or may not be associated with neurology
(v) Cervical cord neuropraxia
(vi) Spinal cord injuries (as the result of unstable injuries)

It is important to appreciate that a plain radiograph may not be enough to exclude unstable injuries and CT and/or MRI may be indicated.

Further reading

Banerjee R, Palumbo MA, Fadale PD. Catastrophic cervical spine injuries in the collision sport athlete, part 1, epidemiology, functional anatomy and diagnosis. *Am J Sports Medicine* 2004; **32**(4): 1077–87.

Banerjee R, Palumbo MA, Fadale PD. Catastrophic cervical spine injuries in the collision sport athlete, part 2, principles of emergency care. *Am J Sports Medicine* 2004; **32**(7): 1760–4.

Cervical spine – cervical ligament and muscle injuries

AA Narvani

Strains refer to muscular or musculo-tendinous stretch injuries, whereas sprains on the other hand are ligamentous stretch injuries. Contusion is localised muscular damage and bleeding is usually caused by a direct blow to the muscle.

These ligament and muscle injuries are extremely common.

Clinical features

- neck pain following "jamming" the neck
- tenderness over the involved structure
- limited range of movement of cervical spine
- absence of neurological/radicular features

Investigation

- Plain radiographs would be normal but important in ruling out fractures and unstable injuries. The following X-ray features may indicate the presence of unstable injuries:
  - (i) vertebral subluxation
  - (ii) vertebral compression fracture
  - (iii) loss of cervical lordosis
  - (iv) interspinous widening
- In addition, in excluding intervertebral disc injuries, a MRI scan may be able to define the ligamentous/muscular damage in greater detail.
- A CT scan can be helpful to exclude bony injuries which could not be diagnosed from plain radiographs.

Treatment

Following exclusion of unstable or bony injuries, treatment involves:

- Analgesia and NSAIDs.
- Soft cervical collar for comfort in the early phase. Prolonged immobilisation is not recommended as it causes atrophy and deconditioning of muscles.
- Physical therapy including manual therapy to the joints, muscle therapy to the muscles, and exercise therapy.

Return to sport

Athletes may be permitted to return to sport when they

- are symptom free
- have achieved full range of movement
- have regained their neck muscle power
- have regained their sport-specific neck function

Further reading

Zmurko MG, Tannoury TY, Tannoury CA, Anderson DG. Cervical sprains, disc herniation, minor fractures, and other cervical injuries in the athlete. *Clinics in Sports Medicine* 2003; **22**: 513–21.

Cervical spine – cervical disc injuries and herniations

AA Narvani

Although acute cervical disc herniations are comparatively rare in athletes, acute and chronic cervical disc disruption without herniation are seen in sports such as American football, wrestling, soccer, other contact sports and high-speed motor car racing (due to the massive G forces on the cervical spine). They are thought to be more common in older athletes.

Pathology

Uncontrolled lateral bending of the neck can result in acute cervical disc disruption. This may or may not lead to nucleus propulus herniation through the posterior annulus. This herniated material may then in turn lead to cord or nerve root compression.

A second pathological process is degeneration of the disc associated with decreased disc height and dehydration of the disc. This is a chronic process with gradual onset and slow progression of symptoms. With time, associated disc herniation may develop.

Clinical features

Symptoms and signs depend on whether or not there is any associated disc herniation.

The following features are seen:

- Varying degree of neck pain.
- Arm pain (usually with disc herniation).
- Neurological features of limbs, occurring as a result of disc herniation, the pattern of which is dependent on the location of the disc herniation.

Investigations

- Plain radiograph (this will initially rule out bony injuries and most of the unstable injuries. It may also reveal the degenerative changes of the cervical spine).
- MRI is the investigation of choice, demonstrating the disc pathology in detail.
- In those where MRI is contraindicated, CT myelogram will also show the disc herniation.

Treatment

Non-operative

- Rest
- Analgesia and NSAIDs
- Immobilisation
- Activity adjustment
- Epidural injections
- Exercise therapy once radicular symptoms improve.

Operative

- Surgery is indicated if there is:
  - (i) myelopathy,
  - (ii) progressive neurological deficit,
  - (iii) failure of non-operative measures.
- Surgery is in the form of decompression ± fusion.

Return to sport

With non-operative treatment, as with muscular and ligament injuries, the athlete is permitted to return to sport once there is complete resolution of symptoms, full pain-free cervical range of motion, and full muscle power. They must also regain complete cervical spine sport-specific function before returning to sports.

Return to sport following surgery is dependent on the type of surgery:

- Following discectomy or decompression on its own, the criteria for return to sports is the same as those of non-operative measures.
- If the decompression/discectomy is accompanied with fusion up to two levels, there must additionally be successful fusion (may require imaging such as CT scan to confirm fusion) before the athlete is allowed to return to sport.
- Athletes with fusions at three or more levels are generally not permitted to return to contact sports even after meeting the above criteria.

Further reading

Scherping SC. Cervical disc disease in the athlete. *Clinics in Sports Medicine* 2002; **21**(1): 37–47.

Zmurko MG, Tannoury TY, Tannoury CA, Anderson DG. Cervical sprains, disc herniation, minor fractures, and other cervical injuries in the athlete. *Clinics in Sports Medicine* 2003; **22**: 513–21.

Cervical spine – fracture/dislocation

AA Narvani

These injuries can be stable or unstable and may or may not be associated with neurological deficits. Cervical injuries where there is actual or potential damage to the spinal cord in association with the structural distortion of the spinal column are referred to as "catastrophic cervical spine injuries".

Twenty to 30% of all spine fractures occur in the cervical spine region. Approximately 10–20% of all spinal traumas are associated with spinal cord injury. Sporting activities account for more than 7% of all the spinal cord injuries and are the second commonest cause of such injuries in the first three decades of life, second only to road traffic accidents. Sporting spinal cord injuries are more common in athletes who are between 20 to 30 years old and are seen in sports such as equestrian, American football, rugby, ice hockey, snow boarding and skiing.

Principles of management

The aims of managing any patient with cervical spine fracture and/or dislocation are (see Banerjee *et al.* (2004) part 1, Further reading):

(i) *Prevention* of damage to uninjured neurological tissue.
(ii) *Realignment* of the spine.
(iii) *Maximisation* of neurological recovery.
(iv) Achievement of *stability*.
(v) *Rehabilitation*.

It has been shown that in a significant number of cases, spinal cord injuries have occurred during the initial management after the initial event. Therefore, the initial management of all athletes with cervical spine injuries according to ATLS, which includes immobilisation, is of vital importance.

Once passed the "initial management", any malalignment of the cervical spine may be corrected by skeletal traction with the aid of:

- Spring-loaded Gardner Wells tongs
- Halo ring

Further management may be non-operative or operative depending on:

(i) Whether there is any *compression of neural* features (as suggested by clinical features and various imaging modalities which include MRI and CT scans).
(ii) *Stability* of the fracture. Stability is defined by White and Punjabi (see Torg, 2002) as the "ability of the spine under physiological loads to maintain relationships in such a way that there is neither damage nor subsequent irritation to the spinal cord or nerve roots and, in addition, there is no development of incapacitating deformity and pain". When this ability is lost, the injury is said to be "unstable".

Although this is a complete and comprehensive definition, clinicians need to be able to assess stability objectively. A cervical spine injury is unstable when it is associated with any one of the following – see Torg (2002) and Banerjee *et al.* (2004), part 1, in the Further reading list:

(a) Dysfunction of all the anterior elements.
(b) Dysfunction of all the posterior elements.
(c) More than 3.5 mm anterior–posterior displacement of one vertebral with respect to the vertebral below.
(d) Angular displacement of more than 11 degrees of adjacent vertebra.

Non-operative management
Stable fractures without any compression of neural tissue may be managed with a rigid cervical brace or halo for 8 to 12 weeks. Injuries that may be treated in this way include:

- Stable compression fractures of the vertebral bodies.
- Undisplaced fractures of the laminae, lateral masses and spinous process.

Reduced unilateral facet joint dislocations may also be treated in a halo vest for 8 to 12 weeks.

Operative management
Surgery is indicated for unstable injuries whether or not there is the presence of any neurological deficits. Surgery is also required in those with neurological deficits and mechanical compression of neural tissue (by definition these are also unstable injuries). Surgery is in the form of decompression (in those with mechanical compression of the neural structure) and stabilisation.

Specific injuries
Cervical spine fracture and/or dislocation injuries may be divided into those that involve the occipitocervical junction and upper cervical spine (down to C2) and those that involve the lower cervical spine (C3 to C7).

Upper cervical spine injuries

Dislocation of the atlanto-occipital joint
These injuries are usually fatal due to respiratory arrest secondary to brainstem compression. In those who survive, management consists of immediate application of the halo vest followed by early surgical internal stabilisation.

Atlas (C1) fractures
These fractures can be divided into:

- Posterior arch fractures
- Anterior arch fractures
- Burst fractures (Jefferson fracture)

They are usually treated by rigid cervical brace or halo vest.

Isolated transverse ligament injuries
Usually caused by a blow to the back of the head, these injuries may involve mid-substance rupture of the ligament or avulsion with a small bone fragment of the lateral mass. Those with substance rupture require early surgery in the form of internal stabilisation. Those that involve bony avulsion may have a trial of non operative management with a rigid cervical brace. Surgery is indicated in those with non-union and persistent instability after 3–4 months.

Odontoid fractures
These are classified into three types.

Type I injuries are avulsion fractures of the tip of the odontoid. These are rare, stable injuries that are not usually associated with any neurological deficit. Most of these are treated with a rigid cervical brace.

Type II injuries refer to fractures through the neck of the odontoid process. These are associated with a high non-union rate. Treatment may be in the form of halo vest immobilisation, however surgery is indicated in those with high risk of non-union (displacement of more than 5 mm, posterior displacement, age >50 years). Surgery is also indicated when union has not been achieved with a halo vest.

Type III fractures extend into the cancellous bone and are associated with a much higher union rate than Type II injuries. Treatment is commonly with halo immobilisation.

Hangman fractures (traumatic spondylolisthesis of C2 (axis))

These injuries are subclassified into three types.

Type I. These are undisplaced or have an anterior translation of less than 3 mm. They are commonly treated with a rigid cervical brace.

Type II. There is anterior translation of more than 3 mm. They are initially treated with halo traction for 3 to 6 weeks followed by a halo vest for up to a further 3 months.

Type IIA. With these injuries there is minimal translation but significant angulation. Treatment involves reduction initially with a halo vest while applying slight compression under an image intensifier (traction is contraindicated). Once reduced, halo vest immobilisation may be continued until healing occurs.

Type III. These injuries involve the posterior facets and are accompanied by unilateral or bilateral facet dislocation at C2–C3. There is significant angulation and translation. Neurological deficits are commonly present. In the vast majority of cases, treatment is in the form of open reduction and internal fixation. Halo vest immobilisation may be required following surgery.

Lower cervical spine injuries

In the lower cervical spine, fractures are more common at C5, C6 and C7 vertebrae and dislocation/subluxations occur most frequently at C4/C5, C5/C6 and C6/C7 interspace.

Posterior ligamentous injury

Disruption of posterior ligamentous complex occurs as a consequence of distraction and flexion forces. It results in the widening of the interspinous process during flexion and may result in unilateral or bilateral facet joint dislocation. Treatment is by surgery in the form of posterior cervical fusion.

Unilateral facet dislocation

The mechanism of injury is flexion and rotation of the cervical spine (classified as distractive flexion injuries) and may be purely ligamentous or involve facet fracture. This can be accompanied with a neurological deficit. Reduction of the dislocation is indicated. This reduction may be achieved by skull traction and, if successful, halo vest immobilisation should be applied for up to 3 months. If reduction cannot be achieved by skull traction then surgery is indicated (open reduction and stabilisation).

It should be noted at this stage that controversy exists on whether or not to obtain an MRI scan prior to attempting the close reduction. This MRI will rule out the presence of herniated nucleus pulposus, which may herniate further when attempting the close reduction and cause a catastrophic cord sequelae.

Bilateral facet dislocation

As with unilateral facet dislocations, the mechanism of injury is flexion and rotation, but neurological deficit is more common with these. They result in more than 50% anterior subluxation of one vertebra over the one below. Although close reduction is comparatively easy, redislocation rate is common with traction or a halo vest. Therefore surgery (open reduction-internal fixation) is usually indicated.

The same controversies regarding MRI scanning (see above) exist.

Vertebral body fractures

Most of these injuries occur as a result of axial loading and compression. There is a wide spectrum of injuries ranging from stable injuries without any neurological deficit to unstable injuries with significant neurological abnormalities. These injuries include the following:

- Simple stable wedge or vertebral end plate compression fractures which are not associated with any neurological deficit. Posterior element soft tissue supporting structures are intact with less than 25% anterior compression. They can be treated non-operatively with external cervical orthotic immobilisation.
- When the compression fracture is accompanied with posterior ligamentous damage, then the injury is unstable. The presence of such injuries may be indicated by anterior compression of more than 50% and the presence of other features of instability (see above). Treatment of such cases involves initial skull traction in order to re-align the spine followed by surgery (stabilisation ± decompression).
- Comminuted burst fractures of the vertebral body, which are usually associated with a retropulsed bony fragment into the spinal canal, which may in turn cause cord injury. Therefore neurological deficit is not uncommon. Imaging in the form of CT and MRI is required to assess the extent of the damage. Initially longitudinal traction is indicated to try to achieve some realignment. This should be followed by surgery (stabilisation ± decompression).
- Teardrop fractures usually result from severe flexion loading of the cervical spine. The teardrop fragment itself is the anterior inferior vertebral body fracture. However, the injury is extensive and usually involves all three spinal columns. Three fracture parts may be seen with these injuries:
  —anterior–inferior teardrop fracture
  —sagittal vertebral body fracture
  —posterior neural arch disruption.
  Highly unstable injuries are commonly associated with neurological deficits. Treatment is by initial traction followed by surgery.

A three-part fracture of the vertebral body can be accompanied with posterior element disruption of the vertebral below. This is highly unstable and frequently associated with neurological abnormalities. Treatment is by initial traction followed by surgery.

Spinous process avulsion fracture

Also referred to as "clay shoveler's" fracture, these are caused by forceful contraction of the trapezius and rhomboid muscles. It is a hyperflexion injury. These are stable injuries and are managed with a cervical brace.

Other isolated fractures

Isolated transverse process fractures, osteophyte fractures and trabecular fractures all tend to be stable and in most cases may be treated non-operatively with a collar.

Return to sport

Cervical spine fracture injuries can have a massive impact. Many athletes must accept that they may not be able to return to contact sport. Those who may return are (see Torg, 2002 in the Further reading list):

- Vertebral body compression fractures that meet *all* following criteria:
  —stable
  —healed
  —with normal neurology
  —pain free
  —with full cervical spine range of movement
  —without ligamentous laxity
  —without posterior bony structure fractures
  —without a sagittal component
- Endplate fractures that meet all the above criteria mentioned for vertebral body compression fractures.
- Isolated spinous process fractures that have healed.

All athletes with all other cervical spine fracture injuries are generally advised against returning to contact sports.

Further reading

Banerjee R, Palumbo MA, Fadale PD. Catastrophic cervical spine injuries in the collision sport athlete, part 1, epidemiology, functional anatomy and diagnosis. *Am J Sports Medicine* 2004; **32**(4): 1077–87.

Banerjee R, Palumbo MA, Fadale PD. Catastrophic cervical spine injuries in the collision sport athlete, part 2, principles of emergency care. *Am J Sports Medicine* 2004; **32**(7): 1760–4.

Torg JS. Cervical spine, cervical spine injuries in adults. In: JC DeLee, D Drez, MD Miller (Eds) *Orthopaedic Sports Medicine, Principles and Practice*, 2nd edn. Saunders, 2002: 791–828.

Cervical spine – cervical cord neuropraxia

AA Narvani

Cervical cord neuropraxia, also known as transient quadriplegia, refers to transient neurological deficits (sensory and/or motor) of limbs as a result of pressure on the cervical spinal cord. Athletes with congenital spinal stenosis are predisposed to this condition. It is seen in sports such as American football, rugby, wrestling and boxing.

Pathology

See Figure 1.

Clinical features

See Figure 1.

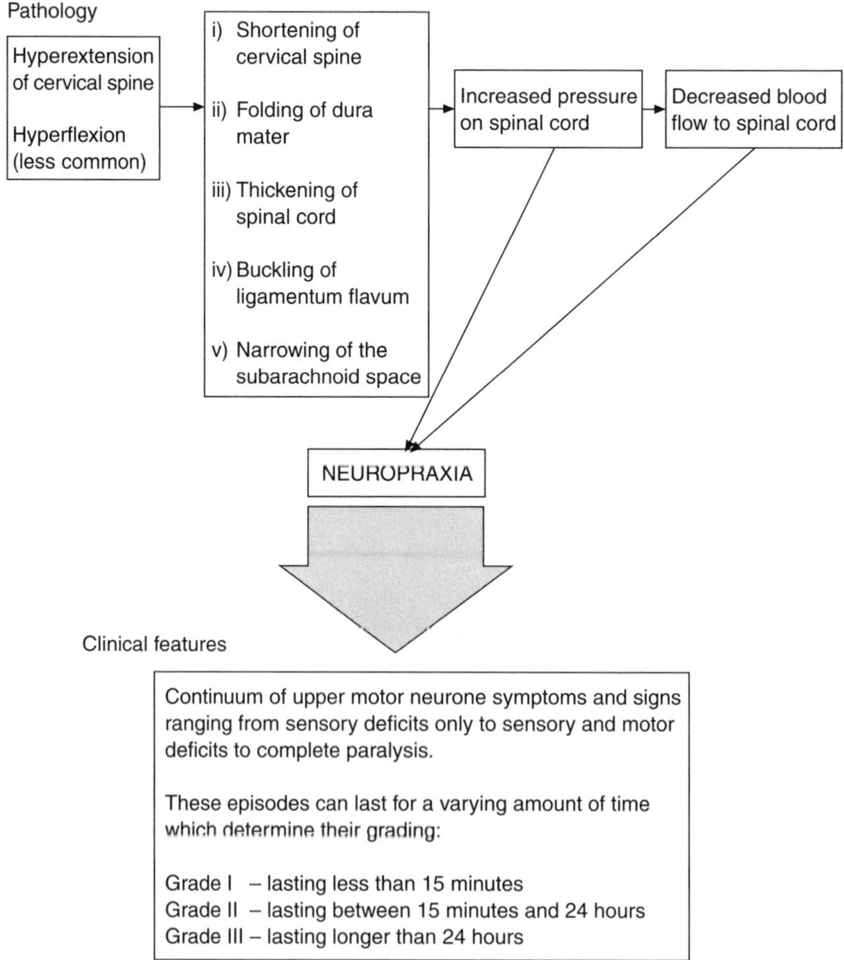

Figure 1 Pathology and clinical features of cervical cord neuropraxia.

Investigations
As well as excluding bony injuries, other unstable injuries, disc herniations, various imaging modalities such as plain radiographs, CT and MRI scans, will help to reveal the presence of cervical stenosis. In the presence of functional stenosis, MRI will illustrate obliteration of local cerebrospinal fluid space in addition to deformation of the cord contour. It may also reveal actual spinal cord injury (signals within the cord).

The Torg ratio, which is measured from plain radiograph, with cervical spine in extension, is a ratio of the distance between the midpoint of the posterior aspect of the vertebral body and the nearest corresponding spinolaminar line to the anterior–posterior width of the vertebral body. A ratio of 0.8 or less is thought to indicate the presence of developmental stenosis.

Treatment
- Treatment is similar to that for nerve root or brachial plexus injuries (see following chapter) with the exception that athletes who have any episodes of cervical cord neuropraxia are generally advised against any further participation in contact sports since risk of recurrence and catastrophic neck injury are significantly greater.
- Role of intravenous steroid administration remains controversial.

Return to sport

See following chapter.

Further reading

Allen CR, Kang JD. Transient quadriparesis in the athlete. *Clin Sports Med* 2002; **1**: 15–27.
Castro FP. Stingers, cervical cord neuropraxia, and stenosis. *Clin Sports Med* 2003; **22**: 483–92.
Kim DH, Vaccaro AR, Berta SC. Acute sports-related spinal cord injury contemporary management principles *Clin Sports Med* 2003; **22**(3): 501–12.

Cervical spine – nerve root/brachial plexus injuries

AA Narvani

First described in 1965, these injuries are also referred to as stingers, burners, cervical pinch syndrome and transient brachial plexopathy. They are common in collision sports, particularly American football but are also seen in rugby, wrestling and boxing.

Pathology
Figure 1 illustrates the pathology of the process.

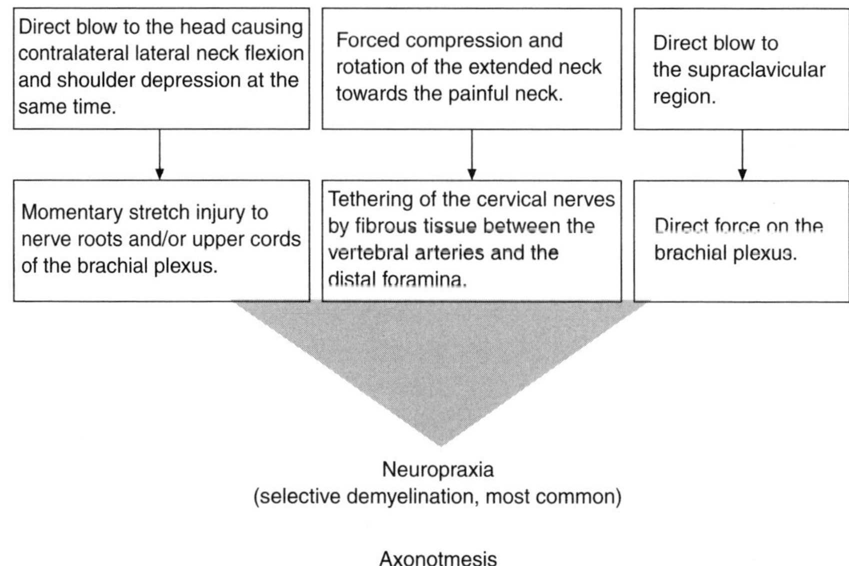

Figure 1 Pathology and features.

Clinical features

- History of injury (see Figure 1).
- Sharp/burning pain in the neck radiating to the shoulder and down the arm.
- Paraesthesia, pins and needles in the arm.
- Weakness of deltoid (C5), biceps (C5, C6), supraspinatus (C5, C6) and infraspinatus (C5, C6).
- "Spurling Manoeuvre" test may be positive. Hyperextension, lateral flexion and rotation of the neck to the side of suspected lesion produces pain down the ipsilateral arm.
- The course of the condition is dependent on the nerve injury type:
  (i) *Neuropraxia*
  There is usually full recovery within 3 weeks of the injury. (Most cases are neuropraxias with symptoms and signs resolving within minutes.)
  (ii) *Axonotmesis*
  Features persist longer than 2–3 weeks.
  (iii) *Neurotmesis*
  Features may not resolve, or if they do resolve, it may take longer than 1 year.

Investigation

Bony and other unstable injuries, disc herniations and cervical stenosis need to be excluded by various imaging modalities, which include plain radiographs, CT and MRI scans.

Electromyographic (EMG) studies are indicated if clinical features persist for more than 3–4 weeks.

Treatment

(i) Initially until symptoms resolve:
- Immediate removal of the athlete from participation.
- Sling.
- Pain management with NSAIDs and physiotherapy.

(ii) Rehabilitation once symptoms resolve:
- Range of movement.
- Muscle strength.

(iii) Prevention of further episodes:
- Neck and shoulder-strengthening programme.
- Sport permitting, use of neck rolls, high-profile shoulder pads.
- Technique adjustment.
- Some athletes may be advised not to return to their sport (see below).

Return to sport

- Following *first* episode, the athlete can return to play only if:
  (i) Symptoms have completely resolved within 24 hours.
  (ii) There is full cervical spine range of movement.
  (iii) There is full recovery of upper limb strength.
  (iv) Other pathological processes have been excluded.
- The above also applies with repeat attacks if the number of episodes has been less than three.
- Athletes with three or more episodes or attacks lasting longer than 24 hours may be advised to consider not returning to future play.

Further reading

Castro FP. Stingers, cervical cord neuropraxia, and stenosis. *Clinics in Sports Medicine* 2003; **22**: 483–92.

Weinburg J, Rokito S, Silber JS. Etiology, treatment, and prevention of athletic "stingers". *Clinics in Sports Medicine* 2003; **21**: 493–500.

Chest injuries

P Thomas

Etiology

These injuries occur when an object penetrates the thorax or due to a crushing force from a collision between athletes at high speed or against a wall or fence. Pneumothorax, haemothorax or haemopneumothorax may develop with or without a flail chest wall segment.

Mediastinal injury occurs usually in motor sports and skiing, from high speed deceleration. This involves injuries of the aorta and myocardium and must be suspected even if the patient appears well at first.

Assessment in the field

The predominant symptoms in a chest injury are pain and dyspnoea.

An assessment must include

- The possible obstruction of the airways by foreign bodies, facial fractures and tracheal injury.
- The chest wall respiratory movements, for instance paradoxical respiration in the presence of a flail segment.
- The air perfusion into the lungs.
- The respiratory rate.
- Position of the trachea and apex beat.
- Cardiovascular assessment.
- Blood pressure, peripheral pulses.
- Jugular venous pressure.

The objective is to establish normal ventilation and cardiovascular function.

Immediate treatment will consist of:

- Analgesia in rib fractures.
- Pericardial aspiration in cardiac tamponade.
- Air and blood evacuation from pleural space.
- Endotrachial tube in respiratory failure.
- Transport to hospital.
- Preparation to treat the effects of developing shock.

Sternum fracture

This is caused by an anterior blow at the sternum. In golf, stress fractures can be seen from a violent muscle contraction during the swing phase. Severe pain appears in inspiration and there may be a gap palpable on examination. Associated cardiac injury such as cardiac contusion or injuries affecting the great vessels must be excluded. Treatment consists of analgesia until healing takes place between 4 to 6 weeks.

Rib fractures

Rib fractures can occur following a direct blow or compression of the chest. The majority of these injuries are undisplaced fractures and most commonly will occur between the fourth through the ninth rib.

Multiple rib fractures may produce "paradoxical respiration" through a flail chest segment. This can be deduced as the affected segment moves in when the chest is expanding.

The assessment will reveal local pain, crepitus, respiration pain and the presence of contusion. Observations will include the appearances of blood during coughing, the rate and quality of breathing sounds. X-rays usually confirm the diagnosis, although injuries with a separation at the costochondral region may not be visible.

Pneumothorax

Pneumothorax is a condition when air is present within the pleura space. It may appear spontaneously and in some patients a background of pulmonary conditions such as asthma, cystic fibrosis or pneumonia may coexist. The cause is usually trauma such as a rib fracture, stab wound or exertion such as running. Air leaked from the lungs progressively reduces the pleural space volume, interfering with lung expansion during inspiration. Symptomatic athletes may require a chest tube. Return to sports which involve collision may be considered after a 4-week period. The athlete with a spontaneous pneumothorax must be carefully advised to alter his or her sport to a collision-free activity. However, if another episode of spontaneous pneumothorax occurs then the individual must be discouraged from continuing any contact sport.

Tension pneumothorax

This is caused by rapid accumulation of air in the pleural space during inspiration, which cannot escape on expiration. The air expansion of the pleural space will inevitably cause displacement of the mediastinum causing compression of the heart, aorta and the uninjured lung. Ventilation and cardiac output could therefore be compromised. In most cases of pneumothorax the air collection at the pleural space increases slowly. The athlete will complain of symptoms of pain, shortness of breath and refer pain to the tip of the shoulder. Observations may confirm an asymmetric lung movement, decreased or absent breath sounds over the affected side and decreased blood pressure and tachycardia. Imaging with repeat X-rays is important since the first X-rays will be negative for a pneumothorax.

The treatment will consist of the insertion of a 12–14 gauge needle in the second intercostal space at the mid-clavicular line. This is followed by insertion of a chest drain.

Haemothorax

Haemothorax refers to the presence of blood within the pleural space from damage of the lung tissue or bleeding from the chest wall veins. The symptoms will include severe pain, dyspnoea, coughing up blood, on occasions cyanosis and shock.

Haemopneumothorax can be treated with an intercostal tube used as chest drain. The early treatment of a haemothorax with a tube connected to low-pressure suction will achieve lung expansion, however continued bleeding may necessitate an open thoracotomy.

Pulmonary contusion

The athlete will be admitted to hospital for observation in case respiratory support will be deemed necessary. Pulmonary contusion usually settles over a period of time without any further intervention being necessary.

Heart injuries

They usually occur following blunt trauma behind the sternum at the right ventricle. Myocardial contusion can lead to arrhythmia and ventricular fibrillation.

Myocardial laceration can cause a pericardial tamponade where increased volume of blood is present in the pericardium compressing the venous return to the heart. The diagnosis will be based on the raised jugular venous pressure, low blood pressure and decreased heart sounds. A large-bore needle inserted through the fourth intercostal space next to the sternum in the pericardium will relieve the pressure immediately. Transfer to hospital must take place as soon as possible because a recurrence of the tamponade will necessitate surgical intervention.

Rupture of the aorta

Motor sports and high-speed downhill skiing are associated with this injury where the intima of the aorta will be ruptured usually at the arch junction.

Associated injuries may include first and second rib fractures. Awareness of this pattern of injury is important since the patient may appear well at first. X-rays may reveal an expanding aortic shadow on the left side, blood over the left lung apex, tracheal displacement, fractures of the first and second ribs. Arteriography must follow. Treatment consists of urgent surgical repair.

Diaphragm rupture

Diaphragm ruptures are compression injuries usually from the abdomen but also from the chest. Diagnosis can be confirmed with a series of X-rays, screening of the diaphragm, CT scan and MRI scan. However, the diagnosis of small tears is difficult and on occasions thoracotomy or laparotomy will be considered. Later on complications may present such as herniation of abdominal contents into the chest. Treatment consists of surgical repair.

Further reading

Erickson SM, Rich BSE. Pulmonary and chest wall emergencies. *Phys Sportsmed* 1995; **23**(11): 95–104.

Zachazewski JC, Magee DS, Quillens WS (Eds) *Athletic Injuries and Rehabilitation.* Philadelphia: WB Saunders, 1996.

Compartment pressure syndromes

P Thomas

Most compartment syndromes involve the lower leg but other sites, such as the thigh and upper limb, could also be affected.

Compartment syndrome results from increased pressure within a confined closed space, which will compromise the blood flow and function of the soft tissues. Acute and chronic forms of a compartment syndrome may exist. Acute compartment syndrome is associated with an injury including soft tissue damage or a fracture. Chronic compartment syndromes present as exercise-related lower leg soreness. The athlete complains of localised tightness with pain during or after exercise, which could last for some time. There are no other findings and peripheral pulses are present and normal. On occasions the complaint may be paraesthesia alongside the anterior ankle and the dorsum of the foot. Precipitating factors include a sudden increase in intensity and duration of the sports activity or in sports such as running or tennis practising on hard surfaces. New equipment such as new footwear must be assessed as they will change the biomechanical balance of the legs and feet.

Anterior compartment pressure syndrome

The anterior compartment comprises the tibialis anterior, extensor digitorum longus and extensor hallucis longus, anterior tibial artery and vein and the deep peroneal nerve.

Symptoms of pain and, in some cases, numbness of the first web space of the foot are the presented symptoms.

Lateral compartment pressure syndrome

Consists of peroneus longus and brevis muscles.

Deep calf compartment pressure syndrome

Comprises the tibialis posterior, flexor hallucis longus and the flexor digitorum longus. The tibialis posterior muscle may be included into its own separate compartment and may produce symptoms that should be distinguished from the medial tibial stress syndrome on the basis of a bone scan and compartment measurements.

Superficial calf compartment pressure syndrome

Includes the gastrocnemius and soleus muscles.

The compartment pressure syndrome pathology may affect more than one compartment and could also be bilateral.

Diagnosis of a chronic compartment pressure syndrome is confirmed by the measurement of the intracompartmental pressures. There are different methods of measuring the compartments. Pressure at rest of less than 10 mmHg, which will increase with exercise but will return to normal within 10 minutes of rest, is the recommended normal range.

Conservative management is active rest, correction of the biomechanics of the legs and feet, physiotherapy massage and stretching/strengthening exercises to adapt to the individual sporting activity and could take several weeks to months before recovery.

Surgery with fasciotomy appears to be the definitive treatment for chronic compartment pressure syndrome pathology.

Further reading

Edwards P *et al.* Exertional compartment syndrome of the leg. *Phys Sports Med* 1996, **24**(4): 31–46.
Mocyersoons JP *et al.* Chronic compartment syndrome. *Acta Orthop Belgica* 1992, **58**(1): 23–7.

Diabetes and exercise

S Parnia

Exercise activity not only plays a major role in the management of people with diabetes but also has a significant role in the prevention of this condition. Thus, in this chapter the recommendations for exercise for patients with diabetes are summarised.

Lifestyle measures and diabetes

For decades now, exercise – along with diet and medication – has been considered one of the major cornerstones of diabetes management, but in recent years major advances have also increased our understanding of the effects of exercise on the regulation of glucose. Studies have demonstrated that lifestyle interventions such as diet and exercise can reduce the incidence of type 2 diabetes in people with impaired glucose tolerance. Additionally, structured exercise interventions in those with type 2 diabetes have shown that exercise is effective in reducing HbA_{1c}, independent of body weight. Other studies have also demonstrated that resistance training (e.g. weight lifting) plays a role in improving glycemic control in type 2 diabetes. Conversely, other large cohort studies have also demonstrated that low aerobic fitness and low physical activity predict increased risk of overall and cardiovascular disease (CVD) mortality in people with diabetes. Therefore, in people with impaired glucose tolerance, a program of weight control is recommended, including at least 150 minutes per week of moderate to vigorous physical activity and a healthy diet with modest energy restriction.

Evaluation of the diabetic patient before recommending an exercise program

It is recommended that before beginning a program of physical activity that is more vigorous than brisk walking, people with diabetes should be formally assessed. Due to the nature of diabetes and its complications, patients should, in particular, be assessed for conditions that might contraindicate certain types of exercise or predispose to injury (e.g. severe autonomic neuropathy, severe peripheral neuropathy or preproliferative or proliferative retinopathy), which require treatment before beginning vigorous exercise, or that may be associated with increased likelihood of cardiovascular disease. The patient's age and previous physical activity level should also be considered.

Pre-exercise assessment: exercise stress testing with and without ECG monitoring Previous guidelines have suggested that before beginning a vigorous or moderate exercise program, an exercise ECG stress test should be done in all diabetic individuals aged >35 years and in all individuals aged >25 years in the presence of even one additional cardiovascular risk factor (Table 1).

However, this recommendation should be balanced out with the fact that the lower the absolute CAD (coronary artery disease) risk, the higher the likelihood of a false-positive test. A recent systematic review has concluded that stress tests should usually not be recommended to detect ischemia in asymptomatic individuals at low CAD risk (<10% risk of a cardiac event over 10 years) because the risks of subsequent invasive testing triggered by false–positive tests outweighed the expected benefits from the detection of previously unsuspected ischemia.

Therefore, some now propose that this test should be particularly directed at those people with diabetes with a 10-year CAD risk of at least 10% (1% per year) and so in the absence of contraindications, maximal exercise testing could be considered in all diabetic individuals in order to assess maximal heart rate, set exercise intensity targets, and assess functional capacity and prognosis. A graded exercise test with ECG monitoring should be seriously considered before undertaking aerobic physical activity with an intensity exceeding the demands of everyday living (more intense than brisk walking) in previously sedentary diabetic individuals whose 10-year risk of a coronary event is >10%. This risk could be estimated directly using the UKPDS Risk Engine (www.dtu.ox.ac.uk/riskengine/download.htm).

Effects of exercise on glycemic control and body weight in diabetes

Studies have demonstrated a strong dose–response relationship between exercise intensity and both cardiorespiratory fitness and HbA_{1c} change. These results would

Table 1 Risk factors for the development of cardiovascular disease in the presence of diabetes.

Diabetes duration >10 years for type 2 diabetes
Diabetes >15 years for type 1 diabetes
Hypertension
Dyslipidemia
Smoking
Proliferative retinopathy
Nephropathy including microalbuminuria
Peripheral vascular disease
Autonomic neuropathy

provide support for encouraging type 2 diabetic individuals who are already exercising at moderate intensity to consider increasing the intensity of their exercise to obtain additional benefits in both aerobic fitness and glycemic control.

Frequency of exercise

The effect on insulin sensitivity of a single bout of aerobic exercise lasts 24–72 h, depending on the duration and intensity of the activity. Because the duration of increased insulin sensitivity is generally not >72 h, it is recommended that the time between successive sessions of physical activity be no more than 72 h. There is some evidence that the effect of resistance exercise training on insulin sensitivity is somewhat longer, perhaps because some of its effects are mediated by increases in muscle mass.

The amount and intensity recommended for aerobic exercise vary according to goals.

- To improve glycemic control, assist with weight maintenance, and reduce risk of CVD, it is recommended to perform at least 150 minutes per week of moderate-intensity aerobic physical activity (40–60% of VO_2max or 50–70% of maximum heart rate) and/or at least 90 minutes per week of vigorous aerobic exercise (>60% of VO_2max or >70% of maximum heart rate). The physical activity should be distributed over at least 3 days per week and with no more than two consecutive days without physical activity.
- Performing >4 hours per week of moderate to vigorous aerobic and/or resistance exercise is associated with greater CVD risk reduction compared with lower volumes of activity.
- For long-term maintenance of major weight loss (>13.6 kg [30 lb]), larger volumes of exercise (7 hours per week of moderate or vigorous aerobic physical activity per week) may be helpful.

Resistance exercise

Resistance exercise improves insulin sensitivity to about the same extent as aerobic exercise. Because of the increased evidence for health benefits from resistance training during the past 10–15 years, the American College of Sports Medicine (ACSM) now recommends resistance training be included in fitness programs for healthy young and middle-aged adults, older adults, and adults with type 2 diabetes. With increased age, there is a tendency to progressive declines in muscle mass, decreased functional capacity, decreased resting metabolic rate, increased adiposity and increased insulin resistance, and resistance training can have a major positive impact on each of these.

Resistance exercise improves bone density, muscle mass, strength, balance and overall capacity for physical activity and therefore is potentially important for prevention of osteoporotic fractures in the elderly.

The ACSM recommends a resistance training regimen for type 2 diabetic individuals whenever possible and so in the absence of contraindications, people with type 2 diabetes should be encouraged to perform resistance exercise three times a week.

Exercise and non-optimal glucose control

Hyperglycemia

When people with type 1 diabetes are deprived of insulin for 12–48h and ketotic, exercise can worsen the hyperglycemia and ketosis. It has been suggested that physical activity be avoided if fasting glucose levels are higher than double the upper limit of normal and ketosis and caution be exercised in the cases where glucose levels are >300mg/dl even if no ketosis is present. In the absence of very severe insulin deficiency, light- or moderate-intensity exercise would tend to decrease plasma glucose. Therefore, provided the patient feels well and urine and/or blood ketones are negative, it may not be necessary to postpone exercise based simply on hyperglycemia.

Hypoglycemia

In individuals taking insulin and/or insulin secretagogues, physical activity can cause hypoglycemia if medication dose or carbohydrate consumption is not altered. This is particularly so at times when exogenous insulin levels are at their peaks and if physical activity is prolonged. Hypoglycemia would be rare in diabetic individuals who are not treated with insulin or insulin secretagogues. Previous guidelines suggest that added carbohydrate should be ingested if pre-exercise glucose levels are <100mg/dl. This applies for individuals on insulin and/or an insulin secretagogue. However, the revised guidelines clarify that supplementary carbohydrate is generally not necessary for individuals treated without insulin or a secretagogue.

Those who take insulin or secretagogues should check capillary blood glucose before, after and several hours after completing a session of physical activity, at least until they know their usual glycemic responses to such activity. For those who show a tendency toward hypoglycemia during or after exercise, several strategies can be used. Doses of insulin or secretagogues can be reduced before sessions of physical activity, extra carbohydrate can be consumed before or during physical activity, or both.

Retinopathy

Exercise and physical activity are not known to have any adverse effects on vision or the progression of non-proliferative diabetic retinopathy or macular edema. This applies to resistance training as well as aerobic training. However, in the presence of proliferative or severe non-proliferative diabetic retinopathy, vigorous aerobic or resistance exercise may be contraindicated because of the risk of triggering vitreous hemorrhage or retinal detachment. Specialist advice should be sought regarding the optimal time to commence exercise following photocoagulation therapy.

Peripheral neuropathy

Common sense indicates that in the presence of severe peripheral neuropathy, it may be best to encourage non-weight-bearing activities such as swimming, bicycling or arm exercises in order to avoid skin breakdown and joint damage.

Autonomic neuropathy

Autonomic neuropathy can increase the risk of exercise-induced injury by decreasing cardiac responsiveness to exercise, postural hypotension, impaired thermoregulation due to impaired skin blood flow and sweating, impaired night vision due to impaired papillary reaction, impaired thirst increasing risk of dehydration, and gastroparesis with unpredictable food delivery. Autonomic neuropathy is also strongly associated with CVD in people with diabetes. People with diabetic autonomic neuropathy should definitely undergo cardiac investigation before beginning physical activity more intense than that to which they are accustomed.

Microalbuminemia and nephropathy

Physical activity can acutely increase urinary protein excretion. The magnitude of this increase is in proportion to the acute increase in blood pressure. This finding has led some experts to recommend that people with diabetic kidney disease perform only light or moderate exercise, such that blood pressure during exercise would not rise to >200 mmHg. There is, however, some data that suggest that the improved diabetes control may improve protein excretion due to its effects on improved glycemic control, blood pressure and insulin sensitivity. Therefore, there may be no need for any specific exercise restrictions for people with diabetic kidney disease. However, because microalbuminuria and proteinuria are associated with increased risk of CVD, it is important to perform an exercise ECG stress test before beginning exercise significantly more intense than the demands of everyday living.

Summary

In summary, lifestyle changes and a structured exercise program may not only prevent the development of type 2 diabetes but may also play a major role in preventing the progression of disease and its complications. However, exercise programs should be tailored to individual needs and the risks of complications as outlined above.

Further reading

American Diabetes Association: Introduction. *Diabetes Care* 2004; **27**(Suppl. 1): S1–S2.

Ruderman N, Devlin JT, Schneider SH, Kriska A (Eds) *Handbook of Exercise in Diabetes*, 2nd edn. Alexandria, VA: American Diabetes Association, 2002.

Sigal RJ, Kenny GP, Wasserman DH, Castaneda-Sceppa C. Physical activity/exercise and type 2 diabetes. *Diabetes Care* 2004; **27**(10): 2518–39.

Disability and sport – overview

AA Narvani

The benefits of exercise for the disabled are even more substantial that those for able-bodied athletes, and include both patho-physiological and psychological factors. Sport and exercise by the disabled improves muscle strength, balance and flexibility as well as decreasing the risk of osteoporosis and cardiovascular disease. Psychological benefits include improved self-esteem and mood, better social integration and perception of self-value. Sport can act as a gateway for a return back to society for many who have become disabled as a consequence of injury. Participation in sports is as much a right for the disabled as it is for able-bodied individuals.

Appreciation of the barriers that exist for the disabled to participate in sports is of vital importance, as are attempts by all to enable such individuals to overcome these barriers. These hurdles include:

- disabled individual
  —picturing him/herself as an athlete,
  —developing enough self-esteem and motivation to participate in sports.
- acceptance by all individuals in the sporting world including:
  —coaches
  —other athletes/team mates
  —sports administrators
  —sports club managers
  —medical staff
- facilities
  —accessibility/transport
  —equipment
  —necessary adaptations
  —changing rooms
  —showers/bathrooms
- financial
  —Participation in sports can be much more expensive for disabled than non-disabled as custom-made equipment is considerably more costly.
  —Adapting sports clubs appropriately and providing special facilities can also be of considerable cost.

While encouraging and enabling the disabled to overcome the above barriers, each individual needs to be advised when choosing a sport. This requires an appreciation of the individual's personality, in addition to a thorough understanding of the particular disability and its special patho-physiology and medical factors (see the chapter on Disability and sport – medical problems). Important factors that must be taken into account when recommending a sport include:

- individual's preference
  —it is important the sport that is chosen is liked by the individual otherwise it would be more difficult and more of an effort to overcome the mentioned hurdles in order to consistently participate in the sport.

- particular disability
  - —physiological limitations as a consequence of the disability
  - —motor and coordination skills
  - —cognitive ability
  - —medical conditions associated with the disability (see the chapter on Disability and sport – medical problems).
- facilities
  - —the choice of sport is also dependent on the availability of all the facilities that are mentioned above.

Further reading

Booth DW, Grogono BJ. Athletes with a disability. In: M Harries, C Williams, WD Stanish, LJ Micheli (Eds) *Oxford Textbook of Sports Medicine*, 2nd edn. Oxford University Press, 1998: 815–34.

Webborn ADJ. Sport and disabilty. In: M Harries, J King, C Williams (Eds) *ABC of Sports Medicine*, 2nd edn. BMJ Books, 2000: 63–7.

Disability and sport – classification

AA Narvani

Ensuring fair competition and a "level playing field", requires a method by which athletes are divided into different groups. This process is of particular importance for disabled athletes as the type and degree of the disability as well as the functional skills of individual athletes can vary over a wide range. The classification system used however must be fair and simple, yet enable the athlete to compete at the highest level irrespective of type and degree of disability.

There are a number of classification systems that are used. Most of these are based on:

- type and degree of the disability
- functional skills
- previous performance

Type and degree of the disability

This classification focuses on the nature of disability and allows athletes with the same disabilities to compete against each other. It involves a medical assessment that makes it an objective classification, but this can make it a more demanding classification as it entails special expertise. Other disadvantages include its tendency to result in too many classifications, and also the fact that some of the variables assessed may not have an important role on the sport's performance. The categories are:

(i) *Athletes who are visually impaired*
Includes those who suffer from:
- diabetes
- tumours
- retinitis pigmentosa
- congenital blindness
- infection

(ii) *Athletes with amputation*
- upper limb
  —below/above elbow
  —most function well without a prosthesis
- lower limb
  —below/above knee
  —most use a prosthesis which is modified for the sport

(iii) *Wheelchair athletes*
- include those with spinal cord injuries/lesions
- further sub-classified according to the level of the spinal cord involvement and the severity of the disability

(iv) *Cerebral palsy athletes*
- different degrees of ataxia, spasticity and athetosis is seen in such athletes
- could be associated with other conditions such as visual, hearing, speech, intellectual impairments and epilepsy

(v) *Athletes with intellectual disability*

(vi) *Athletes who suffer from deafness*

(vii) *Les autres*
- includes athletes who do not fit in the above categories

Functional skills

Also referred to as the sport-specific classification, this is based on assessment of an athlete's ability to do specific skills in their particular sport, as well as an evaluation of their strength, power, balance, coordination and joint range of movement. It requires assessors to have a thorough understanding of the specific sport and the disability. It usually does not result in an extensive number of classes and the variables assessed do have a role on the sporting performance. There is the worry, however, that training may play a part in the classification and result in an athlete being placed in a higher classification than he or she should really be.

Performance

The classification scheme places athletes with similar "best recent" previous performances together. It is a relatively simple classification that does not require special expertise to administer. This system could, however, be exploited by athletes who may cheat by "holding back" at some competitions in order to contest against athletes with greater limitations at other more significant competitions. In addition, some athletes may lose motivation for training hard as they may feel that this would only result in a more difficult competition.

In summary, classification systems are a necessity; however, as can be seen from the above, there is no one ideal system. For many occasions, the various classification systems may need to be combined.

Further reading

Booth DW, Grogono BJ. Athletes with a disability. In: M Harries, C Williams, WD Stanish, LJ Micheli (Eds) *Oxford Textbook of Sports Medicine*, 2nd edn. Oxford University Press, 1998: 815–34.

Disability Sports, Classification Systems. Published on the Internet. Available online at http://edweb6.educ/kin866/cfsystems.htm.

Disability and sport – medical problems

AA Narvani

The medical problems encountered by the disabled athlete can be of a different nature to those faced by other athletes. The reasons for this include the altered physiology and biomechanics as well as the special equipment used by the athlete. It is of vital importance that all members of the medical team dealing with the disabled are aware and appreciate these differences.

Wheelchair athletes

Specific problems faced by such athletes could be divided into those that are related to the cause of the disability, such as spinal cord injury, and those that are related to wheelchair use.

Spinal cord injury related

Thermoregulation

- The problem is worse with quadriplegics and high paraplegics as a result of autonomic system dysfunction.
- There may be sensory deficits resulting in absent afferent input for the thermoregulation centre.
- The efferent arm of the system can also be affected as a result of reduced vasometer and sudometer responses.
- Hyperthermia can occur with exercise in hot climates. Attempts to reduce the risks of it occurring include:
  —decreasing exposure to extreme temperature and sunlight as much as possible
  —reduced clothing
  —ensuring adequate hydration
  —preparation and acclimatisation
  —using cooling systems such as sprays and cold wet towels

- Hypothermia can be a issue with sports undertaken in cold, wet and windy conditions. Preventive measures include:
  —adequate clothing
  —keeping dry
  —use of blankets
  —hydration

Autonomic dysreflexia

- This is a medical emergency occurring as a result of increased reflex sympathetic discharge.
- Seen in spinal cord injury athletes with lesions at or above splanchic outflow at T6 level.
- Can be triggered by trauma, infection, inflammation, bladder distension and physiological stress.
- Features include:
  —raised systolic blood pressure
  —peripheral vasoconstriction
  —severe headache
  —in severe cases could be complicated by stroke, seizures, myocardial infarction and arrhythmias
- Management involves prevention and elimination of the triggering factors, elevation of head and trunk, blood pressure monitoring and pharmacological treatment if it remains persistently raised.

Pressure sores

- Occur as a result of prolonged pressure over an insensitive area leading to local ischemia and subsequent disruption of the skin.
- Another contributing factor in wheelchair athletes is the high position of the knees with respect to the buttocks resulting in raised pressure over the buttocks.
- Common areas include sacrum, ischial tuberosity, posterior aspect of the knee, shoulder blade and foot.
- Preventive measures are of extreme importance and include:
  —padding of the surfaces in contact with pressure areas
  —regular skin checks
  —regular "weight shifts" (position changes)
  —keeping the skin dry

Bowel and bladder complications

- Autonomic system dysfunction can lead to impairment of urinary tract's neurological control resulting in urinary stasis, urinary tract infection (UTI) and renal calculi.
- Measures which could be taken to reduce the risk of UTI include:
  —intermittent catheterisation
  —particular attention to hygiene
  —hydration
  —availability of catheterisation facilities and accessible bathroom facilities

Blunted cardiovascular response in exercise

- Sympathetic system dysfunction, secondary to lesions above T1, can result in decreased maximum heart rate response in exercise.

Compromised ventilatory capacity

- Respiratory response in exercise may be reduced due to absent innervation of the intercostal muscles resulting in their dysfunction.

Wheelchair-associated injuries

Upper limb injuries are not uncommon in wheelchair athletes, most frequent of which appears to be shoulder and hand injuries.

Hand and wrist injuries

Common problems include:

- Callosities, blisters and cuts
  —may be prevented by gloves, taping, padding of rims
- Sprains of finger and wrist joints
- Nerve entrapments

Shoulder injuries

Wheelchair athletes often sustain overuse injuries to shoulders. These include:

- Impingement syndrome and/or rotator cuff tears (see the chapter on Shoulder – impingement syndrome).
  —muscular imbalance seen in wheelchair athletes is a contributing factor to rotator cuff-related pathology (there appears to be a relative weakness of adductors in comparison with abductors in wheelchair athletes resulting in a high riding humerus and tighter subacromial space)
- ACJ pathology (see the chapter on Shoulder – Acromioclavicular joint injuries).

Elbow injuries

- Throwing-related elbow injuries are encountered by wheelchair sports that involve throwing (see the chapter on Elbow – throwing injuries).

Nerve entrapment

- median nerve (carpel tunnel syndrome is thought to occur in over 70% of the wheelchair users)
- ulnar nerve (compression in Guyon's canal and elbow region in throwing athletes)
- radial nerve

Athletes with amputation

- These athletes can encounter stump and prostheses-related problems. It is of vital importance that the prostheses fit properly since an ill-fitting prosthesis will result in skin blisters, abrasions, ulceration and infection.
- Altered biomechanics and increased ground reactions with prostheses may also result in premature degeneration of the joints.
- Thermoregulation may also be sub-optimal due to the reduced surface area available for heat loss. This can lead to overheating and excessive sweating, which can further compromise the fit of the prosthesis by causing it to slip.

Visually impaired athletes

- Many injuries sustained by visually impaired athletes occur following falls and collision.
- Sports that can result in elevation of the intraocular pressure, such as weight lifting and diving, should be advised against in those with glaucoma.
- Similarly those with a detached retina should avoid contact sports.

Athletes with deafness

- Inability to communicate with such athletes can lead to the athlete's lack of awareness of strategies to prevent injuries. Therefore, it is important that all those involved in the care of athletes with hearing difficulties can establish some form of communication with them.

Cerebral palsy

- Specific problems faced by individuals with cerebral palsy who participate in sporting activity is dependent on the associated disorders and their severity (these include visual, hearing, speech and intellectual impairments, epilepsy). Many are wheelchair users as well.

Further reading

Gottschalk FA. The orthopaedically disabled athlete. In: JC DeLee, D Drez, MD Miller (Eds) *Orthopaedic Sports Medicine, Principles and Practice*, 2nd edn. Saunders, 2002: 521–31.

Malanga GA. Athletes with disabilities. Published on the Internet, eMedicine. Available online at http://www.emedicine.com/SPORTS/topic144.htm.

Schilling ML. Disability sports – sports medicine/athletic training. Published on the Internet. Available online at http://edweb6.educ/kin866/resschilling2.htm.

Webborn ADJ. Sport and disabilty. In: M Harries, J King, C Williams (Eds) *ABC of Sports Medicine*, 2nd edn. BMJ Books, 2000: 63–7.

Disability and sport – equipment

AA Narvani

The impact of equipment on a disabled individual's life style is enormous, particularly as far as sport is concerned. In many circumstances, equipment may be the only factor that determines, first, whether or not a particular individual participates in sports and, second, the type of sport in which he or she might wish to become involved. Vast amounts of money and resources are spent on sports equipment for able-bodied athletes. It is of vital importance that as much attention is also paid to equipment for the disabled, since the impact of this can be of greater significance than for able-bodied athletes. Technology has made enormous progress in the sporting world, allowing tennis players to serve at speeds over 150 miles per hour, and racing drivers to cruise along at 225 miles per hour, have crashes at that sort of speed and survive with relatively few injuries. This technology must also be utilised to its full potential in order to minimise the "barriers" for the disabled as well as maximising their performance within the rules and regulations.

Broadly speaking, the equipment used by the disabled athlete can be divided into the following categories:

- wheelchairs
- prosthetics
- other sport-specific specialised equipment

Wheelchairs

Over recent years, there has been a significant increase in the number of wheelchair sports. The desired properties of the wheelchair are dependent on the particular sport, therefore special adaptations are usually required with each field. There are, however, some universal fundamental properties all types of wheelchairs need to possess. These are:

(i) *stability*
(ii) *efficiency*
(iii) *manoeuvrability*

In general, wheelchairs can be classified into four major types:

(i) General sports wheelchairs
(ii) Racing wheelchairs
(iii) Throwing wheelchairs
(iv) Motorised chairs

General sports wheelchairs

Although these have features that distinguish them from "everyday" wheelchairs, many athletes employ these for their everyday use. Specific features include:

- they usually do not have push handles and armrests
- front wheels are commonly of a small diameter, allowing the athlete to turn easily
- hand rims are moderately large, improving efficiency by enabling the athlete to start, accelerate, change direction and stop with least effort
- they are practical for travel as they can be dismantled with relative ease
- they usually have a camber angle of 12 to 15 degrees (this is the angling that brings the top of the wheels nearer to each other and the bottom further apart, resulting in increased stability and contributing to the efficiency of the wheelchair)

Racing wheelchairs

In such wheelchairs, manoeuvrability and, to some degree, stability is sacrificed for velocity. Special features include:

- most have only three wheels (faster but less stable than four wheels)
- large rear-wheel diameters
- small rear-wheel cross-sectional diameter
- they commonly possess a lower body position
- the body position also leans forward more
- light weight yet strong frame
- increased camber

Throwing wheelchairs

These include wheelchairs that are used for throwing javelin, discus and shot. The crucial factor with these is the increased stability required to provide the athlete with a rigid base when throwing. Features include:

- many do not have any wheels
- the seats may be hard and rigid to ensure maximum transfer of energy to the thrown object
- as high a body position as possible and permitted

Motorised chairs

These are designed for athletes who do not possess the ability to use general sport wheelchairs. The motor and battery make them of considerable weight and less practical for transport.

Prosthetics

Prosthetics have revolutionised many sports. Although use of prosthetics is more common with lower limb amputees, the number of sports involving upper limb prostheses is increasing.

Lower limb prostheses

- Many of these are based on the design of Van Phillips and Dale Abildskov, which involves carbon fibre material cut into an L-shaped foot attached to a prosthetic socket above and to a sole below. The idea is to simulate the spring action of the normal foot by the prosthesis returning to its original shape upon removal of load, therefore putting spring into a step.
- May or may not have axial joints for articulation.
- May consist of specialised suspension systems.
- Many sports require their own specific adaptations, for example:
  —Swimmers can choose prostheses with a fin rather than a foot design
  —Cyclists may require a pedal binding system
  —Skiers need prostheses that can be directly linked to the ski binding
  —Climbers benefit from prostheses with a high friction sole to improve grip

Upper limb prostheses

Advances in technology have resulted in the design of specialised upper limb prostheses for a wide range of sports including basketball, cycling, hockey, volleyball, golf, swimming and tennis. Broadly, upper limb prostheses can be divided into three main categories (however, special adaptations have to be made for each specific sport):

(i) Passive function prosthesis
- most frequent type used by athletes

(ii) Mechanical prosthesis
- consists of pulleys and cables

(iii) Myoelectric prosthesis
- Prosthesis receives the translated EMG signals of the residual limb

Other sport-specific specialised equipment

It is beyond the scope of this chapter to cover all the adapted equipment utilised by the disabled athlete. These specialised equipments allow the disabled to compete as other athletes, improve their performance and reduce the risk of injury.

Further reading

Cheskin M. Paralympic athletes, equipped for success. In *Motion* 2004; **14**(3). Published on the Internet. Available online at http://www.amputee-coalition.org/inmotion/may_jun_04/paralympic:html.

Gottschalk FA. The orthopaedically disabled athlete. In: JC DeLee, D Drez, MD Miller (Eds) *Orthopaedic Sports Medicine, Principles and Practice*, 2nd edn. Saunders, 2002: 521–31.

Kim JT. Disability sports – equipment – wheelchair design. Published on the Internet. Available online at http://edweb6.educ/kin866/reskim1.htm.

Malanga GA. Athletes with disabilities. Published on the Internet. eMedicine. Available online at http://www.emedicine.com/SPORTS/topic144.htm.

Drugs in sport – overview

B Lynn

Several chapters will be devoted to aspects of drug abuse in sport. However, right from the outset it is important to stress *education*. The best way to ensure that those involved in sport do not resort to performance-enhancing drugs or procedures is by creating the correct climate. The fundamental issue is to ask what is sport about? If it is not about fair competition, then really it has lost its value. This is certainly true for the individual. If you know you only won because you cheated, what is the point? Hence education programmes, such as the "100% Me" in the UK, are important in the fight against drug cheating. A key role for sports doctors and other health professionals is in education about health risks – which for many drugs are only too real (see the chapters on anabolic steroids and on blood doping).

Winning by cheating may be viewed by some as simply about obtaining a lot of money (and peer popularity). So highly-paid professional sports are likely to need to be policed particularly closely. Here education is still important, but this time educating the audience. While people are still happy to pay money to watch drug cheats, then there is clearly a major job of public eduction waiting to be done.

Anti-drugs policies operate within an administrative and legal framework that has changed dramatically over the last few years. The formation of the World Anti-Drugs Agency (WADA) has provided both the stimulus and the machinery for moving policy forward. We now have internationally agreed systems for penalties and for the regular review of the banned list. We have a Court of Arbitration in Sport. We have a major research programme concerned with improving information about performance-enhancing drugs and how best to detect them. Not everyone is signed up. However, all the Olympic sports are, plus many of the professional ones (e.g. FIFA for association football). The pressure is on the other professional sports as never before. Examples like real testing and real penalties in pro baseball in the USA are good to see! More information on the administrative framework for drugs in sport is given in a later chapter on this topic.

Testing continues to improve and to be carried out in a more fair and rigorous manner. This is now such an important area, with a major role for sports doctors, that it will be covered in detail in a separate chapter. However, one point is worth stressing here and that is the need for effective out-of-competition testing. Many of the most abused drugs have effects that are significantly longer than the time for which they can be detected. So sports that really want to deal with drugs such as anabolic steroids or erythropoietin need to test potential winners before competition, either with home or training ground visits. And these visits must be unannounced!

The main classes of drugs that are abused are stimulants, anabolic steroids, erythropoietin (plus illegal blood doping), hormones affecting growth and muscle function, and opiate painkillers. The classes as listed by WADA are given in Table 1. Other substances that are banned for specific sports are alcohol and beta blockers. Steroids get their own chapter in this book, as do blood doping and erythropoietin. Other banned substances will be briefly discussed in this chapter.

Stimulants

These are the traditional performance enhancers and are based either on adrenaline (epinephrine) or amphetamine. They need to be taken at the time of the event and so can be detected readily by testing during competitions. A problem has been cough and cold remedies that include significant amounts of adrenaline-related compounds. Fortunately, pseud-ephedrine has now been removed from the banned list. Many others remain, however. It is essential that sports doctors advise clearly on what is allowed and what is not. A useful resource for this is the web-based Drug Information Database (DID) run by UK Sport. More on this below. A rather different stimulant is caffeine. There used to be a threshold for this, but it has now been removed altogether from the list (but keep an eye on the DID – drugs can be re-instated!). Another stimulant, Modafinil, has also been the cause of positive drug tests.

Table 1 WADA 2005 prohibited list – summary of classes of substance and methods banned to different extents.

Substances and methods prohibited at all times (in- and out-of-competition)

Prohibited substances
S1. Anabolic agents
S2. Hormones and related substances
S3. Beta-2 agonists
S4. Agents with anti-oestrogenic activity
S5. Diuretics and other masking agents

Prohibited methods
M1. Enhancement of oxygen transfer
M2. Chemical and physical manipulation
M3. Gene doping

Substances and methods prohibited in-competition
Includes S1 to S5 and M1 to M3 defined above, as well as:
S6. Stimulants
S7. Narcotics
S8. Cannabinoids
S9. Glucocorticosteroids

Substances prohibited in particular sports
P1. Alcohol
P2. Beta-blockers

From: *The 2005 Prohibited List*, published by World Anti-Doping Agency, www.wada-ama.org.

Hormones

Various hormones that affect growth or muscle function have been abused and are on the prohibited list, including growth hormone, human chorionic gonadotrophin (hCG) and insulin. Growth hormone has been used to increase muscle growth and reduce body fat. The evidence that it is performance enhancing is quite weak. However, it is thought that the main abusers may use it in combination with anabolic steroids and possibly insulin. No controlled trials of these combination treatments have been carried out. However, there are no legitimate reasons for a sports person to be taking growth hormone and there are health risks (e.g. cardiac effects). The ban therefore appears logical, even though it is not at present enforced by any recognised test. Suitable tests can be developed, however, based on abnormal levels of endogenous compounds that are directly affected by growth hormones (for example Insulin-like Growth Factors (IGFs) and IGF binding proteins). Therefore, a test could be introduced at any time, and on past policy this would *not* be pre-announced. Human Chorionic gonadotrophin (hCG) is used by males to boost testosterone production from the testes. It thus acts like taking testosterone, the natural anabolic steroid, and can increase muscle size and strength. Abuse of hCG is thought to be widespread. It can be detected in urine so standard testing procedures can pick up hCG abuse.

Opiate painkillers

Morphine and related narcotics are banned. Only codeine is allowed. Again, these are likely to be in the body at the time of competition so detecting them with testing at events is straightforward.

Diuretics

These are banned as they can cause a urine sample to become very dilute, thus making illegal compounds harder to detect.

Other banned compounds

Beta blockers are banned in competition in sports like shooting as they reduce tremor. They are not banned in most sports, and interestingly are allowed in snooker. Steroids of the glucocorticoid family are generally allowed out of competition, but are banned in competition. However, preparations for skin use are not banned. And steroid inhalers are permitted as long as a Therapeutic Use Exemption (TUE) has been obtained. A TUE requires application in advance using a standard form and with appropriate medical support and information. This is an important system that ensures that where a banned drug is essential for medical purposes it is still possible for an individual to compete. More information on TUEs will be given in the chapter on the administrative framework for drugs in sport.

The complexities of anti-doping regulations and the cost of effective testing programmes can lead to an attitude that says, well maybe we should just let people do what they want to improve performance. After all, the sport would still be entertaining. But a moment's reflection shows that the fight against drug cheats is worth it. Why are we entertained by sport? Why do we encourage our children to play sports? It is to improve our and their lives, to broaden our humanity. Cheating, often with health-damaging drugs, is the antithesis of these things. If we want sport to continue as a vehicle for improving ourselves and our society, then we must educate people so that drug cheating becomes marginalised further. And we must be vigilant – and pay the price in money terms and in inconvenience – to ensure that no one, for monetary or other motives, undermines one of the great human endeavours.

The ultimate horror that awaits any laissez-faire attitude is gene doping. This is the use of gene therapy methods to artificially alter an individual's physiology to improve performance. This route could lead to sport as a gene-fuelled freak show. Some of the issues involved in gene doping are discussed in a separate chapter. But let us hope this problem can be defeated by a combination of education and scientific methods for detecting the practice.

Further reading

Drug Information Database (DID), Publishing on the Internet. Available online at http://www.didglobal.com/page/choose%20country.

Mottram DR (Ed) *Drugs in Sport*, 3rd edn. Routledge, London, 2003.

100% Me. Published on the Internet. Available online at http://www.100percentme.co.uk.
Prohibited list of drugs and methods. Published on the Internet. Available online at http://www.wada-ama.org/en/prohibitedlist.ch2.
WADA. Published on the Internet. Available online at http://www.wada-ama.org/en/.

Drugs in sport – the administrative framework: doping control procedures

B Lynn

The legal and administrative framework for anti-doping programmes has much improved in recent years due to international cooperative action. The key event was the setting up in 1999 of an independent body, the World Anti-Doping Agency (WADA). This body is jointly funded by the Olympic movement and national governments. It has moved rapidly to bring uniformity into policy and practice across all sports and all countries. A detailed WADA code covering anti-doping policy has been adopted by all major sports organisations except a small number of professional sports. This code now forms the basis of a UNESCO Convention that is being ratified by governments. So we now have a robust legal basis for the effective policing of drug abuse in sport.

Within each sport, international governing bodies supervise anti-doping policy. These bodies have all signed up to the WADA code. Within many countries there are national anti-doping agencies, often set up as independent bodies (e.g. the USADA), and practical anti-doping action is provided by national bodies for individual sports.

Key points from the WADA code

The WADA code runs to 44 pages, but much of this is commentary explaining the individual articles. After some initial definitions there are three main sections. The largest deals with doping control (see the next paragraph), then two shorter sections deal with education and research and with the responsibilities of signatories such as national governing bodies and international associations.

Doping control in the WADA code

Article 2 covers rule violations and article 2.1.1 restates what was already the accepted principle, i.e. "It is each athlete's personal duty to ensure that no Prohibited Substance enters his or her body." Rule violations related to trafficking, failure to provide whereabouts information and tampering with doping control are also covered. Article 3 covers the important issue of burden of proof. Crucially it is not necessary to establish doping "beyond reasonable doubt". A lesser criterion is given: "to the comfortable satisfaction of the hearing body". This is more than just a "balance of probabilities", but as already stated, less than "beyond reasonable doubt". WADA's role in taking over publication of the Prohibited List is covered in article 4. This section also covers standardisation of procedures for therapeutic use exemptions. Articles 5 and 6 cover aspects of testing and analysis. The accreditation of laboratories becomes the responsibility of WADA. Article 7 covers the tricky area of results management. Who tells who what and when! When the A sample has given an adverse result the athlete is informed by the anti-doping organisation involved and can request that the B sample be checked. Provisional suspension from competition can be imposed before the B sample results are available. Various safeguards are set out in detail. Exactly who is responsible for publishing details of the violation is not set out in the code. Article 10 covers sanctions against the athlete and here the simple rule is: 2 years' suspension for first violation and lifetime ban for a second. This was one of the most contentious compromises in the code. But in the end there was agreement that it was best to have a single "across the board" rule that would be simple to administer and difficult to appeal. Article 13 deals with appeals and sets up a Court of Arbitration for Sport (CAS) to which international-level competitors can appeal. Interestingly, it is also possible for the IOC or WADA to appeal a result. This might be important if it appeared that a national body had only placed a minimal sanction on a star athlete.

Therapeutic use exemptions (TUEs)

An important role for sports doctors is to ensure that any necessary medication involving a prohibited agent is notified to the relevant authority via the TUE machinery and to prepare the necessary accompanying documentation. Procedures vary a little between sports. The procedure for athletics (track and field) is typical. A TUE application must be made at least 21 days before a competition and lasts for a specified period (whose duration depends on the condition). A slightly different form is used for beta-2 inhalers and for non-systemic application of corticosteroids (i.e. inhaled, local injection, etc.). For international-level competitions, and for international-level athletes in any competition, the form must be submitted to the international governing body, i.e. in this case the IAAF. For national-level competitors, the form goes to the relevant National Federation. The form requires the notifying medical practitioner to justify not using a different medication that is not on the banned list (e.g. a non-steroidal anti-inflammatory rather than a steroid). Appropriate documentation is required (including test results, images, etc.) plus dosage information. If a TUE is denied, the athlete can appeal, if necessary all the way to the Court of Arbitration in Sport.

There are some variations from sport to sport, so it is necessary to be familiar with any special rules that may apply. For example, in football, FIFA rules allow a TUE to be submitted only 48 hours before a match, or even to be brought along to any doping test. Finally, remember that insulin is on the prohibited list, and even long-standing diabetics require a current TUE.

Doping control procedures

This section deals with some of the important "nuts and bolts" aspects of drug testing in sport, including sample collection rules and laboratory methods. Only the collection and analysis of urine samples will be covered.

Samples may be collected at events "in competition" or during training "out of competition". At major events a team from the relevant anti-doping agency will set up a doping control station and generally test all winners plus a random sample of non-winners. Subjects for out-of-competition testing generally include only elite level performers likely to figure in national championships or international events. WADA, in its out-of-competition testing, also looks out for athletes showing unexpected increases in form.

At doping control the subject urinates into a suitable container under observation from a member of the doping control team. This is necessary as attempts have in the past been made to substitute someone else's urine. The sample is divided between two containers, A and B. The samples are taken to an accredited laboratory, of which there are now 33 worldwide. There the B sample is stored and the A sample is analysed. Key analytical methods are gas chromatography, high-pressure liquid chromatography, mass spectroscopy (combined with gas chromatography) and immunoassay.

The running of doping control is likely to become more standardised with the introduction of ADAMS (Anti-Doping Administration and Management System). This is a web-based software package developed by WADA to allow sports organisations to manage doping control in a standardised, secure way. It will also allow WADA to collect statistics on violations more efficiently. In addition, it has a module that allows athletes to log their whereabouts over the Internet, a very useful aspect of the software.

Summary

(1) The formation of the World Anti-Doping Agency has established an almost universally accepted set of rules for dealing with doping violations, the WADA code.

(2) Key features of the code are
   (a) it is only necessary to provide evidence "to the comfortable satisfaction of the hearing body",
   (b) a standard 2 year ban is imposed for a first violation, a lifetime ban for a second.

(3) Therapeutic use exemptions (TUEs) allow athletes to compete when receiving for medical purposes a substance on the banned list.

(4) Doping control procedures involve the supervised collection of a urine sample and its analysis by a WADA accredited laboratory using the latest analytical methods.

Further reading

IAAF information on TUEs. Published on the Internet. Available online at http://www.iaaf.org/antidoping/index.html.

Verroken M, Mottram DR. Doping control in sport. In: DR Mottram (Ed) *Drugs in Sport*. Routledge, London, 2003, Chapter 11.

WADA Code: Published on the Internet. Available online at http://www.wada-ama.org/en/dynamic.ch2?pageCategory.id=250.

Drugs in sport – anabolic steroid abuse

B Lynn

Steroid hormones fall into four groups:

- Glucocorticoids (e.g. cortisone)
- Mineralocorticoids (e.g. aldosterone)
- Female sex steroid hormones (oestrogens, progesterone)
- Male sex steroid hormones (testosterone)

In sport it is testosterone and related natural and synthetic steroids that are taken for the *anabolic* (muscle-building) action. However, the main actions of testosterone are on the male reproductive system:

- Development of male secondary sexual characteristics
- Control of spermatogenesis
- Feedback to hypothalamus to regulate FSH, LH

Testosterone has the standard four-ring steroid structure with two additional methyl groups, making it a 19 carbon steroid. In the body it is synthesised in the testes, ovaries and adrenal cortex. An isomer, epitestosterone, is always synthesised at the same time in the ratio 12:1, testosterone:epitestosterone. Some testosterone is converted into oestradiol in the body by a process called aromatisation. This only becomes of interest when excess amounts of testosterone are present. Under these conditions enough oestradiol can be produced to cause feminising effects in males (see below).

Plasma levels
Males – 0.6 mg/dl
Females – 0.03 mg/dl

In the blood it is mostly bound to SHBG – sex hormone-binding globulin. Nevertheless, enough of the compound is filtered into the urine to make urine testing straightforward. Testing using gas–liquid chromatography and mass spectroscopy is now technically very sophisticated. It is possible to look not just at single compounds but at the pattern of precursors and metabolites. This is important in testing for some steroids that occur naturally in small quantities (e.g. nandrolone) and for assessing the testosterone:epitestosterone ratio. It is also possible to examine carbon 12 to carbon 13 isotope ratios and in this way reveal a synthetic origin for naturally occurring compounds.

Actions and effects

Testosterone acts on intracellular, cytoplasmic receptors. The receptor–hormone complex then translocates to the nucleus where it acts on DNA transcription. Steroid hormones thus have a direct action on patterns of protein synthesis in cells. Early controlled trials of anabolic steroids demonstrated rather small effects on muscle strength. However, a well-controlled recent study using large doses, closer to those used by steroid abusers, clearly shows significant increases in muscle bulk and strength. It also shows that these effects are additive to the effects seen with intense strength training (Bhasin *et al.* 2001). A 10-week programme of testosterone at supra-physiologic doses gave a 16% increase in strength on a squat test. The same treatment combined with intense strength training produced a 38% rise in strength.

What is the extent of abuse?

First some history. Figure 1 shows the winning distances in the women's shot put in Olympic Games from 1952 to 2004. For comparison, the winning heights for the high jump are plotted, with both expressed as a percentage of the 1952 level. In the 1950s and early 1960s both events show a steady increase, probably reflecting the growth in athletics participation amongst women. From the early 1960s the shot put winning distance starts to increase rapidly until, by 1972, it is a remarkable 40% above the 1952 value. At this point the trend levels off. After 1988 the winning distance does something remarkable – it falls in every subsequent Olympics until it is now back to close to the high jump trend.

So what does this graph represent? Two events were probably crucial. In 1976 the IOC introduced testing for steroids. But most important of all, in 1989 the Berlin Wall came down and East and West Germany merged. From papers discovered after the fall of the wall, a major nationally sponsored programme of steroid administration was revealed (Ungerleider 2001; Franke and Berendonk 1997). All the shot put winners in the years 1968–1988 were from eastern Europe, with one exception. Notice the dip in 1984? This was the Los Angeles Olympics that were boycotted by the Russians and East Germans.

So what is the extent of steroid abuse now? With effective testing, both in and out of competition, the level of abuse has certainly fallen in recent years. If the shot put trends are typical it may even be that top-level Olympic sports now have a relatively low level of abuse. But positives still occur. And the discovery in 2003 of THG (Tetrahydrogestrinone, a previously unknown steroid) in urine samples from several top sprinters, American football players and baseball players shows that problems still

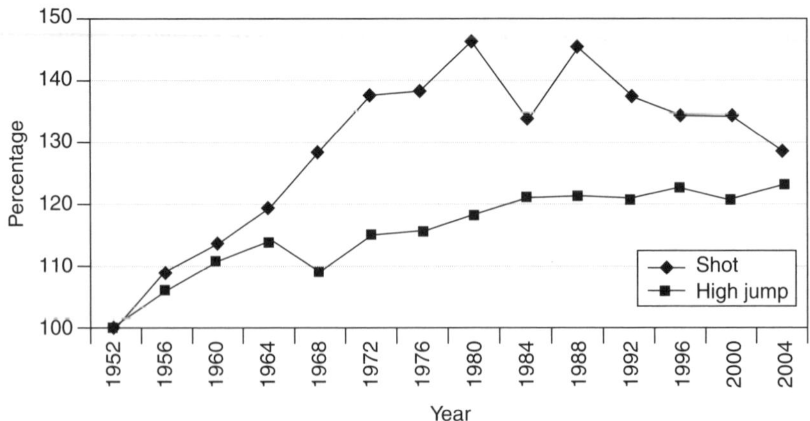

Figure 1 Women's shot put and high jump winning value as % 1952 value for Olympics 1952–2004.

exist. Steroid abuse is not only a problem in sport. Abuse is widespread in body-building with magazines openly on sale that minimise, or even ridicule, the health risks. And anabolics are widely available over the Internet. Surveys in the early 1990s in the UK show about 10% of gym users admitted using steroids. In surveys in the US, including among high school children, higher figures have been reported.

The health risks and side effects

- Cardiac myopathy
- Liver toxicity and liver cancer
- Male sterility, gynaecomastia
- Masculinisation in females
- In children, stunting of growth
- Other side effects: acne, baldness, aggression

NB: Despite what the adverts say, all anabolic steroids are androgenic.

The cardiac and liver problems represent major health risks. A recent examination using echocardiography in power lifters and weight lifters indicated an unhealthy thickening of the left ventricular wall in those using steroids. And importantly, very little recovery in those who had stopped using steroids for at least 1 year (and on average 2 years) (Urhausen *et al.* 2004). This lays to rest another myth amongst abusers that any bad effects will rapidly reverse on stopping use.

Is there excess mortality among anabolic steroid users? The answer, at least in Finnish power lifters, appears to be yes. Pärssinen *et al.* (2000) traced 62 champion power lifters from the period 1977–82. At a 12-year follow up, eight were dead (13%). This was five times the mortality in a matched control group.

Other banned substances related to AAS abuse

The beta-2 agonist Clenbuterol has been abused for its supposed anabolic action and is on the prohibited list. Anti-oestrogen compounds are banned as they are used to control feminising side effects of taking large amounts of testosterone. It is one of the paradoxes of AAS abuse aimed at developing a muscular body that sterility results, plus breast growth in males! The latter is due to conversion of excess testosterone to oestradiol in the body, with the inevitable consequences. Anti-oestrogens can inhibit this effect. The only male competitors likely to be taking them are AAS abusers, hence they are banned and urine samples are checked for them.

Summary

- Testosterone and related compounds have anabolic as well as androgenic actions.
- They are abused by those aiming to increase muscle bulk – so the problem is in power events (sprints, shot put, etc.).
- Widespread abuse in past – much more and effective testing now.
- Major health risks and side effects.
- Effects such as cardiac myopathy do not reverse on stopping taking the steroids.

Further reading

American Swimming Coaches Association web site. 1999 interview with East German swimmer Birgit Heukrodt who was given steroids when competing in the early 1980s. Published on the Internet. Available online at http://www.swimmingcoach.org/articles/9904/9904-6.htm.

Bhasin S, Woodhouse L, Storer TW. Proof of the effect of testosterone on skeletal muscle. *J Endocrinol* 2001; **170**: 27–38.

Franke WW, Berendonk B. Hormonal doping and androgenization of athletes: a secret program of the German Democratic Republic government. *Clin Chem* 1997; **43**: 1262–79.

George AJ. Androgenic anabolic steroids. In: DR Mottram (Ed) *Drugs in Sport*, 3rd edn. Routledge, 2003; Chapter 5.

Knight J. Two pieces on THG and on Don Catlin's Olympic Analytical Lab in Los Angeles. *Nature*; **425**: 752 (23 Oct 2003) and **426**: 114–15 (13 Nov 2003).

Parssinen M, Kujala U, Vartiainen E, Sarna S, Seppala T. Increased premature mortality of competitive powerlifters suspected to have used anabolic agents. *Int J Sports Med* 2000; **21**: 225–7.

Ungerleider, S. *Faust's Gold. Inside the East German Doping Machine*. St Martin's Press, 2001

Urhausen A, Albers T, Kindermann W. Are the cardiac effects of anabolic steroid abuse in strength athletes reversible? *Heart* 2004; **90**: 496–501.

Drugs in sport – blood doping, erythropoietin and altitude training

B Lynn

The basic idea is to raise the oxygen-carrying capacity of the blood and so improve performance in events involving aerobic exercise, i.e. any events lasting more than 1–2 minutes. This can be done by increasing the haemoglobin (Hb) content in the blood either by legal means (altitude training) or illegal means (blood doping or "boosting" or use of the hormone erythropoietin).

We have 3×10^{13} red blood cells, containing a total of 900 g of haemoglobin. Red cells last on average 120 days, so we need to replace 1/120 every day, i.e. 2.5×10^{11} cells, or 3 million every second! This massive production of red cells takes place in the bone marrow.

Table 1 shows the normal ranges of haemoglobin and haematocrit.

Table 1 Normal ranges of Hb and haematocrit.

	Men	Women
Hb, g/dl	14–16	12.5–15
Haematocrit	42–50%	38–47%

Definitions:
Hb: Amount of this oxygen-carrying protein within red blood cells. Units g/decilitre blood (decilitre = 100 ml).
Haematocrit: Proportion of red blood cells to the total blood volume (= packed cell volume or PCV).

Blood doping

This is the direct method. Blood, or more usually concentrated red cells, is transfused via an intravenous catheter. If blood cells from a donor are used this is heterologous transfusion. Alternatively the athlete's own blood can be collected, stored, then transfused back – this is autologous transfusion. Either way, careful storage of red cells is necessary. Blood boosting definitely works, although estimates vary of the extent of improvements in performance. A recent review concludes that endurance performance is typically improved by 2–3% (Gledhill *et al.* 1999) but other studies have shown maximal oxygen uptake (VO_2max) up by 13% (Robinson *et al.* 1982).

Although blood doping clearly works, and so demonstrates the usefulness of boosting blood oxygen-carrying capacity for endurance events, there are a number of difficulties. If heterologous transfusion is used, then great care needs to be taken over tissue matching. In addition, there is always the risk of getting a blood-borne infection such as AIDS or hepatitis. Autologous transfusion means long periods out of competition as it takes 4–6 weeks to recover from a blood donor session. In addition, the effects of the donation begin to wane within 3–4 weeks. There have been some cases and plenty of rumours of blood doping in sport. It would not be surprising if rumours of blood boosting occurred as a significant number of people need to be involved in the process of taking blood, storing it, re-infusing it and checking haematocrits. The extent of blood doping is not known, but recent evidence from professional cycling indicates that it is a significant problem. Raids by Spanish police as part of Operation Puerta found blood transfusion equipment and stored blood. The start of the 2006 Tour de France was affected in a major way with the last-minute withdrawal of several top riders.

Erythropoietin (EPO)

EPO is a hormone that is released from the kidney in response to tissue hypoxia, and travels to the bone marrow. It is a large peptide (or small protein) comprising 165 amino acids with a large number of attached carbohydrate residues (it is 30% glycosylated). In the bone marrow it stimulates production of pronormoblasts (immediate red blood cell (erythrocyte) precursors) from CFU-E cells (committed unipotential colony-forming unit – erythroid). Pronormoblasts in turn develop into normoblasts. The normoblasts start to lose their nucleus and become reticulocytes. The reticulocytes enter the blood system and finally develop into red blood cells with no nuclear material visible at all.

Recombinant human EPO is used to treat anaemia associated with kidney failure, e.g. for those on dialysis, and so is widely available, although pretty expensive. EPO-induced increases in blood Hb appear, like blood doping, to increase performance in endurance events (Birkeland *et al.* 2000).

It is important not to get Hb too high. The effect of blood viscosity on haemodynamics means the heart works harder, and so there is an increased risk of heart problems. Pathologically-elevated red cell counts also lead to a higher risk of clots. But many people who live at altitude have elevated Hb without any circulatory or cardiac problems – but maybe have made compensating adaptations. A spate of unexplained sudden deaths in cyclists in late 1980s was attributed to the arrival of EPO on the scene. There have also been problems with side effects in some long-term dialysis patients.

Some sports (e.g. cycling) set upper limits on haematocrit (50% for male competitors) and ban on health grounds (i.e. risks due to increased blood viscosity). But 1% of the normal population (and 20% of native highlanders) have haematocrits at or above this level. It is also claimed that haematocrit tests are subverted by masking with plasma expanders. If you expand the plasma volume, then the proportion of red cells (the haematocrit) will fall, even though the total number of red cells is still much elevated. Measuring total blood volume is not an easy thing to do, so expanding plasma volume is a straightforward way to avoid detection in a haematocrit test.

Cyclists apparently get by the haematocrit test by having saline infusions shortly before being tested at the start of events. The short-term boost to blood volume may also aid performance! Others use high molecular weight expanders. But these are easily detected over a long period, as almost the entire Finnish cross-country skiing team found to their cost at the world championships in 2001! (Seiler 2001).

Detecting EPO use

It is possible to distinguish recombinant EPO from endogenous EPO, and this can even be done in urine samples. Unfortunately, EPO has a short life in the body and is only detectable for 1–2 days. As blood cells last 120 days, single tests at the time of competition are useless. Interestingly, a longer lasting version of EPO is now available for clinical use – darbepoetin or Aranesp. This is effective for longer, so patients (or athletes) need fewer injections and this is more convenient and cheaper. It does make it easier to detect, however, and this version of EPO was in fact successfully detected in competitors in the 2002 Winter Olympics.

Another approach to EPO detection is to count the number of immature red cells (reticulocytes) in the blood. This rises in a characteristic way with EPO supplementation and the effect is detectable for several weeks (Parisotto *et al.* 2001). This test is now being used widely by anti-doping agencies.

It is also possible to look at iron metabolism. Hb contains iron and the body has well-developed transport and storage systems for iron so that enough is available to constantly produce the red cells we need. If EPO stimulates red cell production then the levels of the iron storage protein, ferritin, fall. At same time the levels of the soluble transferrin receptor (needed to get iron into developing red cells) rise in response to the increased demand. So by looking at the ferritin:transferrin ratio you get quite a good indication of red cell production rates. Unfortunately, you can mask these changes by increasing the iron and folic acid intake in a diet. It may be possible to track transferrin receptor mRNA levels – these rise up to 40 times with EPO use – but no one has a test based on this yet.

With better testing, the problem of EPO abuse may now wane. Even though the effects of EPO (up to 120 days) outlast the test detection duration (14 days) this is in part compensated by the need to take EPO over a period to get a significant effect. Also, the peak boost does not last 120 days, and the effectiveness falls throughout this period (presumably why the Festina cycling team was toting EPO around in the 1998 Tour de France, an event that lasts 3 weeks). Given these dynamics a strategy of random tests in the run up to major competitions looks the way to go. It will be interesting to see how many sports in how many countries develop such a programme!

Altitude acclimatisation

Living at altitudes above about 2000 m leads to enough tissue anoxia to stimulate EPO release and red cell production. For example, a group who spent 30 days at the top of Pikes Peak in Colorado had average increases in Hb from 13.7 on arrival to 16.2 at departure, with parallel increases in haematocrit (from 43–48%). These are similar to the increases seen with blood doping or EPO use. However, on return to sea level, little if any increase in endurance performance is found. The reasons are complex. Firstly, it is not possible to train at maximum intensity at altitude just because the atmospheric oxygen levels are lower. Secondly, the adjustments of the circulation to altitude involve more than just an increased Hb. Hyperventilation, a normal response to the lowered oxygen level, leads to increased carbon dioxide excretion and eventually to a reduction in the buffering power of the blood. This may reduce performance levels as lactic acid produced during high-intensity exercise will not be so well neutralised. There may also be reductions in blood volume and shifts in the Hb dissociation curve, changes that may impair performance. Note, however, that for competitions held at altitude, suitable acclimatisation is essential.

To get round some of these problems coaches have developed the "live high, train low" approach. You live and sleep up the mountain, but travel down to sea level to train. This option is now available to those of us who do not live conveniently close to a suitable mountain – the nitrogen tent or house. Athletes live in nitrogen tents with the oxygen level reduced to 15–16% (equivalent to being at 2500 m altitude). They can therefore train in the normal way, but should get a useful boost in blood Hb due to the time spent at simulated altitude. There will still be problems with other, disadvantageous, circulatory adaptations. Data on the efficacy of this approach are not very extensive. Preliminary results from the nitrogen house set up by the Australian Institute of Sport have stimulated interest. They found no increase in Hb, but claimed there were small increases in performance levels. The possibility of placebo effects cannot be ruled out!

Summary

Increasing blood haemoglobin levels to the very top end of the normal range appears to increase aerobic exercise capacity significantly. Such effects are obtained with direct blood transfusions or with EPO injections.

Both procedures are banned. Detection based on haematocrit is being superseded by new EPO tests. The new tests look adequate to eliminate EPO abuse.

Altitude (real or simulated) acclimatisation is not the same as blood boosting as the overall changes to blood and circulation are more complex, and deliver smaller, if any, advantages in terms of sea-level performance.

Further reading

Birkeland KI, Stray-Gundersen J *et al.* Effect of rhEPO administration on serum levels of sTfR and cycling performance. *Med Sci Sports Exerc* 2000; **32**(7): 1238–43.
Gledhill N, Warburton D, Jamnik V. Haemoglobin, blood volume, cardiac function and aerobic power. *Can J Appl Physiol* 1999; **24**: 54–65.
Mottram DR (Ed). *Drugs in Sport*, 3rd edn. London: Routledge, 2003.
Parisotto R, Wu M *et al.* Detection of recombinant human erythropoietin abuse in athletes utilising markers of altered erythropoiesis. *Haematologica* 2001 **86**(2): 128–37.
Robinson RJ *et al.* The effect of induced erythrocythemia on hypoxia tolerance during exercise. *J Appl Physiol* 1982; **53**: 490.
Seiler S. Doping disaster for Finnish ski team: a turning point for drug testing? *Sportscience* 2001; **5**(1). Published on the Internet. Available online at sportsci.org/jour/0101/ss.html.

Diving – hyperbaric medicine

B Lynn

The aquatic environment presents special challenges, with the twin dangers of high pressure and cold. Hypothermia will be covered in a separate chapter. Here we will concentrate on the medical problems of diving that relate to pressure. The focus will be on sport diving, i.e. dives of relatively short duration. We will not deal with saturation diving, where commercial divers stay at high pressure for many days. Finally, the tricky question of who should be dissuaded from diving due to a pre-existing medical condition will be considered.

Diving can either be done by simply holding one's breath, or by breathing from a gas tank (SCUBA diving). Some problems are common to both forms of diving (e.g. acute barotrauma from collapse of air-filled spaces), while others are particular to the particular type of dive.

Breath-hold diving, snorkelling

The duration of a breath-hold dive is limited by the build up of CO_2 (hypercapnia) and/or lack of oxygen (hypoxia), although after training the limit can become the collapse of lung capacity to reserve volume. In untrained individuals breath-holds typically last about 30 s and are limited by the build up of carbon dioxide. If one hyperventilates first, then longer dives are possible, now limited by hypoxia. Trained breath-hold divers (e.g. Ama, pearl divers) can dive for 5 min without hyperventilating or using supplementary oxygen.

Hyperventilation is dangerous

Breath-hold after hyperventilation can cause problems at depths as little as 2 m, and accidents can occur even in a swimming pool. The main problem is fainting due to cerebral hypoxia on ascent. The lack of CO_2 drive means that the dive lasts longer and more oxygen is used. At depth, the increased pressure keeps the oxygen partial pressure at adequate levels. However, during ascent, as the total pressure falls, so does the oxygen partial pressure. It can easily fall below the level required to maintain consciousness. Prolonged hyperventilation may also occasionally cause problems due to the effects of hypocapnia on the brain.

SCUBA diving

The SCUBA apparatus delivers gas to the lungs at ambient pressure. So for example, if you are 10 m down, the ambient pressure is twice atmospheric, and gas is delivered at that pressure. There is thus no risk of lung collapse or hypoxia, etc. At depth, gas becomes more dense, so increases respiratory work. Helium lowers the density, but due to its high thermal capacity, increases heat loss.

Barotrauma

Barotrauma is the general term for any injury caused by pressure change.

Pulmonary barotrauma

Any lung space that does not equilibrate, e.g. tuberculous cavity, bulla or air trapped due to constricted brochioles in chronic obstructive pulmonary disease, will be subject to major volume changes. Problems usually occur on ascent. Air trapped at high pressure must be able to exit as it expands. The biggest change in volume occurs close to the surface (remember Boyle's Law, volume halves in the first 10 m as pressure doubles, then only falls by another quarter over the next 20 m and so on). If air cannot readily get out, perhaps due to an asthma attack, then the expanding gas will cause major trauma to the lungs. If a rapid ascent from depth is necessary, e.g. if air runs out, then it is *essential to breathe out.* Pneumothorax and air emboli can occur in these situations.

Barotrauma can also affect the ears and the sinuses. The ears will be discussed below.

Respiration at high pressure

Nitrogen

There are two problems with nitrogen.

(1) Solubility, especially in fat. Typically 7 litres of nitrogen is dissolved in fat at rest, but at 20 m (3 atm) this will rise to 21 litres and will obviously be much more at greater depths. All this extra nitrogen has to be blown off during ascent. If ascent is too quick, then nitrogen bubbles form and we get decompression sickness (see below).
(2) Nitrogen narcosis. Nitrogen is very mildly anaesthetic even at 1 atm. "Rapture of the depth", a sort of reversible drunkenness, sets in at 30 m. At 100 m the anaesthesia leads to unconsciousness. At these depths divers use helium mixes.

Oxygen

The oxygen partial pressure in compressed air reaches 1.6 atm at 70 m, a level that causes acute toxicity. Chronic toxicity occurs at much lower pressures, 0.6 bar (20 m), and compressed air is not generally used beyond 50 m (1.2 bar).

Carbon monoxide (CO)

CO is a common contaminant with compressors. A level of only 0.1% (1000 ppm) gives 14% COHb leading to breathlessness, headache, etc. at normal pressure. At 40 m, the partial pressure would be up fivefold, and a lethal level of COHb would occur. Problems can appear during ascent. At depth, the partial pressure of O_2 is high and this can provide enough dissolved oxygen to allow reasonable oxygen delivery to the tissues. But during ascent, as O_2 partial pressure falls, COHb is relatively slow to break down and severe anoxia can develop. Limits for CO in diving air are 5 ppm in the UK and 20 ppm in the USA. Best practice is to use CO filters just in case.

Decompression sickness – DCS, "the bends"

As mentioned earlier, large volumes of nitrogen dissolve in tissues when under high pressure. Some of this gas may form bubbles on ascent. Bubbles lodging in the tendons, ligaments and joint capsule cause painful restriction of movement (the bends). Bubbles forming in the pulmonary circulation cause respiratory distress ("the chokes"). Bubbles can also lodge in the spinal cord and brain causing major neurological symptoms. Finally, bubbles in the inner ear can cause vertigo – not something you want to happen when under water!

Predisposing factors for DCS are exercise, being female, age and possibly obesity. Onset may not be instant. Fifty per cent of cases do occur within 1 hour of ending the dive, but 10% take more than 6 hours. DCS may come on on the flight home due to the low pressure in the plane (NB: astronauts get this going from atmospheric to sub-atmospheric pressure on space walks). The general rule is not to fly home until 24 hours after the last dive.

DCS is classified as Type I, musculoskeletal; or Type II, neurological and/or pulmonary.

Neurological DCS

The spinal cord is most commonly affected with the development of segmental pain, weakness, paraplegia and incontinence. Cerebral problems are also frequent (frontal, parietal lobes most commonly).

Treatment of DCS

Standard treatment is immediate recompression followed by gradual decompression. Added O_2 helps. Recompression usually leads to immediate symptom relief. Avoidance is best by careful adherence to tables for decompression, i.e. waiting on ascent for time appropriate to depth and duration of dive.

Ear problems – commonest diving diseases

Because it is important to avoid any blockage of the external auditory meatus there are cases of otitis externa apparently caused by over-syringing.

Barotrauma of descent. External ear

If the external canal is blocked, trapped air compresses, and epithelial oedema, bleeding and ear drum damage ensue. Obviously divers should never use ear plugs!

Barotrauma of descent. Middle ear

Open the eustachian tube (yawn, etc.) to clear ears, equalise pressure. One needs to do this more frequently at the start (Boyle's law again – biggest volume change near the surface). If left too late, then the eustachian tubes may "lock". Middle ear tissues swell, bleed, and the eardrum perforates. Predisposing factors: mucus, allergies. Treatment: leave to heal, check hearing at regular intervals, should recover fully.

Barotrauma of ascent. Middle ear

Air admitted to middle ear on descent must be able to get out again. Sometimes it does not. Effects are painful but usually short-lived. Predisposing factors: recent barotrauma of descent; decongestants. Note, barotrauma of the middle ear can lead to inner ear problems, hearing and/or vestibular. Clinical feature: tinnitus, vertigo.

Other diseases associated with prolonged high pressure

Dysbaric osteonecrosis. Not common in sport divers. Caisson workers more at risk. High-pressure neurological syndrome (HPNS) seen only at extreme depths, >200 m. Tremors occur, then loss of consciousness. HPNS limits deep diving.

Medical screening for sports diving

Diving organisations require some degree of health screening before allowing someone to dive. This may take the form of self-certification (present UK system), or an actual medical certificate from a qualified physician may be required. Anyone with a wide range of conditions is required to get medical clearance. There are several conditions that are pretty much incompatible with safe diving. Excellent advice is available on the UKSDMC web site and "standards" are published for the more common situations encountered (see Table 1)

Rules vary from country to country and organisation to organisation. The following information is based on UKSDMC advice. Epilepsy is a no-no, unless subjects have been off medication and had no fits for 5 years. Diabetes is just about OK –

Table 1 Conditions for which the UKSDMC has published advice ("standards").

Cardiovascular	General	Neurological	Respiratory
Arrhythmias	Diabetes mellitus	Epilepsy	Asthma
Pacemakers	Dysbaric illness	Head injury	Pneumothorax
Revascularisation	Hyperlipidaemia	Multiple sclerosis	
Exercise testing	Obesity	Neurological disease	
Hypertension	Ophthalmological problems		
Intracardiac shunts	Pregnancy		
Previous myocardial infarction	Depression		
Prosthetic valves			
Anticoagulants			

Source: http://www.uksdmc.co.uk/index.html.

must be well controlled, low HbA, no hypos in the last year and no systemic disease. Cold- or exercise-induced asthma is a complete bar. Well-controlled allergic asthma is allowed. Exercise testing is not required, but a decent level of fitness is necessary. Diving is not like a game of tennis. If you get tired after a few sets, you can just stroll off the court and have a sit down. If you get fatigued 30m down then you are a danger to yourself and your diving buddies. The large commercial dive training organisation PADI has the requirement to be able to walk 1 mile in 12 minutes (brisk walking speed). Hopefully it will become clear during training if swimming fitness is adequate.

Further reading

Brubakk A, Neuman T. *The Physiology and Medicine of Diving*, edited by A Brubakk and T Neuman. WB Saunders, 2003.

Edmonds C *et al. Diving and Subaquatic Medicine*, 4th edn. London: Arnold, 2002.

PADI Medical statement. Published on the Internet. Available online at http://www.padi.com/english/common/courses/forms/pdf/10063-Ver2-0.pdf.

UK Sports Diving Medical Committee (UKSDMC). Published on the Internet. Available online at http://www.uksdmc.co.uk/index.html.

Ear, nose, throat conditions in athletes

N Munir

Acute and chronic sports-related ENT conditions are common and clinicians involved in sports medicine should be apt at managing these. The aim of this chapter is to provide a succinct overview of the commonest conditions rather than to provide an exhaustive text on the subject.

The use of protective face gear is not mandatory in most sports. Hence, faces are usually exposed and susceptible to injury, particularly in sports such as football, rugby, boxing and skiing.

General management

All head and neck injuries should initially be managed as closed head injuries with appropriate evaluation of airway, breathing, circulation and cervical spine. Brisk bleeding is often a feature of head and neck injuries due to the rich blood supply of this region. Such bleeding should not distract the medical attendant from prompt, systematic evaluation of the patient. A thorough history and examination are imperative.

Nose

The nose is particularly susceptible to injury due to its prominent central location and low breaking strength of its skeletal support. Nasal injury may result in a combination of soft tissue injury, nasal bone fracture, septal dislocation/fracture, septal haematoma or cerebrospinal fluid (CSF) leak.

Nasal trauma often occurs in conjunction with other maxillofacial injuries and these need to be carefully excluded. The usual symptoms of nasal injury are epistaxis, a noticeable cosmetic deformity with or without nasal airway compromise. Periorbital and subconjunctival ecchymosis may also be present.

At the initial assessment it is important to note the nature of the injury, any previous trauma and whether the nasal deformity is old or new. The nasal airway needs to be examined and the nasal septum assessed for any obvious deformity or a septal haematoma. Soft tissue swelling and tenderness may make adequate assessment difficult unless seen almost immediately after the injury. In such cases, if uncomplicated, it would be pertinent to reassess the patient in 5–7 days, allowing time for the soft tissue swelling to subside.

Radiological investigations are usually not required in uncomplicated nasal injuries, but have a role to play in cases where additional facial injuries are suspected.

Management

Soft-tissue injuries

Wounds should be cleaned thoroughly. Abrasions are best left open to heal. Steristrips may be used to close small lacerations; larger lacerations should be sutured. The patient's tetanus immunisation status should be assessed and appropriate cover provided.

Epistaxis

Nasal injuries are often accompanied by epistaxis. The vast majority settle with application of direct pressure. Persisting epistaxis in the presence of a nasal fracture may settle following closed fracture reduction. In cases where epistaxis fails to resolve by these measures nasal packing may be required to arrest the bleeding.

Nasal bone fracture

Nasal fractures are classified based according to the direction and degree of the causative force. They are characterised as frontal or lateral injuries. Uncomplicated fractures without a cosmetic or functional deficit do not require any treatment. In cases of simple displaced fractures closed reduction under local or general anaesthetic can be carried out. This should be carried out either immediately after the injury before onset of gross soft tissue swelling or 5–7 days after the injury allowing for soft tissue swelling and distortion to subside. Fracture reduction should not be delayed for longer than 2 weeks after the injury, as the bones start to fix after this period and manipulation can be very difficult if not impossible. More extensive injuries may require open reduction under general anaesthesia. In cases of malunion of nasal bones a formal septorhinoplasty will be required.

Septal haematoma

Trauma can tear blood vessels in the perichondrium leading to a subperichondrial collection of blood which dissects the perichondrium away from the septal cartilage. The haematoma may be unilateral or bilateral. Cartilage, devoid of its own intrinsic blood supply, is dependent on the perichondrium for nutrition. Cartilage necrosis starts to occur if the haematoma is left untreated for more than 48 hours. The usual presentation of a septal haematoma is progressive nasal obstruction following nasal trauma, with or without epistaxis. On examination a large, soft, bluish/red swelling may be noted in the nasal airway. The swelling may be confused with nasal polyps, a deviated nasal septum or hypertrophied turbinates. The definitive treatment is adequate drainage of the haematoma and reapposition of the perichondrium to the cartilage. In early cases, needle aspiration may suffice, however, once an organised clot has formed a formal incision and drainage is required. If left untreated a septal abscess and cartilage necrosis follow, resulting in cosmetic ("saddle nose deformity") and functional deficit.

CSF leak

The cribriform plate is extremely thin and prone to damage in nasal trauma. CSF leak should be suspected in the presence of clear rhinorrhoea following nasal injury. Diagnosis can be confirmed by testing for glucose content of the rhinorrhoea (similar to serum levels) or checking for Beta 2 transferrin (protein present in perilymph and CSF). Most CSF leaks heal spontaneously. Persistent leaks, however, require surgical repair. The patient is at risk of developing pneumococcal meningitis until the leak stops and they should be explicitly made aware of this risk. The role of prophylactic antibiotics is disputed.

Ear

Auricular haematoma

The pinna is an unprotected appendage readily accessible to trauma. Blunt injuries, common in boxers and wrestlers, produce shearing forces disrupting the adherence of auricular perichondrium to the underlying cartilage. The subperichondrial space becomes filled with blood, thus depriving the cartilage (without an intrinsic blood supply) of nutrition. If left untreated infection, fibrosis and cartilage necrosis ensue, causing auricular deformity ("cauliflower ear"). Treatment involves complete evacuation of the haematoma and reapposition of the perichondrium to the cartilage. The aim is to prevent deformity of the auricle. A pressure dressing should be applied to prevent re-collection.

Tympanic membrane perforation

The commonest cause of tympanic membrane perforation is otitis media. However, sports-related blunt trauma or barotrauma from swimming/diving can also result in tympanic membrane perforation. The patient may be asymptomatic, or may complain of hearing loss, vertigo, bloody or serous ottorrhoea, or ear discomfort exacerbated by wind or cold weather. Most traumatic perforations heal spontaneously within weeks. The ear canal should be kept dry until the perforation has healed. In cases where the perforation fails to heal spontaneously, a tympanoplasty may be considered if the patient is symptomatic.

Swimmer's ear

Swimmer's ear is a term commonly used to describe a localised bacterial infection affecting the external auditory canal (otitis externa). The condition is not exclusive to swimmers. The main pathogens are *pseudomonas aeruginosa*, *staphylococcus aureus* and *proteus*. The clinical history is one of initial discomfort or itching of the external auditory canal rapidly progressing to tenderness and pain. In severe cases, the pain may be constant and worsened by even the slightest manipulation of the auricle. The patient may also complain of a sensation of fullness and reduced hearing as a result of canal occlusion secondary to oedema. On examination, the canal appears erythematous and oedematous. There may be eczematous changes evident. All patients with otitis externa should be advised to keep their ears dry and avoid instrumentation with cotton buds, etc. Mainstay treatment is topical aural medication containing a combination of antibiotics (e.g. neomycin), steroid and a wetting agent (e.g. propylene glycol), buffered to an acidic pH. In more severe cases, aural toilet with or without insertion of an aural wick may be necessitated to augment the topical therapy.

Throat

Sports-related laryngeal injuries are fortunately very rare. The larynx is formed by a complex arrangement of cartilage, nerves and muscles covered by a mucous membrane lining. Laryngeal cartilage can be fractured or dislocated resulting in a serious life-threatening airway compromise, hence such injuries should be recognised early and treated promptly. While severe injuries are usually clearly evident, less severe injuries may present with hoarseness/change in voice, dysphagia, odynophagia and anterior neck pain. Clinical findings may include dyspnoea, stridor, surgical emphysema, haemoptysis and soft tissue swelling/ecchymosis on the anterior neck. Management of the patient should be as per ATLS guidelines with airway protection and maintenance being the most important immediate concern. Cervical spine injury must also be suspected and excluded in these cases. Clinicians dealing with such cases should be apt at providing initial acute airway management.

Further reading

Norris RL, Peterson J. Airway management for the sports physician. *The Physician and Sportsmedicine* (Online) 2001; **29**(10).

Roland NJ, McRae RDR, McCombe AW. *Key Topics in Otolaryngology*, 2nd edn. BIOS Scientific, 2001: 177–9.

Romeo SJ, Hawley CJ, Romeo MW, Romeo JP. Facial injuries in sports: a team physician's guide to diagnosis and treatment. *The Physician and Sportsmedicine* (Online) 2005; **33**(4).

Elbow – lateral epicondylitis (tennis elbow)

AA Narvani

This condition was first described in 1873. It is the most common cause of lateral elbow pain in adults and some reports estimate it to affect between 7 to 10% of the adult population at any one time. It is more common in patients 30–60 years old who perform some type of repetitive motion with their upper arm, but it can affect athletes of any age. Its incidence is equal among males and females.

Pathology

Lateral epicondylitis is thought to represent a repetitive overuse injury to common wrist extensors at the lateral epicondyle. The pathology appears to be at the origin of the tendinous origin of the extensor carpi radialis brevis; however, tendinous origins of the extensor carpi radialis longus and the extensor digitorum communis may also be involved. In most cases there is partial or complete tears of the extensor tendon with disruption of the normal collagen architecture with ingrowth of fibroblastic and granulation tissue. Acute and chronic inflammatory cells are often absent. This appearance has been referred to as micro-tearing followed by incomplete healing.

Predisposing factors

Long duration and increased intensity of arm use predisposes to the described tendinopathy. Therefore, this condition occurs more commonly in patients whose profession places a high demand on their upper extremity. Other factors which may be important include inadequate or compromised musculoskeletal conditions, incorrect techniques and genetic predisposition.

Clinical features

There is pain over the lateral epicondyle which may extend proximally or over the forearm. Initially this pain may be elicited by activities of daily living and made worse by lifting, gripping or repetitive wrist activity. This may be followed by rest pain once the pathological changes become more extensive.

On examination, typically there is localised tenderness over the extensor mass just distal to the lateral epicondyle. This is made worse by resisted wrist extension or passive wrist flexion.

Investigations

Plain X-rays are normal in the majority of the patients with lateral epicondylitis, but some patients may have calcification in soft tissue adjacent to the epicondyle. X-rays do, however, help to exclude other pathologies. The use of ultrasound in diagnosis of lateral epicondylitis is not widespread yet (it can demonstrate a degree of tendon damage and increased blood flow over the extensor mass).

Differential diagnosis

Other causes of lateral elbow pain include posterior interosseous nerve entrapment, synovitis, loose bodies, osteochondral defects, postero-lateral impingement and cervical radiculopathy.

Treatment

The steps in the management of lateral epicondylitis, as with other tendinopathies, involve:

(1) Control of pain and inflammation
(2) Promotion of healing process

(3) Restoration of flexibility and strength
(4) Restoration of general fitness
(5) Control of force loads and correction of predisposing factors
(6) Surgery if above fail

Control of pain and inflammation
This includes protection, rest, ice, compression, elevation, medication (NSAIDs) and other modalities. Corticosteroid injections have therapeutic and diagnostic values, but recurrence of symptoms is not uncommon. Modalities used include ultrasound, heat/cold modalities, shock-wave therapy, laser, iontophoresis, acupuncture and massage therapy.

Promotion of healing process
This may be achieved by rehabilitative exercises, massage therapy, high-voltage electrical stimulation, extracorporeal shock-wave therapy and absence from abuse. Long-term studies are, however, lacking with many of these techniques.

Restoration of flexibility and strength
Physical therapy involves stretching the extensors followed by light progressive, pain-free active and isometric strengthening.

Control of force loads and correction of predisposing factors
Counterforce bracing may have a role in some patients. It is thought to offload the wrist extensor origin during repetitive activity. It should be applied approximately 5 cm distal to the epicondyle. Correction of predisposing factors involves assessment of technique and equipment (i.e. grip size).

Return to sport

If it is a first-time injury, proper care and sufficient healing time before resuming activity should prevent permanent disability. Healing time can be between 3 to 12 weeks depending on the severity of the injury.

Further reading

Bisset L, Paungmali A, Vicenzio B, Beller E. A systematic review and meta-analysis of clinical trials on physical interventions for lateral epicondylalgia. *British Journal of Sports Medicine* 2005; **39**(7): 411–22.

Whaley AL, Baker CL. Lateral epicondylitis. *Clin Sports Med* 2004; **23**(4): 677–91.

Elbow – medial epicondylitis (golfer's elbow)

AA Narvani

Although less common than lateral epicondylitis (tennis elbow), this condition can be seen in those athletes who are involved in golf, tennis, squash, baseball, cricket, javelin throwing, American football, weight lifting and all other throwing and racquet sports. It is more common in the second to fifth decades of life, but can occur in other age groups as well. With the majority of athletes, this condition involves the dominant arm.

Pathology

Like lateral epicondylitis, medial epicondylitis is thought to represent a repetitive overuse injury. The pathology is at the origin of the flexor–pronator musculotendenous region of the medial epicondyle with pronator teres and flexor carpi radialis being affected more often than palmirus longus, flexor digitorum superficialis and flexor carpi ulnaris. In most cases there is partial or complete tears of the flexor tendon with disruption of the normal collagen architecture with ingrowth of fibroblastic and granulation tissue. Acute and chronic inflammatory cells can be absent. This appearance has been referred to as micro-tearing followed by incomplete healing and degeneration which may be referred to as tendinopathy.

Predisposing factors

As with other sports injuries these can be classified as:

(1) Sports related:
- Participation in sports that require high demand on the upper extremity, i.e. racquet and throwing sports.

(2) Athlete related:
  (i) Previous injury
  (ii) Inadequate management and recovery from previous injury
  (iii) Inadequate or compromised musculoskeletal condition (muscle weakness, poor flexibility, lack of fitness)
  (iv) Genetic predisposition

(3) Technique related:
- Poor technique (excessive grip tension, poor forehand and serve in tennis, incorrect golf swing).

(4) Training related:
- Recent history of increase in intensity and duration of training, lack of warm up.

(5) Equipment related:
- Wrong grip size
- Old tennis balls
- Too tight strings

Clinical features

- Pain over the medial epicondylitis
  —Made worse by gripping, repetitive wrist activity and lifting
  —Varying severity
- Localised tenderness over flexor mass, just distal to the medial epicondyle.
  —Made worse by
    —passive wrist extension
    —*resisted* wrist flexion and forearm pronation.
- There may be a reduced range of movement of the elbow joint.
- There may be features of ulnar nerve dysfunction (in up to 20% of the athletes).
- Ulnar collateral ligament injury must be excluded as it could coexist, particularly in throwing athletes.

Investigations

Plain radiograph

- normal in majority of athletes
- may show calcification
- will aid to exclude other pathologies (see next chapter on Throwing injuries).

Ultrasound and MRI

- As well as helping to exclude other pathologies, these investigations may demonstrate features of tendinopathy.

Differential diagnosis

These include:

- Elbow related:
  —Elbow ulnar collateral ligament injury
  —Posterior olecranon impingement
  —Stress fractures
  —Osteoarthritis
  —Loose bodies
  —Osteochondral defects
  —Medial epicondyle apophysitis
- Nerve related:
  —Cervical radiculopathy
  —Ulnar nerve neuropathy

Treatment

The steps in the management of medial epicondylitis as other tendinopathies involve:

(1) Control of pain and inflammation
(2) Promotion of healing process
(3) Restoration of flexibility and strength

(4) Restoration of general fitness
(5) Control of force loads and correction of predisposing factors
(6) Surgery if above fail

Control of pain and inflammation

This includes protection, rest, ice, compression, elevation, medication (NSAIDs) and other modalities. Corticosteroid injections have therapeutic and diagnostic values, but recurrence of symptoms is not uncommon (must be extremely careful not to inject the ulnar nerve). Modalities used include ultrasound, heat/cold modalities, shock-wave therapy, laser, iontophoresis, acupuncture and massage therapy.

Promotion of healing process

This may be achieved by rehabilitative exercises, massage therapy, high-voltage electrical stimulation, extracorporeal shock-wave therapy and absence from abuse. Long-term studies are, however, lacking with many of these techniques.

Restoration of flexibility and strength

Physical therapy involves stretching the flexors followed by light progressive, pain-free active and isometric strengthening.

Control of force loads and correction of predisposing factors

As with lateral epicondylitis, counterforce bracing may have a role in some athletes. It is thought to offload the wrist flexor origin during repetitive activity. It should be applied approximately 5 cm distal to the epicondyle. Correction of predisposing factors involves assessment of technique and equipment (see above).

Surgery

Surgery may be offered to those athletes who are still symptomatic despite 3 to 6 months of *adequate* non-operative programme when all other causes of elbow pain have been excluded. There are a number of techniques but most involve identification and excision of torn and scar tissue, which may be followed by some form of repair of the healthy tendon. As well as identifying and protecting the ulnar nerve, it may be necessary to perform ulnar nerve decompression or transposition.

Return to sport

As with other sports injuries, return to sport is permitted once the athlete is pain free, able to achieve a full range of movement and has regained enough strength to perform their sport-specific activities. With non-operative management, return to play usually takes 6 to 12 weeks. Return to play following operative management may take 3 to 6 months.

Further reading

Ciccotti MC, Schwartz MA, Ciccotti MG. Diagnosis and treatment of the medial epicondylitis of the elbow. *Clinics in Sports Medicine* 2004; **23**: 693–705.

Elbow – throwing injuries

AA Narvani

With throwing sports, excessively large forces are generated at the elbow joint. Therefore, elbow injuries are not uncommon in athletes who participate in sports that involve throwing, such as cricket, baseball, some track and field sports and American football, especially for those with poor technique. As the frequency of participation in many of these sports is increasing, sports clinicians' appreciation and understanding of "throwing elbow injuries" is of vital importance.

Pathology

Throwing may be divided into five phases, which are:

- Wind up
- Early cocking phase
- Late cocking phase
- Acceleration
- Deceleration

In late cocking and early acceleration phases, the elbow is placed under tremendous valgus forces, which also result in large compressive forces on the lateral radiocapitellar articulation (as much as 500N). Such forces can cause damage to medial, lateral and posterior compartments of the elbow.

Figure 1 illustrates the different conditions encountered by the throwing athlete. Ulnar collateral ligament injury of the elbow, posterior olecranon impingement, olecranon stress fracture, medial epicondyle apophysitis and osteochodritis dissecans are described in this chapter while medial epicondylitis and ulnar nerve dysfunction are described elsewhere.

Ulnar collateral ligament injuries

Ulnar collateral ligament consists of an anterior bundle, a posterior bundle and a transverse bundle. The anterior bundle plays a vital role in providing medial stability to valgus force in the range of 30 to 120 degrees of flexion. It is therefore subjected to extremely high forces during the late cocking and the acceleration phase of the throwing motion. As a result, ulnar ligament injuries occur in sports that involve a throwing motion. It is also seen in many racquet sports. Its injury can occur by two mechanisms, either an acute rupture of the ligament (which can occur with elbow dislocation) or repetitive stress causing micro-trauma in the ligament. These two mechanisms can cause a spectrum of ulnar collateral ligament injuries.

Clinical features

Presentation may be chronic, acute or acute on chronic.

- Athletes may recall an acute injury that started the symptoms. This acute injury may have caused elbow dislocation.

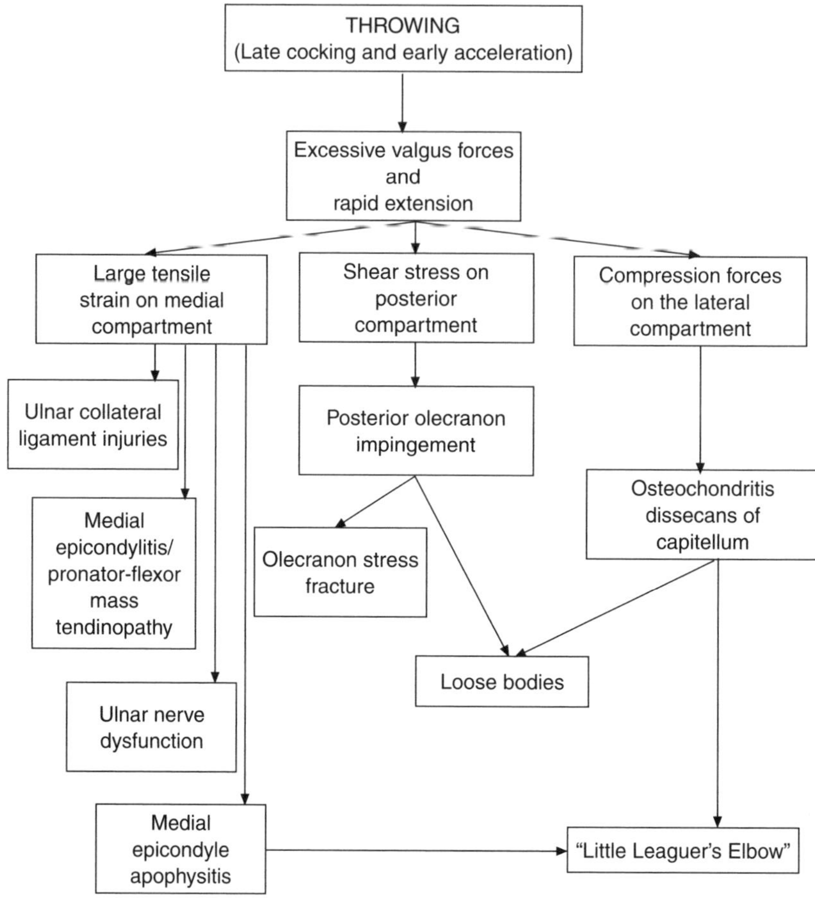

Figure 1 Elbow conditions in throwing athletes.

- Medial pain during throwing (in most athletes in the acceleration phase).
- In most athletes pain usually improves with rest.
- May complain of popping in elbow while throwing.
- Medial elbow tenderness.
- Valgus stress to the elbow flexed 20–30 degrees reproduces the pain and causes medial joint opening (up to 1 mm medial joint opening is normal).

Investigations

Plain radiograph

- In acute setting will exclude elbow dislocation and/or fractures.
- May demonstrate an avulsion fragment.
- Will aid to exclude other causes of elbow pain.
- Stress radiographs, with valgus stress, will demonstrate increased medial opening.

Ultrasound

- Dynamic ultrasonography may have a role in evaluating injuries to ulnar collateral ligament but it is operator dependent.

MRI

- With contrast, this is the investigation of choice and will demonstrate any presence of damage to the ulnar collateral ligament and whether or not this damage is partial or a full thickness tear.
- MRI will also aid to exclude other injuries.

CT

- As well as helping to exclude some of the other injuries, CT arthrogram can also be useful in illustrating the ulnar collateral ligament injuries.

Treatment

Non-operative

- Short-term elbow rest (usually 3 to 6 weeks but may be longer).
- NSAIDs
- Once pain is controlled:
  —Range of movement exercises
  —Supervised and progressive return to throwing

Operative

- Surgery is indicated:
  —In throwing athletes with complete tear (in order for the athlete to return to their throwing sports).
  —In those throwing athletes with incomplete tears in whom adequate non-operative management has failed.
  —In non-throwing athletes who remain symptomatic despite adequate non-operative measures.
- In most athletes, surgery involves reconstruction of the ulnar collateral ligament using palmaris longus tendon autograft.

Return to sport

With non-operative treatment, return to play is permitted once athletes have completed their rehabilitation programme pain free. This may take anything from 6 weeks to 6 months.

With operative treatment, the athlete is usually allowed to return to play 9 to 12 months following surgery.

Posterior olecranon impingement

This is not an uncommon condition among throwing athletes and occurs as the valgus extension force to the elbow during throwing leads to impingement of the posteromedial olecranon tip against the olecranon fossa. These repeated impingements will, in time, cause soft tissue hypertrophy and osteophyte formation, which will further worsen the impingement. As the condition progresses, these osteophytes may fracture and form loose bodies.

Clinical features

- Postero-medial elbow pain in acceleration phase of throwing.
- Athlete may not be able to extend the elbow fully.

- Tenderness in the posterior medial tip of the olecranon.
- Repeated forced hyperextension and valgus force to the elbow provokes posteromedial pain (Valgus Extension Overload test).

Investigations
- Plain radiograph may show presence of osteophytes, loose bodies or fractures.
- Bone scan, CT or MRI will help to exclude stress fractures.

Treatment
Non-operative
- Short-term elbow rest
- NSAIDs
- Once pain is controlled:
  —Range of movement exercises
  —Supervised and progressive return to throwing

Operative
- Surgery is indicated in those athletes who do not respond to non-operative treatment. The option in these athletes is arthroscopic or open excision impinging soft tissue and osteophytes ± removal of the loose bodies.

Return to sport
Throwing athletes are allowed to return to play once they are pain free and have achieved full range of movement and strength. Following surgery, this may take 3 to 4 months.

Olecranon stress fractures

Repeated impingement of the olecranon in throwing athletes (see above) can lead to stress fractures.

Clinical features
- Posterior elbow pain in acceleration phase of throwing. Pain can persist after throwing.
- Localised tenderness over the fracture site.

Investigations
- Although plain radiograph may show the fractures in some athletes, it may be normal in other athletes with stress fractures.
- Bone scan, CT or MRI are the investigations of choice if stress fractures are suspected clinically.

Treatment
Non-operative
- Rest from throwing.
- Once pain is controlled:
  —Range of movement exercises
  —Muscle strengthening exercises
  —Supervised and progressive return to throwing

Operative

- Surgery is indicated in those athletes who do not respond to non-operative treatment. Surgical options in these athletes include:
  —Open internal fixation
  —Arthroscopic internal fixation
  —Excision of olecranon tip

Medial epicondyle apophytis

In skeletally immature throwers, the medial epicondyle appears to be weaker than the ulnar collateral ligament, therefore the repetitive valgus force encountered during throwing results in its apophyseal fragmentation or avulsion rather than rupture of the collateral ulnar ligament. These injuries are thought to be most common in 9 to 12-year-old athletes, especially in young baseball pitchers, but are also seen in sports such as tennis (serving) and javelin throwing. Together with osteochondritis dissecans of the capitellum (see below), these injuries form a group of conditions that are sometimes referred to as "little leaguer's elbow".

Clinical features

- Medial elbow pain
  —Usually in the dominant arm
  —Commonly insidious onset
- Impaired throwing and performance (reduced throwing effectiveness and distance)
- Swelling
- Localised tenderness
- Decreased range of movement of the elbow joint

Investigations

Plain radiograph

Antero–posterior, lateral, right and left oblique views and may need to compare with films of the uninjured side.

- May reveal:
  —Enlargement of the elbow
  —Apophyseal irregularities
  —Apophyseal fragmentation
  —Apophyseal separation
  —Epicondyle beaking
- Will aid to exclude other causes of medial elbow pain.

Bone scan, CT and MRI

- Can be helpful in those with very subtle plain film features as well as excluding other causes of elbow pain.

Treatment

This may be both non-operative or operative.

Non-operative
- Rest from throwing (4 to 6 weeks)
- Ice
- NSAIDs
- Splint immobilisation for undisplaced or minimally displaced medial epicondyle avulsion fractures.
- Once pain is controlled:
  —Range of movement exercises
  —Supervised and progressive return to throwing.
- Activity modification and correction of any predisposing factors that could have contributed to the condition (i.e. poor technique, rules concerning intensity of throwing and training in young athletes, education of coach and athlete).

Operative
- Open reduction internal fixation is indicated in those young with significantly displaced medial epicondyle avulsion fractures.

Return to sport

Young athletes are allowed to return to throwing once they are pain free, and have achieved full range of movement and strength. This return must be cautious and gradual in order to prevent recurrent injury. The time taken for return to play is dependent on the exact pathology and can range from a few weeks to a whole season.

Osteochondritis dissecans of capitellum

This condition, seen in adolescent throwing athletes, also belongs to the group of conditions sometimes referred to as "little leaguer's elbow". It occurs as a consequence of the compressive forces between the radial head and the capitellum during throwing, which in turn are thought to disturb the subchondral blood supply. The end result is osteochondral injury which may be associated with loose body formation.

Clinical features

- Elbow pain
  —Commonly insidious onset.
- Impaired throwing and performance (reduced throwing effectiveness and distance).
- Localised tenderness.
- Flexion contracture and decreased range of movement of the elbow joint.

Investigations

Plain radiograph
- May reveal:
  —Rarefaction
  —Irregular ossification
  —Subchondral rarefied crater in the capitellum
  —Enlarged radial head
  —Loose bodies

Contrast tomograms, CT, MRI and arthroscopy

- Can be helpful in evaluating the lesions of the articular surface and subchondral bone in detail.

Treatment

This may be both non-operative or operative.

Non-operative

- Rest from throwing
- Ice
- NSAIDs
- Splint.
- Once pain is controlled:
  —Range of movement exercises
  —Supervised and progressive return to throwing
- Activity modification and correction of any predisposing factors that could have contributed to the condition (i.e. poor technique, rules concerning intensity of throwing and training in young athletes, education of coach and athlete).

Operative

- Indications for surgery are:
  —Presence of loose bodies
  —Presence of mechanical symptoms
  —Persistent symptoms despite adequate non-operative management
- Surgical options include:
  —Arthroscopic
    —Removal of loose bodies
    —Abrasion chondroplasty
    —Capitellum drilling
  —Open
    —Removal of loose bodies
    —Abrasion chondroplasty
    —Capitellum drilling
    —Humeral osteotomy

Further reading

Bradley JP, Petrie RS. Elbow injuries in children and adolescents. In: JC DeLee, D Drez, MD Miller (Eds) *Orthopaedic Sports Medicine, Principles and Practice*, 2nd edn. Saunders, 2002: 1249–64.

Caine EL, Dugas JR, Wolf RS, Andrews JR. Elbow injuries in throwing athletes: a current concept review. *Am J Sports Medicine* 2003; **31**(4): 621–34.

Dugas JR, Andrews JR. Throwing Injuries. In: JC DeLee, D Drez, MD Miller (Eds) *Orthopaedic Sports Medicine, Principles and Practice*, 2nd edn. Saunders, 2002: 1236–49.

Whiteside JA, Andrews JR, Fleisig GS. Elbow injuries in young baseball players. *The Physician & Sportsmedicine* 1999; **27**(6).

Epilepsy and exercise

S Parnia

Until recently, people with epilepsy had been strongly discouraged and even prohibited from participating in sports activities. This advice had traditionally been based upon a largely common-sense and conservative approach as regards the potential theoretical risks of participation in sports. The reasoning behind this advice included the concern that the occurrence of a seizure during certain exercises could pose substantial risk to the participant. In addition, it had been argued that repeated or severe head injury during contact sports could exacerbate seizures in a patient known to have epilepsy. Although these concerns and risks still remain, the latest evidence suggests the need for a more reasoned and less conservative approach, which leads to few restrictions overall. This chapter reviews clinically relevant aspects of the relationship between epilepsy and exercise.

Seizures, epilepsy and the risk of injury during seizures

Seizures may result from any event leading to a transient alteration in brain function and a sudden interruption in the brain's highly complex electro-chemical activity. Epilepsy is a condition in which seizures recur spontaneously, and it is estimated that more than 300,000 people in the UK (one in 200) suffer with this condition. As regards the risk of exercise in people with epilepsy, the type of seizure experienced by patients influences their potential exposure to harm.

Seizures are classified as either generalized or partial seizures and assessing each seizure type provides the basis for understanding how harm may occur during a seizure.

Generalized seizures

Generalized seizures are expressed globally throughout the brain at their onset and are of several different types. Generalized tonic–clonic seizures, previously termed grand mal, begin with generalized tonic limb extension, resulting in unprotected falling and followed by rhythmic clonic jerks. Atonic seizures consist of sudden loss of muscle tone with unprotected falling, which can result in serious injury.

Absence seizures consist of brief (typically 3–10 s), motionless, non-distractible staring, but balance is usually maintained. Therefore, absence seizures do not cause falling injuries.

Partial seizures

Partial seizures begin in one focal part of the brain and cause symptoms appropriate to the part of the brain in which they originate. Simple partial seizures begin in such a small part of the brain that consciousness is not altered. These are thus unlikely to cause unanticipated injury to sports participants.

Complex partial seizures are defined by alteration (but not loss) of consciousness, usually of 1 to 2 minutes' duration, followed by a few minutes of confusion. Complex partial seizures are likely to render the participant unable to participate for at least a few minutes. Seizures that begin as partial seizures may generalize, with the same implications as primary generalized seizures noted above.

Potential of athletics to exacerbate seizures

Athletic participation can be associated with factors that could alter seizure threshold, including repeated head injury during contact sports, excessive aerobic exercise, hyperventilation and changes in drug metabolism.

Repeated head injury

Despite the concern that repeated head injury during contact sports could trigger seizures there is little evidence to support this. One reason for a lack of evidence may be the fact that most patients are dissuaded or prohibited from participating in contact sports and thus there is little experience on which to base this judgement.

Aerobic exercise

Aerobic exercise occasionally causes seizure exacerbations, but on average it improves seizure frequency during prospective formal evaluation. There are rare case reports of patients whose seizures are "triggered" by exercise, but this is generally not a significant problem. Overall, aerobic exercise has great benefit to general health and may reduce seizure frequency. Therefore, it is recommended for most patients, although it must be recognized that it will trigger seizures in a few individuals.

Hyperventilation

Hyperventilation triggers absence seizures when performed at rest during a routine EEG, so it has been feared that it could trigger seizures during exercise-induced hyperventilation; however, there is no evidence to support this. Exercise-induced hyperventilation may even produce a refractory period that can delay the activating effects of resting hyperventilation. Therefore, absence seizures are not usually exacerbated by exercise-induced hyperventilation.

Drug metabolism

Physical training induces hepatic microsomal enzymes, and this may be particularly important for patients who are taking antiepileptic drugs, such as phenytoin. Therefore, it is worthwhile to consider that patients with exercise-triggered seizures could have altered pharmacokinetics that may lead to alterations in the dose of medication required to control their seizures.

Sports as a cause of seizures and epilepsy

There is little evidence that repeated head injury associated with contact sports predisposes to epilepsy. It has been observed that what appear to be seizures can immediately follow a severe head injury, yet these typical concussive convulsions are not actually seizures. There is also some epidemiological evidence that head injury may cause epilepsy, but the association is only significant for severe head injury. In the most severe case of military-related, penetrating-missile head injury, epilepsy may occur in up to 50% of cases. However, there is no consistent report of increased risk of subsequent epilepsy from typical mild head injury in the general population. A typical sports-related head injury is so mild that it is extremely unlikely to be associated with epilepsy based on severity, and the paucity of reports of epilepsy following participation in contact sports such as boxing suggests that it is uncommon.

Risk–benefit analysis of sports participation

The decision for anyone to participate in sports is whether the benefit outweighs the risk and for an individual with epilepsy this is highly dependent on the athletic activity, the type of seizures, the likelihood of seizures, and whether any comorbid conditions are present.

Specific recommendations for athletic participation

There is little evidence of increased risk of participation in sports, and clear evidence of benefit. However, there is clearly increased risk for some patients and some sports. This emphasizes the paramount importance of individualizing the decision for each patient.

Water sports (swimming, rowing, boating, canoeing, rafting, sailing, fishing, scuba diving)

Water sports present a particularly difficult problem because of the known increased risk of drowning due to seizures. Yet, it is generally recommended that water sports be permitted with appropriate precautions. The risk of drowning during a seizure is extremely low with close supervision in the shallow, clear water of a swimming pool, and therefore patients should generally be allowed to swim with direct visual supervision. Rowing, boating of any type, and fishing pose a risk from falling into open water during a seizure. Therefore, patients should always wear floatation devices and these activities should be avoided if seizures are frequent.

Scuba diving is prohibited for patients with active epilepsy and is not recommended even if their seizures are controlled by anti-epileptic medication. The medical committee of the British Sub-Aqua Club (BSAC) has produced a factsheet outlining the issues and risks. For example, it states that people taking anti-epileptic medication are more likely to experience "nitrogen narcosis" than those not on any medication and this might put them at risk in the water.

The BSAC suggests that people should be seizure free and off medication for 5 years (or 3 years if seizures only occur during sleep) before they consider scuba diving.

Competitive underwater swimming and diving pose problems similar to scuba diving and should be avoided.

Sports at heights (sky diving, hang gliding, flying, climbing, bungi jumping, gymnastics, horseback riding)

Sky diving, hang gliding and free climbing would place a patient at considerable risk if a seizure were to occur, and should be discouraged. Epilepsy presents no specific additional risk as regards bungi jumping. Gymnastics may pose a risk for activities that involve swinging from parallel bars or other acrobatic activities for some patients, but other activities are not discouraged. There is significant risk of injury due to falls during equestrian sports, so horseback riding should generally be avoided for patients with active epilepsy.

Contact sports (boxing, football, American football, hockey, rugby)
There are no strict prohibitions on contact sports for patients with epilepsy, because there is no evidence that repeated mild blows to the head exacerbate seizures. It seems prudent to advise against them only when seizures are newly diagnosed and their course for a given patient has not been defined.

Aerobic sports (running, track and field, ice skating, skiing)
There are no prohibitions to aerobic exercise and there is evidence that it reduces seizure frequency and improves self-image. Appropriate head gear and safe practices should be followed during ice skating and skiing. A consideration for skiers is whether a seizure might occur on a ski lift and whether the patient would fall out of a lift chair.

Wheeled sports (cycling, rollerblading, skateboarding)
There are no specific prohibitions for wheeled sports. It is prudent to restrict these activities, however, if seizures are frequent or of as-yet-undetermined frequency.

Summary

Epilepsy is a very individual condition so choices about whether or not to participate in particular activities or sports need to be made on an individual basis, depending on the type and frequency of seizures and the level of control with medication. For example, people whose epilepsy is completely controlled may not need to take the same precautions as those who still have seizures. Choices should be realistic not restrictive. Most activities can be made safer by adopting simple safety measures to help minimize any potential risk.

Ideally, all decisions should be made with the full involvement of the person who will be affected by them. It is important that children of school age who have epilepsy are included in the full range of activities unless their seizures prevent this.

Further reading

Dubow JS, Kelly JP. Epilepsy in sports and recreation. *Sports Med* 2003; **33**(7): 499–51.

Fountain NB, May AC. Epilepsy and athletics. *Clin Sports Med* 2003; **22**(3): 605–16.

Howard GM, Radloff M, Sevier TL. Epilepsy and sports participation. *Curr Sports Med Rep* 2004; **3**(1): 15–19.

Exercise physiology – circulatory and respiratory systems

B Lynn

This section will concentrate on the important circulatory and respiratory adjustments that are needed for aerobic exercise. In fact, this common way of looking at exercise physiology is really quite wrong. To quote Barcroft (writing in 1937): "The condition of exercise is not a mere variant of the condition of rest, it is the essence of the machine." Thus, in many ways the norm, in the world in which our bodies evolved, must have been exercise, and in studying exercise physiology we are really studying the situation for which our bodies, including our circulatory and respiratory systems, evolved.

Respiration in exercise

Breathing

Pulmonary ventilation increases with exercise intensity from around 6 l/min up to 100–150 l/min. For light to moderate exercise the increase is mostly in tidal volume, with respiratory rate increasing at higher exercise intensities. The relation with oxygen consumption is linear for light to moderate exercise with 20–25 litres needing to be breathed to extract each litre of oxygen. So someone exercising at a level where oxygen consumption is 3 l/min will be breathing about 60 l/min, ten times the resting level. At moderate to high exercise levels, pulmonary ventilation increases faster than oxygen consumption.

Even at VO_2max, pulmonary ventilation is not at the level that can be attained during voluntary hyperventilation and tidal volume never gets close to vital capacity. However, the high cost of supplying the breathing muscles themselves with oxygen and the fatigue of these muscles probably sets limits during real exercise that are less than the maximum possible.

Quiet breathing at rest involves principally the diaphragm during inspiration and elastic recoil of the lung tissues during expiration. During exercise, additional inspiratory movement is produced by contraction of the external intercostals and the scalene muscles. Also, contraction of some abdominal muscles assists by providing a stable base for the diaphragm. Expiration also now involves active muscle action from the internal intercostals and some abdominal muscles. At high pulmonary ventilation inspiration is also assisted by the so-called "accessory" muscles, mainly sternocleidomastoid and the pectorals.

During exercise, breathing may become coupled to locomotion. This is true for rowing, cycling and running (and rather obviously swimming!). On a cycle ergometer it is not uncommon to see sudden switches from 1 breath every 3 revolutions, to 1 every 2, then even 1 breath per revolution close to VO_2max.

Control of breathing

During exercise, pulmonary ventilation reaches levels far above anything that can be achieved by administering high CO_2 and low O_2 gas mixtures. This observation immediately indicates that the normal control mechanisms (carbon dioxide/pH acting on central chemoreceptors and anoxia acting peripherally) provide only part of the story during exercise. It appears that neural feedback from the muscles themselves plays some part. Both proprioceptors and small fibre receptors sensing local chemical and vascular changes appear to be involved. The rapid doubling of breathing that occurs immediately at the start of exercise is certainly driven by peripheral or central motor control signals. Finally, the linking of respiratory rhythm to locomotor time pattern also indicates that there must be coupling between motor control signals and the respiratory centre.

Gas exchange and transport

Gas exchange at the lungs works well during respiration. Carbon dioxide, with its high lipid solubility, crosses readily from circulation to alveolar air. Oxygen crosses sufficiently rapidly to maintain complete arterial saturation except in some highly trained athletes with high oxygen consumption where a modest degree of oxygen desaturation has been observed. In the muscles, gas exchange is aided by the increased diffusion gradient due to low tissue pO_2 and high pCO_2 that exists when muscle is metabolising hard. Diffusion of oxygen is aided in S and FR fibres by the presence of myoglobin, responsible for their red pigmentation.

The circulation in exercise

The heart

Cardiac output increases from its resting value of around 5 l/min to as much as 30 l/min in a trained athlete. The increase is nicely linear with oxygen consumption, as this increases from about 0.25 l/min to 5 l/min. How a sixfold increase in CO is compatible with a 20-fold increase in oxygen consumption will be explained below. Cardiac output is the product of heart rate and stroke volume and both increase during exercise. The heart rate increase falls with age, with maximum heart rate in adults estimated usually by the formula 220 − age. So in young fit subjects heart rates of 200 per second are seen. The increase in heart rate follows a reduction in vagal drive to the pacemaker at lower levels of exercise. At higher exercise levels, the sympathetics and adrenaline push the heart rate up further, and speed up the conducting system. Overall heart rate in a young unfit individual may increase threefold while in a trained athlete the increase may be fourfold. The stroke volume increases less, by about 50% and mostly at low to moderate intensity exercise levels. The increase partly reflects increased venous return and better filling in the normal Frank–Starling manner. The increased venous return is largely a consequence of the muscle pump. There is also increased contractility of the ventricles due to activation of the sympathetic nervous system and release of adrenaline. Over a long exercise period (>20 min) when oxygen consumption is at a steady level there is usually a continuing upward drift in heart rate accompanied by a drop in stroke volume. The reduction in exercise capacity in patients on beta blockers is largely because these drugs limit heart rate rises.

Muscle and non-muscle peripheral vasculature

In the periphery, a massive vasodilatation occurs in the active muscles. Partial compensation occurs with vasoconstriction in viscera. Blood flow to essential organs, such as the brain, is preserved and, obviously, blood supply to the heart is also massively increased. This pattern is largely orchestrated by (1) the sympathetic nervous system and (2) the local dilator actions of metabolites diffusing from muscle fibres.

Skin blood flow and thermoregulation

The degree of cutaneous vasodilatation during exercise is regulated to allow the heat generated by active muscles to be dissipated. This means, for exercise at any level in a hot environment and for high-level exercise at almost any environmental temperature, substantial cutaneous vasodilatation occurs.

Regulation of the circulation including blood pressure regulation

During exercise, diastolic blood pressure stays approximately stable or may fall a bit while systolic blood pressure rises substantially. Clearly pulse pressure is markedly up, while average blood pressure is usually up a bit. An exceptional situation is isometric exercise, where long-lasting contractions will increase the peripheral resistance in muscle, thus causing a large rise in average blood pressure. Systolic blood pressures above 250 mmHg are not uncommon during resistance exercises such as bench presses.

The baroreceptor reflex still operates during steady exercise and is one of the control factors. Another important factor is feedback from small fibre "ergoreceptors" in active muscles. These converge with other relevant inputs in the brainstem to regulate sympathetic and parasympathetic outputs to the heart and the circulation.

Factors limiting maximum oxygen consumption

Maximum oxygen consumption (VO_2max) is an excellent measure of aerobic fitness. It depends on many factors including the performance of the circulatory and respiratory systems and the capacity of the muscles to use oxygen. At VO_2max oxygen consumption is up about 20-fold. Breathing will have increased by about this amount. Heart rate is up only sixfold, but the greater arterio-venous difference in concentration plus the additional proportion of blood going to the muscles means that oxygen-carrying capacity is up 20-fold.

VO_2max appears to be principally determined by the ability of the circulation to get oxygen to the tissues. In some highly trained individuals there appears to be a limitation on oxygen transport in the lungs. Such individuals have a modest desaturation at high exercise levels and if given higher than atmospheric oxygen to breathe, show increased VO_2max. This does not happen in most individuals. The capacity of the muscle to use oxygen appears to be quite a lot higher than the capacity of the circulatory system to supply it. The circulatory limitations thus appear to be (a) the ability of the heart to pump blood and (b) the ability of blood to carry oxygen. The limiting nature of the oxygen carriage is shown by the fact that increasing blood haemoglobin concentration, by blood doping or taking erythropoietin, does lead to significant increases in VO_2max. The limiting nature of cardiac output is demonstrated by the increases in VO_2max seen with aerobic training.

Summary

- Pulmonary ventilation increases 20 times or more during exercise.
- Cardiac output increases up to sixfold in exercise with most of the increase due to increased heart rate.
- Maximum oxygen consumption (VO_2max) is limited by the ability of the blood to carry oxygen and of the heart to pump blood.

Further reading

Astrand P-O, Rodahl K, Dahl HA, Stromme SB. *Textbook of Work Physiology*, 4th edn. Champagne, Illinois: Human Kinetics, 2003; Chapters 5 and 6.

Exercise promotion

B Lynn

Many people now have a sedentary lifestyle that increases the risk of many diseases and reduces quality of life. There has been a reduction in physical activity in all aspects of our lives – at work, at home, in the ways we travel. Consequently, the encouragement of more physical activity has become a public health objective in most developed countries. How we can achieve that objective, and particularly the role of the sports doctor, is the subject of this chapter.

Two strategies for increasing our physical activity look promising. Firstly, can we build a modest level of physical activity – but enough to contribute to health – into everyday activities? For example, encourage the use of stairs instead of lifts or promote walking or cycling for short journeys. In this area, the role of health professionals is essentially supportive. The second strategy is to increase enjoyable forms of exercise, many of which will involve sports participation. This is an area where medical input can be more influential.

Exercise prescriptions for at-risk individuals

In the primary care area it is essential to identify individuals who are particularly at risk due to a sedentary lifestyle. Key factors include (a) being overweight, and (b) poor blood lipid profile. The use of various counselling techniques, often coupled to exercise prescriptions, to get such individuals started has been tried in the primary care area. Results have been variable with problems keeping people exercising over long periods, i.e. in really changing ingrained sedentary behaviour (e.g. see Taylor 2003; Hillsdon *et al.* 2005). A recent Canadian study added simple fitness testing to the usual primary care mix and found maintained increases in activity over 12 months (Petrella *et al.* 2003). The effect of having some objective feedback on progress appeared to help in motivation. For individuals with a number of chronic conditions, exercise programmes can also be effective in limiting the progress of the disease. Exercise programmes have long been encouraged for patients recovering from heart disease. But such programmes also help with diabetes, arthritis, depression, osteopenia and a range of other chronic illnesses. In these situations it is important that the development of appropriate clinical exercise programmes with proper medical oversight is encouraged.

Physical activity often falls to very low levels in older individuals. This is an area where the health message about the benefits of physical activity has been getting through. It is difficult to frighten a young person with good health into exercising to improve their health in the future. But for older people, this message is clearly seen as much more relevant. Recent surveys in the UK show an interesting trend for older people to be increasing their participation in leisure-time physical activity, whereas the trend in younger age groups is still downward (Figure 1).

Access to sports facilities

The provision of accessible sports and exercise facilities is something for which sports medicine professionals have long argued. But sports medicine perhaps has its most important role in ensuring that as many people as possible do feel safe in using such facilities. It is important that suitable reassurance is given about exercise during pregnancy, after illness, etc. Where appropriate it should be possible to organise electrocardiogram (ECG) and other testing, including exercise stress testing.

Finally, it is important also to be aware of the arguments about screening. In some countries, participation in organised sport is only allowed following a medical check up. Whilst this is appropriate for at-risk individuals, the case for such pre-participation screening for all has not been made. For healthy individuals, a simple screening questionnaire such as the PAR-Q (Physical Activity Readiness Questionnaire) is adequate. It is essential to stress all the time that life is not risk free. And one of the

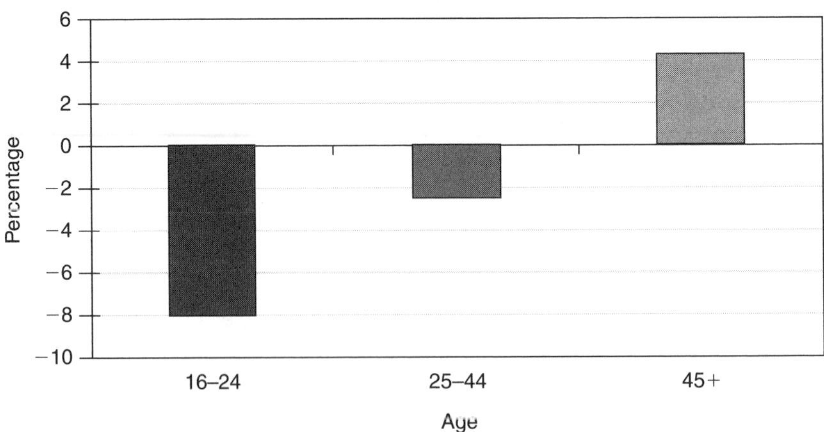

Figure 1 Trends in participation in at least one sport, game or physical activity in the 4 weeks before interview by age. Data from General Household Survey of Great Britain, sampling approximately 15,000 individuals in 8000 households selected by postcode. The younger age categories have shown a fall in participation over the last 15 years, whereas the older groups have shown an increase.

most risky things you can do is *not* exercise. There are certainly tragic cases of sudden deaths during sports. But the numbers of such deaths is very small compared with the premature morbidity associated with lack of exercise (Maron 2000). It is noteworthy, however, that the small risk of sudden death during or immediately following a bout of vigorous exercise is higher in those unaccustomed to such exercise. Therefore good advice is always to build up any exercise programme slowly.

Key points

- Support changes in the built environment and in transport that may provide extra physical activity opportunities.
- Support strategies to increase involvement in leisure time exercise and sports.
- Provide necessary medical support for exercise programmes for patients with chronic diseases or the frail elderly.
- Argue for the minimum barriers to exercise, for example no need for medical screening in healthy individuals.

Further reading

Fox K, Rickards L. Sport and leisure. Results from the sport and leisure module of the 2002 General Household Survey. London: HMSO, 2004. Published on the Internet. Available online at http://www.statistics.gov.uk/lib2002.

Hillsdon M, Foster C, Thorogood M. Interventions for promoting physical activity. The Cochrane Database of Systematic Reviews 2005 Issue 1. Art. No.: CD003180.pub2.

Maron BJ. The paradox of exercise. *N Engl J Med* 2000; **343**: 1409–11.

Petrella RJ, Koval JJ, Cunningham DA, Paterson DH. Can primary care doctors prescribe exercise to improve fitness? The Step Test Exercise Prescription (STEP) project. *Am J Prev Med* 2003; **24**: 316–22.

Taylor A. The role of primary care in promoting physical activity. In: J McKenna, C Riddoch (Eds) *Perspectives on Health and Exercise*. Basingstoke, UK: Palgrave Macmillan, 2003, Chapter 8.

The PAR-Q screening form is available from the Canadian Society for Exercise Physiology. Published on the Internet. Available online at http://www.csep.ca/forms.asp.

Eye injuries in sports

AA Narvani

Eye injuries are extremely common in sports. Sports account for up to 40% of all eye injuries requiring hospital admission. Thirty per cent of all eye injuries in children are sports related. Furthermore, in about 30% of all eye injuries, there may be serious damage to the intraocular structures. Sports that are particularly associated with eye injuries include those that require use of racquets, bat, ball and those with body contact. Examples of such sports include boxing, martial arts, squash, hockey, baseball, cricket, tennis, rugby, American football, soccer, hurling, fencing and badminton.

Assessment of athletes with eye injuries

The most important responsibility of clinicians faced with athletes who have suffered eye injuries, other than excluding and treating life-threatening conditions, is to distinguish those with serious eye injuries from those with minor injuries. This is of vital importance, as those with serious injuries require urgent and immediate referral to ophthalmologists. In order to make this differentiation, clinicians must rely on accurate and thorough clinical assessment.

History

A thorough history should emphasise the following points:

- pain
  —onset and timing
  —severity
- mechanism of injury
  —Broadly speaking, there are four main mechanisms in injury which include:
    —blunt trauma (most common)
    —penetrating injuries
    —injuries involving chemicals
    —radiation injuries
- impaired visual acuity
- blurred vision
- double vision
- flashing lights
- floaters
- halos around lights
- photophobia
- previous eye problems
- use of eye protection

Examination

This should be complete, systematic and include:

- Assessment of visual acuity
  —eye chart
  —newspaper-sized prints
- Assessment of visual field
  —impairments may be caused by retinal, optical nerve and central nervous system injuries
- Assessment of eyelids
  —bruising
  swelling
  —laceration
  —bleeding
- Assessment of eye surface
  —corneal foreign bodies
  —corneal abrasions

  - —both of the above can become more obvious with fluorescein drops as they stain (if there is suspicions of ruptured globe, fluorescein should not be applied)
- Assessment of anterior chamber
  —hyphaema implies blood in the anterior chamber and indicates serious injury
- Assessment of pupils
  —size
  —shape
  —irregularity
  —symmetry
  —reactivity (including consensual light reflex which is pupil constriction when light is directed to the other pupil)
- Funduscopic assessment
  —Absence or alteration of *red reflex* can imply serious injuries such as intraocular bleeding and retinal detachment
  —retina oedema
  —retina haemorrhage
  —vitreous haemorrhage (secondary to retina tears) may result in inability to see the fundus
- Assessment of eye movements
- Assessment of the orbit
  —inspection and palpation
  —swelling
  —bruising
  —laceration
  —bleeding
  —proptosis
  —enophthalmos
  —tenderness
  —crepitus
  —bony step offs
  —altered sensation around the orbit
  —fractures of the lateral wall of the orbit can result in trismus and pain with mouth opening
- Cranial nerve examination

Once the injury is evaluated, then a valid decision can be made on whether the athlete requires urgent referral to ophthalmologists. Indications for urgent referral include:

- Penetrating injuries
- Radiation injuries
- Chemical injuries
- Impaired visual acuity
- Impaired visual field
- Double vision
- Photophobia
- Flashes/floaters/halos around light
- Significant pain

- Proptosis/enophthalmos
- Substantial subconjunctival swelling
- Extensive subconjunctival haemorrhage
- Hyphaema
- Any pupil abnormality (including size, shape, irregularity, asymmetry, reactivity)
- Embedded foreign body
- Laceration (corneal, eyelid)
- Any abnormalities with funduscopic examination (see above)
- Suspected globe rupture
- Abnormal eye movements

Specific injuries

Orbital fractures

This can involve the floor (most common), walls or roof of the orbit. Mechanism of injury is usually blunt trauma. These can be associated with significant structural damage including injuries to cornea, retina, optic nerve, lens and eyelids and result in the orbit content herniating through the orbital defect.

Clinical features include pain (worse with eye movements), swelling, impaired/double vision, impaired eye movements. Other associated injuries must be excluded. Imaging in the form of plain radiograph and CT are indicated.

Athletes should be referred urgently to ophthalmologists. Treatment of isolated injuries includes use of antibiotics and surgery in those with trapped soft tissue in the bony defect, fractures involving more than 50% of the orbital floor, or enopthalmos greater than 2 mm.

Eyelid lacerations

These may be caused by both blunt and penetrating injuries. Exclusion of other eye injuries is of vital importance. Laceration itself may involve the lid margins or be extra-marginal. Initial management of the isolated lacerations include cleaning the wound as well as keeping it moist and ensuring corneal lubrication. This should be followed by repair of the laceration and in most cases this is best performed by an ophthalmic surgeon.

Subconjunctival haemorrhage

The vast majority of these just require reassurance as they disappear within a few days. However, they might imply more serious eye injury. When extensive or combined with the above features, ophthalmologist referral is necessary.

Corneal abrasions/foreign body

There is commonly a history of being struck in the eye. Usual features include pain, a feeling of foreign body in the eye, and blurred/decreased vision. Eversion of the eyelid may reveal a retained foreign body. Most corneal abrasions cannot be seen by the naked eye and are best visualised following application of fluorescein, which stains them. This is more comfortable after introduction of anaesthetic eye drops. Examination must also include assessment for features of more serious injuries (see above).

Uncomplicated corneal abrasions are usually treated with pain relief, prophylactic antibiotic eye drops and regular follow up. Use of eye patches have been popular in the past, however recent randomised control trials (see Weber 2005 in the Further reading list) suggest that they do not offer any benefits in terms of pain relief and healing.

Foreign bodies in the cornea can be removed with use of a moistened cotton-tipped swab. Ophthalmologist referral is necessary when the foreign body cannot be removed and when it is completely embedded in the cornea.

Hyphaema

This refers to bleeding in the anterior chamber. The bleeding is secondary to tearing/rupture of the iris and ciliary vasculature. This bleeding can lead to raised eye pressure and acute glaucoma by obstruction of the aqueous fluid outflow. Mechanism of injury is usually a direct blow but it can also be caused by some haematological disorders, tumours, vitreous haemorrhage and diabetes. Athletes could complain of impaired/blurred vision, and photophobia. In some athletes, the condition can only be diagnosed following slit lamp assessment, which also allows detection of other associated injuries. A clear fluid level is seen.

The presence of hyphaema is an indication for urgent referral to ophthalmologists as it could be associated with significant structural damage and complications. Once other pathologies and injuries are excluded, treatment is dependent on the severity and includes rest, avoidance of aspirin, and NSAIDs and regular monitoring.

Retinal detachment

There are three different types of retinal detachment. The most common, and certainly the type seen in sporting injuries, is "rhematogenous" retinal detachment. This occurs when a tear in the retina allows the liquid vitreous to enter the potential space beneath the retina, enlarging the initial tear, and resulting in detachment of the retina.

Athletes present with visual impairments, "curtain-like" loss of vision, flashes of light and floaters. Funduscopic assessment can reveal the retinal tear.

The athlete should be urgently referred to an ophthalmic surgeon as surgical repair is indicated.

Injury prevention

Prevention of eye injuries must be among the priorities of those dealing with the athlete. All athletes should have screening assessment, which should include a thorough examination, to exclude any eye disease or any visual impairment. Fair play and following the rules should be encouraged by all involved. Appropriate eye protection should be used. The American Society for Testing and Materials (ASTM) has made recommendations for selected protective eyewear in a number of sports (see Rodriguez *et al.* (2003) in Further reading). The material of choice for both frame and lenses (both prescription and non-prescription) is polycarbonate. This is a highly impact-resistant plastic, much stronger than most other materials in the market, and has the capability of absorbing ultraviolet light. It is important to appreciate that eye glasses and contact lenses do not provide appropriate protection.

Further reading

Moeller JL, Rifat SF. Identifying and treating uncomplicated corneal abrasions. *The Physician and Sports Medicine*, 2003; **31**(8).
Rodriguez JO, Lavina AM, Agarwal A. Prevention and treatment of common eye injuries in sports. *American Family Physician* 2003; **67**(7): 1481–8.
Weber TS. Training room management of eye conditions. *Clinics in Sport Medicine* 2005: **24**: 681–93.

Female athlete – the triad

B Lynn

The last 100 years has seen increasing participation in elite sports by women. A number of sports injuries appear to be more common in women (e.g. anterior cruciate ligament problems). There are also issues related to exercise during pregnancy. However, a rather unexpected problem has dominated this area – an inhibitory effect of intense training on reproductive function and a parallel reduction in bone mineral density. These two changes are associated with under-eating, hence the triad:

Osteopenia – menstrual disturbances – disordered eating

Incidence

The clearest indication is irregularity or cessation of menstrual periods – oligomenorrhea or amenorrhea (Table 1). Early indications may be luteal phase shortening. Incidence of menstrual disorders is higher in athletes and dancers than in the general population. It is clearly associated with low body weight, particularly low body fat levels. For example, it is more common in lightweight rowers than heavyweights and is a particular problem in dance and gymnastics where slim body shape is important. Menstrual problems are also seen in weight-sensitive sports such as endurance running, but are not so common in swimming or power events.

Table 1 Definitions of menstrual disturbances.

Amenorrhea	Cessation of menstrual periods for at least 3 months or less than 3 cycles per year
Oligomenorrhea	Cycles at intervals greater than 35 days or less than 6 cycles per year
Luteal phase deficiency	Shortening of the luteal phase to less than 10 days

What is the linkage between the three elements?

Under-eating to reduce body weight appears to be the fundamental cause, leading to a fall in adipose tissue mass. This might appear a good thing, but we now know that adipose tissue has important endocrine functions. In particular, adipose tissue secretes leptin, a polypeptide hormone. If adipose tissue mass falls, so does leptin secretion. Leptin plays an important biological role in control of reproduction and lack of leptin stops reproduction when food is scarce. In female athletes with very low fat mass there is hypothalamic "switch off" of GnRH (gonadotrophin-releasing hormone) and so of reproduction. The consequent fall in oestrogen leads to bone mineral loss, just as it does at the menopause. The relation between mineralisation and menstrual function has been demonstrated many times now – but is still a relatively recent finding – the first studies were only in the mid 1980s.

An example is the work of Warren *et al.* (2002) on dancers. In dancers with normal menstrual cycles the foot bone density is much higher than normal – a consequence of the high-impact exercise to which the foot is subjected during dancing and a highly desirable health gain. However, there is no sign of this benefit in dancers with menstrual disturbance. In skeletal structures that are not subjected to high impacts (e.g. the spine) there is a clear difference between dancers with normal menstrual function and normal bone density, and those with amenorrhea who have markedly reduced bone density. Dancers who change their eating habits and restart menstruation do not appear to regain all the lost mineral, and other studies have given the same picture. Some recovery can occur – but it is not complete.

A closer look at leptin

The discovery of leptin has been one of the amazing advances of the last decade. We had known for years that adipose tissue levels affected appetite in a negative feedback manner – the "adipostat". We had no idea what the signal was until the leptin gene was found to be the cause of obesity in a congenitally obese mouse strain. The gene codes for a large peptide hormone that is released from adipose tissue and acts on the centres in the hypothalamus that control feeding – and reproduction. In fact it is probably its action in permitting reproduction that is biologically important. You do not want to be pregnant or lactating in times of food shortage!

The leptin story continues to develop. It is now known that leptin has effects on bone resorption and formation that are independent of other hormonal factors – and may in part involve the sympathetic nervous system. Importantly, it has been found in animal models that leptin can block the bone loss that occurs (a) in a bone-unloading experiment and (b) following ovariectomy. So it appears that some of the female triad effects on bone mineralisation may be due directly to leptin insufficiency, and not just due to falls in oestrogen levels. Finally, leptin appears to have an important role in maintaining an effective immune system. Lymphocytes have leptin receptors and individuals lacking leptin have very low levels of several cytokines. The implications of this for low-body-fat athletes are obvious, but have yet to be followed up.

Treatment

Train less and eat more! But this is not popular with athletes or coaches. There needs to be a greater awareness of long-term risks, followed by a supportive approach involving the athlete and their entourage. In some instances oestrogen supplementation can be appropriate (oral contraceptive pill, or HRT of post-menopausal type). However, these treatments have side effects. In practice the effects of oestrogen supplementation have been disappointing, although some increased mineralisation has been shown. An obvious strategy is leptin supplementation. This has been shown to work in women with amenorrhea associated with strenuous exercise (Welt *et al.* 2004). Presumably only cost is limiting further trials (leptin costs around £100 per mg and approximately 10 mg/day was used in the published trial).

Prevention

Ideally we need to change the mind set in some sports/dance areas away from ultra-thin profiles. Otherwise athletes and coaches need to be informed so that they can spot early signs. Then education about the serious long-term, partly irreversible, effects of bone loss is required.

Key points

- Female athletes in weight-sensitive sports may have menstrual disturbance and bone mineral loss associated with under-eating.
- Key cause appears to be very low body fat mass and consequential low circulating levels of the hormone leptin.
- Reduction in training levels and/or increased eating leads to recovery of normal menstrual function but is not paralleled by a full recovery of bone mineralisation.
- Athletes need to be educated about the risks of osteopenia and informed so that early signs of menstrual dysfunction are noted and appropriate action taken to prevent bone mineral loss.

Further reading

Martin A *et al.* Leptin modulates both resorption and formation while preventing disuse-induced bone loss in tail-suspended female rats. *Endocrinology* 2005; **146**: 3652–9.

Otero M *et al.* Leptin, from fat to inflammation: old questions and new insights. *FEBS Letters* 2005; **579**: 295–301.

Otis CL, Drinkwater B, Johnson M, Loucks A, Wilmore J. American College of Sports Medicine position stand. The Female Athlete Triad. *Med Sci Sports Exerc* 1997; **29**: 1–11.

Shell ER. *The Hungry Gene*, Atlantic Books, 2002: A marvellous journalistic account of leptin's discovery and application to treating obese children (and lots of other interesting stuff on the obesity/slimming industry).

Warren MP, Brooks-Gunn J, Fox RP, Holderness CC, Hyle EP, Hamilton WG. Osteopenia in exercise-associated amenorrhea using ballet dancers as a model: a longitudinal study. *J Clin Endocrinol Metab* 2002; **87**: 3162–8.

Welt CK *et al.* Recombinant human leptin in women with hypothalmic amenorrhea. *N Engl J Med* 2004; **351**: 987–97.

Female athlete – exercise during pregnancy

B Lynn

Pregnancy should not mean confinement. New guidelines from the American College of Obstetrics and Gynecology reflect current best practice in recommending that significant levels of exercise should continue during pregnancy in order to maintain cardiovascular fitness and muscle condition (Artal 2003). Clearly any serious pre-existing medical condition must be taken carefully into account, as must any problem developing during pregnancy. Overall, the benefits of maintaining fitness outweigh any risks from continuing to exercise.

Certain changes are, however, necessary. In the second and third trimester, exercising lying supine is to be avoided as the uterus can press on the vena cava and reduce venous return to the heart. Contact sports should be avoided, as should scuba diving. For competitive athletes, a break from competition is inevitable as performance will be diminished as weight is gained. However, training can continue, but should be at a reduced level.

There are clear benefits from maintaining fitness. Labour is on average shorter in physically active mothers. Also in gestational diabetes, exercise can contribute to normalising blood glucose levels.

Pregnancy offers a golden opportunity to improve maternal health. It is notoriously difficult to persuade sedentary individuals to start exercising regularly (just as it is hard to persuade smokers to stop and to persuade those with a bad diet to eat their fruit and veg). Becoming pregnant is an event that stimulates people to look hard at their lifestyle and try to make healthy changes. So it is a good time to point out the advantages for mother and baby of taking regular exercise (and stopping smoking, etc). We certainly need to try this as at present quite the opposite usually happens. For example, a recent survey in the USA found that on average pregnant women take only around half the exercise of age-matched non-pregnant women (Peterson *et al.* 2005).

After birth, assuming no problems, a full exercise programme can be undertaken immediately. Not too many new mothers will want to rush straight out to the gym, so a gradual resumption of full training will be the norm. There is no evidence that high levels of physical activity affect lactation as long as maternal nutrition is adequate.

Further reading

Arena B, Maffuli N. Exercise and pregnancy. In: N Maffuli *et al.* (Eds) *Sports Medicine for Specific Ages and Abilities.* Edinburgh: Churchill Livingstone, 2001; Chapter 15.

Artal R, O'Toole M. Guidelines of the American College of Obstetricians and Gynecologists for exercise during pregnancy and the postpartum period. *Br J Sports Med* 2003; **37**: 6–12.

Petersen AM, Leet TL, Brownson RC. Correlates of physical activity among pregnant women in the United States. *Med Sci Sports Exerc* 2005; **37**: 1748–53.

Fitness testing

B Lynn

It is often useful to have a good measure of aerobic fitness and the usual one is VO_2max, the maximum oxygen consumption. Fitness is an excellent predictor of future health. Fitness measures also have a role in monitoring rehabilitation and can be used to assess when return to competition is possible. Finally, fitness measures can be useful in monitoring the effect of fitness programmes, for example as part of an exercise prescription, and can help motivate subjects.

For young healthy individuals, VO_2max can be measured directly using a maximal exercise test. However, before such a test the subject's history needs to be checked to ensure there are no health issues that might make such a test dangerous. A simple questionnaire such as the PAR-Q is generally sufficient (see Petrella *et al.* 2003).

Maximal tests can involve stepping, running on a treadmill or cycling. The subject starts exercising at an easy level, then the work rate is stepped up until a maximum heart rate is obtained and the subject cannot perform the next work rate. Measurement of expired gases and their volume allows VO_2max to be determined. There are several well-established protocols that are given in exercise physiology texts. VO_2max can also be estimated without actually measuring VO_2. An example is the shuttle test where subjects do repeat sprints between markers with speed increasing each time. The relation between final speed and VO_2max has been determined for test populations and these relations can be used to provide a good estimate for VO_2max.

A good estimate of VO_2max can also be obtained using submaximal tests and such tests are normally used with older subjects and where the highest accuracy is not required. Many different submaximal tests have been described. Most submaximal tests involve modifications of maximal tests and use stepping, treadmill walking/running or cycling and are carried out in the gym or the exercise lab. These tests depend on measuring heart rate at defined submaximal work levels. An estimate is then made of the subject's maximal work rate based on their age-related maximal heart rate. VO_2max is estimated from the relation between work rate and oxygen consumption determined for the appropriate population and exercise modality.

There are a large number of submaximal protocols available. Some involve making two or three heart rate measures at rising work rates, then graphically extrapolating to maximum heart rate to estimate maximum work capacity. Other tests use a single exercise level and heart rate and interpolate into previously determined data on oxygen consumption in relation to heart rate. A popular method uses stepping or cycling and calculates VO_2max using the Astrand–Rhyming nomogram. Quite simple step tests can give good results and when linked to a computer can give an instant printout of VO_2max. Such a test has been used in a large primary care survey in Canada (Petrella *et al.* 2003).

VO_2max can also be estimated from standard exercise patterns and heart rate. For example, the Rockport test involves walking as quickly as possible for 1 mile, then estimating VO_2max from the time taken and the final heart rate. Such tests are suitable for relatively unfit individuals.

What does a given VO_2max mean? Key here is to compare with population norms. Generally we need to allow for body weight, gender and age. Average data are given

Table 1 VO_2max (ml O_2min^{-1} kg body wt^{-1}) for UK population. Data from Allied Dunbar National Fitness Survey, 1990.

Age range	16–24	25–34	35–44	45–54	55–64
Males	55 (15)	49 (17)	46 (16)	42 (13)	36 (15)
Females	40 (13)	38 (13)	35 (12)	31 (12)	27 (10)

95% confidence intervals in brackets. Total number of subjects, 1471.

in Table 1. It is important not to "over-interpret" individual data. Population norms reflect the subjects that were tested and the methodology used. So it is important that the individual matches the population and uses a comparable method. However, trends in VO_2max, where the same method is used successively, can be quite reliable whatever particular method is used.

Summary

- VO_2max is the accepted measure of aerobic fitness and is the best indicator of cardiovascular and other health risks.
- A wide range of submaximal tests is available and these allow safe and accurate estimation of VO_2max.
- Trends in VO_2max can give reliable indications of fitness trends, for example during rehabilitation.

Further reading

Allied Dunbar National Fitness Survey, Health Education Authority and the Sports Council, UK, 1992.

Par-Q and you. Canadian Society for Exercise Physiology, 2002. Published on the Internet. Available online at http://www.csep.ca/forms.asp.

Petrella R, Koval JJ, Cunningham DA, Paterson DH. Can primary care doctors prescribe exercise to improve fitness? The Step Test Exercise Prescription (STEP) project. *Am J Prev Med* 2003; **24**: 316–22.

Forearm and wrist conditions

P Thomas

Compartment syndrome of the forearm

This can occur in the flexor compartment of the forearm in strength training sports and canoeing. The symptoms include increased pain, and diagnosis is confirmed by compartment pressure measurement. Treatment consists of coaching modalities, rest and physiotherapy, but if this fails, then surgical fasciotomy may be required.

Scaphoid fracture

This injury usually occurs by a fall on the outstretched hand. Pain and tenderness will appear at the anatomical snuff box of the thumb. X-rays could appear negative during the first 2 weeks. A bone scan is positive as early as 48 hours following the injury. The treatment will consist of a plaster cast to be kept on for 6 weeks. On removal of the plaster cast, X-rays are required to confirm healing, since a non-union is a significant risk in this type of fracture and this will lead to avascular necrosis of the proximal scaphoid. Scaphoid non-unions can be dealt with surgically.

Fracture of the hook of the hamate

This fracture is associated with golf or sports using a racquet or a bat. Injuries can be due to direct force to the hypothenar part of the hand or from overuse. Cause is usually by mis-hitting the ball or hitting the ground. Special view X-rays should include an oblique view with the forearm supinated and the wrist dorsiflexed. Bone scans will be positive and a CT scan will be necessary if X-rays are not revealing the fracture. A plaster cast will be applied for 6 weeks. Surgical excision of the hook of the hamate is very effective and the athlete can return to sport 6 weeks after surgery.

Kienbock disease

The patient will present with wrist pain, decreased range of movement and decreased grip following trauma or even without any history of an injury altogether. Later on osteoarthritic changes and lunate collapse will be present. Treatment in the early stages will consist of joint levelling procedures but later on salvage procedures with permanent limitation of the range of movement of the wrist will be the outcome.

Dislocations of the carpal bones

The lunate is the most commonly subluxed or dislocated wrist bone usually after a forced dorsiflexion. Manipulation under anaesthetic is successful at the early stages. A perilunate dislocation is a traumatic condition where the carpal bones are dislocated and disassociated around the lunate, which itself remains intact into the wrist joint. Careful history taking, X-rays and the early involvement of the orthopaedic surgeon is the appropriate management.

Distal radius and Colles' fracture

This is a fracture of the distal radius with dorsal angulation of the distal fragments and impactions. Other patterns of fractures may exist. Treatment is based on manipulation under anaesthetic and a plaster cast for 6 weeks. In different fracture types, insertion of K-wires or open reduction and internal fixation of the distal radial fracture may be necessary.

Triangular fibrocartilage injuries (TFC)

TFC is the expansion of the radial carpal fibrocartilage, which lies between the ulna and the carpus. Forced dorsiflexion and supination with adduction or abduction can cause damage of the TFC. Anatomical variation of a longer ulna can be associated with an impingement and risk of an injury. Arthrography or an MRI scan can reveal the diagnosis. Treatment with rest and immobilisation in a brace for 6 weeks may relieve symptoms. Arthroscopic surgical excision will lead to return to sport in 8 weeks.

De Quervain's

This is a stenosing tenosynovitis affecting the abductor pollicis longus and extensor pollicis brevis. The left thumb of a right-handed golfer is at risk because of the hyper-abduction which is required during the swing. Pain persists on testing abduction and extension of the thumb. Localised tenderness and swelling may be also observed. Finkelstein's test is positive.

Treatment consists of rest; splinting and steroid injection into the sheath is effective. In chronic cases with recurrence and fibrosis surgical decompression is recommended.

Intersection syndrome

Inflammation is present at the crossing point of the abductor pollicis longus and extensor pollicis brevis with the radial wrist extensors, extensor carpus radialis longus and brevis. The surgical decompression of the long extensor tendons at the forearm will provide relief.

Impingement syndrome

A repetitive wrist dorsiflexion in young gymnasts produces pain at the dorsum of the wrist due to capsulitis of the dorsal wrist soft tissue. Treatment consists of rest and splinting, leading to a 3-month absence from the sport.

The presence of an exostosis on the dorsum of the distal radius and scaphoid in young gymnasts confirmed by a CT scan can lead to surgical treatment with cheilectomy of the exostosis.

Further reading

Mellion MB *et al.* (Eds) *The Team Physician's Handbook*. Philadelphia: Hanley and Belfus, 1997.

Nicholas JA, Hershman EB, Posner MA (Eds) *The Upper Extremity in Sports Medicine.* Mosby, 1990.

Gender verification

B Lynn

Gender verification has been a contentious area and one where the medical profession has played a major part in defining policy. It is a female issue because testing has only been applied to women competitors. There are known cases of males competing as females, but most are in the distant past and none have been revealed by formal gender verification tests. Gender testing by examining chromosomes was introduced by the IOC in 1968 and abandoned in 1999. The history of gender testing offers a fascinating insight into sports politics and the problems of getting the medical viewpoint across (Ferguson-Smith 1998).

The problem is the small numbers of women with the wrong chromosomes. Genetically, females are XX and males XY. The presence of the Y chromosome leads to development of testes, production of testosterone, and subsequent development of all the male equipment. In the absence of a functioning Y chromosome or testosterone, the individual develops outwardly as female. Abnormalities are uncommon, but during the period of genetic testing unusual chromosome patterns were seen in around 1 in 400 female athletes.

The critical question is whether such abnormalities give a competitive advantage. The commonest reasons for retaining female appearance in the presence of a Y chromosome are (1) androgen insensitivity and (2) failure of the testes to develop due to another reason (gonadal dysgenesis). In such cases there is clearly no competitive advantage, so such individuals are allowed to compete as female. But this was not the case in much of the 1970s and 1980s, and it required extensive lobbying by medical groups to get these problems recognised, and to put in place the necessary counselling needed for affected individuals. At the time of writing, the IOC position is still "provisional", although there is much pressure to make the abandonment of genetic verification tests permanent (Dickenson *et al.* 2002).

The protection against cheating by males masquerading as female now rests on the observations of drug control officers. At drug control a urine sample must be produced under observation by the doping control officer. It is felt that this makes it very unlikely that a male competitor could successfully pass themselves off as female.

Finally, the IOC position regarding trans-sexuals has also now been clarified (IOC 2004). Anyone undergoing sexual reassignment after puberty should be treated as the reassigned gender. Thus, males assigned to female now compete as women (and females assigned to male compete as men). The key conditions are that (a) appropriate surgery has been completed, (b) hormone therapy for the assigned sex is taking place and (c) it is at least 2 years since gonadectomy. Note that transvestites with male physiology who live as females are not allowed to compete as females.

Further reading

Dickinson BD, Genel M, Robinowitz CB, Turner PL, Woods GL. Gender verification of female Olympic athletes. *Med Sci Sports Exerc* 2002; **34**: 1539–42.

Ferguson-Smith MA. Gender verification and the place of XY females in sport. In: M Harries,

C Williams, WD Stanish, LJ Micheli (Eds) *Oxford Textbook of Sports Medicine*, 2nd edn. Oxford University Press, 1998: 355–67.

Report of The Executive Board of the International Olympic Committee (IOC) 7 May 2004. Published on the Internet. Available online at http://www.olympic.org/uk/organisation/commissions/medical/full_story_uk.asp?id=841.

Groin pain

AA Narvani and EE Tsiridis

Groin pain affects about 5% of the patients referred to sports clinics but accounts for far greater loss of time from sport overall. The diagnosis of groin pain, however, remains a major problem and is a source of frustration for both the athlete and the therapists. The difficulty with the groin issue is partly because a wide variety of the conditions that involve many different specialties (orthopaedics, rheumatology, general surgery, urology, gynaecology and internal medicine) can cause groin pain. This in recent years has been recognised and a multidisciplinary approach for its management has been recommended.

Aetiology

Groin pain may originate from muscles, tendon, bones, bursae, fascial structures, nerve, joints, intra and retro-peritoneum organs. Some of the more common conditions that cause groin pain include adductor strains, iliopsoas-related pathology, abdominal hernias, osteitis pubis, stress fractures, referred pain and acetabular labrum tears.

Adductor strains

Adductor strains are thought to occur in 30 to 50% of the patients who present with groin pain.

Clinical features

Onset of the groin pain may be acute or insidious. The patient usually provides a history of pain at the site of the adductor longus associated with activities involving rapid adduction of the thigh, for example by kicking across the body. On examination there is localised tenderness at one particular point on the pubic bone over the insertion of the muscle. Pain is exacerbated on resisted adduction and passive abduction.

Investigations

Plain X-rays may show calcification around the origin of the muscle on the pubic bone. Ultrasound imaging can be useful in delineating the lesion, as can CT or MRI. Investigations may be unnecessary since this is mainly a clinical diagnosis.

Treatment

Treatment involves reducing the inflammation using the RICE regime. After the initial phase of inflammation has subsided, patients can begin gentle stretching and progressive strengthening exercises. This should not be commenced too early as there is a risk of developing chronic tendinopathy. Once the patient achieves a complete range of movement with full strength, then activities involving rapid change of direction can be started. Cardiovascular fitness must be maintained in this period and attention must also be paid to correction of the predisposing factors such as muscle strength imbalance or incorrect technique.

Return to sports

If it is a first-time injury, proper care and sufficient healing time before resuming activity should prevent permanent disability. Healing time can be between 3 to 8 weeks depending on the severity of the injury.

Osteitis pubis

This condition is characterised by sclerosis and bony changes about the pubic symphysis. These are thought to be as a result of cyclic loading of the pubic symphysis that occurs in sports such as running and jumping. It is suggested that this is the main cause of groin pain in about 5 to 10% of the patients.

Clinical features

Patients may present acutely or more often subacutely or by gradual onset. The pain is on the anterior aspect of the pubic bone, however it may radiate to the suprapubic area or into the groin. Pain is exacerbated by kicking, running, jumping and twisting. On examination there is usually tenderness over one or both pubic tubercles and over the pubic symphysis. Squeeze test is very sensitive (patient's knees are flexed to 90°, the examiner's hand is placed between the patient's knees and the patient performs a strong isometric, bilateral adductor contraction; this will exacerbate the bony tenderness).

Investigations

Plain X-rays may show resorption or sclerosis of the bone adjacent to the pubic symphysis. Increased uptake over the pubic tubercle may be seen with radionucleide bone scan. CT may display abnormalities of the bony structure and MRI will demonstrate bone marrow oedema in the body of the pubis.

Treatment

This is a self-limiting condition. Treatment involves rest and NSAIDs. Some clinicians consider corticosteroid injection if patients do not progress with conservative measures. Once the patient is pain free, there should be a progressive return to activity supported by manual therapy and stretching and strengthening programmes.

Those minority athletes who do not benefit from non-operative measures may be candidates for surgical intervention. This involves wedge resection of the symphysis or arthrodesis with or without metalwork.

Return to sport

Patients will get better, however the recovery period may be as long as 6 months.

Hernia

Inguinal hernias occur in athletes as in the general population, sports hernia, however, refers to a condition of chronic groin pain caused by weakness of the posterior inguinal wall, and, in many patients, without a clinically obvious hernia. There are reports to suggest that this condition could be the cause of groin pain in about 50% of the patients; however there are other studies that acknowledge that many of the patients with osteitis pubis are misdiagnosed as suffering from sports hernias. Gilmore's groin is a similar condition in which the torn conjoint tendon is associated with a tear in the external oblique aponeurosis, resulting in a dehiscence between the inguinal ligament and conjoint tendon.

Clinical features

Sports hernias tend to occur in athletes who participate in sports that require repetitive twisting and turning at speed. There is local pain and tenderness which is made worse if the patient half sits up while local pressure is maintained over the area of the conjoint tendon. There may be a palpable cough impulse and occasionally an obvious swelling.

Investigations

Ultrasonography can demonstrate the defect in the medial posterior inguinal wall but it is very operator dependent. Herniography is the most useful investigation even though it is technically demanding.

Treatment

Non-operative management usually results in a prolonged clinical course; therefore, once the diagnosis of hernia is made, surgical repair is the main option.

Return to sport

Postoperatively, most athletes return to sport within 6 to 12 weeks following surgery, after specific rehabilitation targeted at abdominal strengthening, adductor muscle flexibility, and a gradual return to activity.

Iliopsoas strain and bursae

Iliopsoas is irritated by repeated activity involving hip flexors and therefore can cause groin pain in runners, jumpers, hurdlers and footballers.

Clinical features

Both bursitis and tendinopathies of the iliopsoas muscle produce a deep groin pain which, because of the deep insertion of the muscle, patients find difficult to localise. There might also be a lack of point tenderness. Pain can be elicited by having the patient flex the hip 90° and then try to flex it further against resistance or by passive stretching with hyperextension at the hip.

Investigations

Although USS and CT may have a role, MRI seems to be the best diagnostic tool.

Treatment
Iliopsoas muscle strains and associated bursitis are managed by anti-inflammatory medication and modalities, together with appropriate stretching and strengthening of the iliopsoas muscle. If a bursitis is present, aspiration of the bursae and injection of local anaesthetic and corticosteroid may be attempted.

Return to sport
Return to sport can take between 2 to 6 weeks depending on the severity of the injury.

Acetabular labrum tears

Acetabular labrum tears have only begun to emerge as a significant cause of groin pain in the last decade. It has been suggested that it could be the cause of groin pain in up to 20% of the athletes who present with groin pain.

Clinical features
There may or may not be a history of trauma. In the presence of a recalled incident, the trauma can vary from a severe type to a very mild one such as twisting or falling. The pain is mainly in the groin, but could be in the trochanteric or the buttock region. It could have an acute onset or be gradual. It is usually associated with a clicking, catching or locking sensation. On examination, the range of the movement of the hip joint is not usually limited but there may be pain at extreme ranges. There are a number of clinical tests but, generally speaking, combined movement of flexion and rotation causes pain in the groin.

Investigations
Although plain radiographs and CT may have a role in excluding other pathologies, there is not a useful tool in the diagnosis of acetabular labrum tears. There are some studies that suggest that magnetic resonance arthrography is both sensitive and specific in detecting labral tears. The gold standard, however, is hip arthroscopy.

Treatment
The natural history of acetabular labrum tear is not known. Conservative management consists of bed rest with or without traction followed by a period of protected weight bearing. Surgery is in the form of arthroscopic debridement of labral tear. Although there has not been a randomised controlled trial comparing conservative management against surgical intervention, there are a number of studies that suggest better results in patients who undergo surgery.

Return to sport
Following arthroscopic debridement of the labral tears, return to sport may take between 3–6 months. Recovery seems to be slower with conservative management.

Further reading

Anderson K, Strickland SM, Warren R. Hip and groin injuries in athletes. *Am J Sports Medicine* 2001; **29**(4): 521–33.

Mandelbaum B, Mora SA. Osteitis pubis. *Operative Techniques in Sports Medicine* 2005; **13**: 62–7.
Narvani AA, Tsiridis E, Kendall S, Chodhuri R, Thomas P. Acetabular labrum tears in sports patients with groin pain. *Knee Surgery, Sport Traumatology, Arthroscopy* 2003; **1**(6): 403–8.
Narvani AA, Tsiridis E, Tai CC, Thomas P. Acetabular labrum and its tears. *Br J Sports Medicine* 2003; **37**(3): 207–11.

Hand injuries

P Thomas

Skier's thumb

Rupture of the ulnar collateral ligament of the first metacarpal phalangeal joint when falling and the hand is still holding the pole. Surgical treatment to repair the ligament is recommended.

Damage of the dorsum ligament with subluxation or dislocation of the base of the thumb

X-rays will confirm the diagnosis. A closed reduction and splint such as thumb spica for 3 weeks is recommended. If conservative management fails or dislocation exists, then surgical management should follow otherwise the pinch-grip function will be compromised.

Bennett's fracture

This is a fracture dislocation at the base of the first metacarpal bone. Manipulation under anaesthetic, possible insertion of K-wires and a plaster cast for 4 weeks is necessary, otherwise degenerative arthritis of the first carpal metacarpal joint may develop.

Mallet finger

It represents a tear of the extensor expansion from the attachment at the base of the terminal phalanx and may be associated with a fracture. The finger is kept flexed and cannot be actively extended at the distal interphalangeal joint. Treatment consists of a splint to keep the joint in extension for a 6–8 week period.

Distal interphalangeal joint dislocations

These are usually stable after reduction. Treatment following reduction consists of splinting in extension for 3 weeks followed by additional 3 weeks of splinting during sport.

Volar plate injuries

These are hyperextension injuries which may be associated with proximal interphalangeal joint dorsal dislocation. Splinting in extension is important to stop a later swan neck deformity. In cases of chronic presentations, surgical management with tenodesis is recommended.

Volar proximal interphalangeal joint dislocation

It is associated with an avulsion of the central slip of the extensor mechanism and radial collateral ligament damage. Surgical management is necessary to stop butonniere fixed flex deformity.

Dorsal proximal interphalangeal joint dislocation

Treatment consists of reduction and extension block splinting when the fracture of the middle phalanx base involves less than 50% of the articular surface. Otherwise surgery with open reduction and internal fixation is appropriate. Return to sport between 6–8 weeks' time.

Flexor profundus tendon avulsion

It occurs usually with a bone avulsion at the base of the distal phalanx. Early and direct repair is the treatment of choice.

Extensor digitorum communis subluxation: the sagital bands of the extensor hood are torn on the radial side of the extensor tendon and the tendon subluxes laterally at the metacarpal phalangeal joint. Patients are unable to extend the finger. If the finger can be extended passively then conservative management enables the finger to be kept at this position. If in acute stages, treatment with a metacarpal phalangeal joint splint in extension for 4 weeks is recommended. In chronic stages, surgical repair is recommended.

Boxer's knuckle

Involves multiple tears of the extensor digitorum communis tendons and dorsal joint capsule at the metacarpal phalangeal joints. Surgical exploration and repair of the defects is recommended with 6 weeks' immobilisation.

Traumatic subluxation of the extensor carpi ulnaris (ECU)

The injury can occur in forceful supination, volar flexion and ulnar deviation in tennis players. Direct repair and immobilisation for 6 weeks is the treatment of choice.

Subungal haematoma

This is the traumatic collection of blood under the fingernail.

Decompression with a needle under sterile conditions would produce immediate relief.

Further reading

Nicholas JA *et al.* (Eds) *The Upper Extremity in Sports Medicine*, Mosby, 1990.
Stover CN *et al.* (Eds) *The Medical Aspects of Golf.* Philadelphia: PA Davis Co., 1994.

Head injury

P Thomas

Head injuries can occur in many sports, usually in contact sport by an accidental collision between two players or a fall onto the ground. In boxing alone, direct blows to the head are allowed between the athletes. In non-contact sports the fall of the athlete to the ground such as when riding or if hit by an object, such as in athletics, golf, etc., could cause a head injury.

The etiology relies on a direct impact force to the head or an indirect force applied to the protective helmet producing linear translation or rotational acceleration or deceleration of the head.

Management at the field of injury

(1) The athlete can continue to play if he/she
- is alert
- is oriented
- does not suffer from amnesia
- does not demonstrate neurological deficits
- is not confused
- can repeatedly place finger at tip of nose
- has normal eye movements

The sixth cranial nerve is the most sensitive and the first to be affected in intracranial injury, impairing the lateral eye movement.

(2) Evidence of amnesia, drowsiness, lack of orientation, neurological deficit will lead to the removal of the athlete from the field for observation.

(3) Knocked out but has regained consciousness, the athlete is removed from the field and observation will take place. During observation, a chart should be methodically kept on:
   (a) If there is any change to the conscious state, then the patient should be transferred to the hospital.
   (b) Orientation, mental status, the knowledge of the score of the game, the place and names of popular public figures.
   (c) Vomiting or nausea will indicate increased intracranial pressure.
   (d) Headache that is getting worse will indicate focal or general cerebral oedema or haematoma.
   (e) Examination of ear and nose for blood, CSF.

(f) Slowing of pulse rate is associated with an increased intercranial pressure.
(g) Increased blood pressure will occur in rise of intercranial pressure.
(h) Eye examination, the pupil size and reaction light in addition to eye movements and the presence of double vision.
(i) Complete neurological examination.

An unconscious athlete or one who is disorientated or with neurological signs needs to be transferred to the local hospital. At the field and during the transfer the cervical spine is protected. The Glasgow score (3 to 15 points) is recorded until transfer to the hospital.

Concussion

"Concussion is a clinical syndrome characterised by immediate and transient post-traumatic impairment of neuro function, such alterations of consciousness, disturbance of vision and equilibrium due to brain stem involvement" (Committee of Head Injury of Neurological Surgeon, USA).

The patient could present with confusion and amnesia but loss of consciousness does not always occur.

Classification following the American Academy of Neurology.

(1) ***Grade 1/mild***
- with no loss of consciousness, no post-trauma amnesia, confusion which lasts less than 15 minutes.

(2) ***Grade 2/moderate***
- no loss of consciousness
- post-traumatic amnesia
- confusion which lasts more than 15 minutes.

(3) ***Grade 3/severe***
- any loss of consciousness
- post-traumatic amnesia
- presence of deteriorating mental state or neurological state deficits.

The American Academy of Neurology suggests return to sport:

- Grade 1 concussion – the same day
- Multiple Grade 1 concussions – 1 week
- Grade 2 concussions – 1 week
- Multiple Grade 2 concussions – 2 weeks
- Grade 3, with brief loss of consciousness only for seconds – 1 week
- Grade 3, prolonged loss of consciousness in minutes – 2 weeks
- Multiple Grade 3 concussion – 1 month.

A worsening headache should be investigated with a CT or MRI scan. A headache that fails to clear within 1 month should also be investigated.

Post-concussion syndrome

This can develop within the first 48 to 72 hours after a trauma. Persistent headaches, vertigo, blurred vision and inability to concentrate are usually the presenting symptoms. The MRI scan is generally normal. The athlete is provided with analgesia for headaches and is not allowed to return to sport until a full recovery has been made.

Skull fracture

A direct impact from an object such as a ball or a cricket bat or a fall onto a hard surface such as an ice rink, may lead to a skull fracture.

X-rays will confirm the diagnosis. Linear undisplaced fractures will heal within 2 or 3 weeks without specific treatment. Depressed fractures can cause brain injury. A careful assessment of brain damage including CT may be necessary. Treatment is dependent on fracture and whether there are any associated bleeds. Neurosurgical opinion may be necessary.

Intracranial haematomas

Extra dural

Bleeding occurs from the middle meningeal vessels between the skull and the dura. The athlete, after the regional injury, may recover well for a few hours until he or she falls into unconsciousness. There may be an increasingly severe headache. Examination will confirm changes in the eye pupil size and other mild neurological changes.

Sub dural

Bleeding occurs from the torn veins at the surface of the brain as a result of a direct impact injury and it presents the most common intracranial injury.

Intracerebral

This is a severe brain injury with immediate or rapid progress to loss of consciousness.

Subarachnoid

Low progressing haematoma with increased headache from torn small surface veins to the brain.

Mixed patterns may exist.

The management of the intracranial haematomas consists of the immediate transfer to a nearby hospital, an urgent CT or MRI scan and in some cases during the transfer a dose of dexomethasone may be recommended.

Chronic brain injury

It is predominantly associated with boxing (punch drunkenness). Progression of the condition is associated with symptoms of slurred speech, tremors, lack of coordination and abnormal gait. The treatment is symptomatic with immediate removal from the sport.

Further reading

KinderKnecat JJ. *Head Injuries in Athletic Injuries and Rehabilitation*. WB Saunders, 1996.
Warren WL Jr *et al.* On the field evaluation of athletic head injuries. *Clinical Sports Medicine* 1998; **17**(1): 13–26

Heel pain

R Sreekumar

Heel pain is one of the commonest complaints of the lower limb encountered in sport orthopaedics practice.

Causes

These could be sub-classified as follows:

Local

- Bone
  —Stress fractures
  —Infection
  —Tumours
- Joints
  —Osteoarthritis
  —Inflammatory arthritis
  —Tumours
  —Osteochondral defects
- Soft tissue (see below)
  —Fascia
  —Bursa
  —Ligament
  —Tendons
  —Nerves
  —Skin conditions
  —Soft tissue tumours

Systemic disease

- Degenerative
- Inflammatory
- Infection

- Malignancy
- Vascular

Referred pain
Radicular pain
Some of the more common causes of heel pain are highlighted in this chapter.

Plantar fasciitis

Anatomy

The plantar aponeurosis arises from the os calcis and consists of three bands – medial, central and lateral segments. The central portion originates from the medial tuberosity of os calcis and is called the plantar fascia. This divides distally into five bands which pass to the proximal phalanges of the lesser toes through longitudinal septa, to the great toe through the sesamoids and into the skin of the ball of the foot through the vertical septa. The plantar fascia along with spring ligament, short and long plantar ligament comprise the ligament system that supports the longitudinal arch. Extension of the toes and the metatarsophalangeal joints tenses the plantar aponeurosis, raises the longitudinal arch and inverts the hindfoot by a mechanism called the windlass mechanism. This is passive and depends on bony and ligamentous structures.

Aetiology

The cause of plantar fascia is still uncertain and is probably multifactorial. The predisposing factors are:

- increased age
- tight tendoachilles
- increase in body mass
- work situations, where the amount of time spent on the feet increases
- hard walking surfaces
- high arched foot as in pes cavus
- increased stretching in a flat foot
- stretching in a pronated foot

Half of all patients with plantar fasciitis have heel spur, but this is not thought to contribute to symptoms.

Pathology

The pathology is considered to be chronic inflammation associated with periosteal inflammation and microtrauma of plantar fascia.

Clinical findings

The consistent and pathognomonic sign is pain in the heel after rest, especially in the morning – "Poststatic dyskinesia". Fascial pain is usually at midstance to take-off while pain at initial heel contact is suggestive of bursitis. Usually the pain reduces with continued activity. Patients also complain of an ache at night or when resting after a period of activity. The pain can be reproduced by having patients stand on tip toe or by passively dorsiflexing the metatarsophalangeal joints.

On palpation, tenderness over the medial tubercle and over the heel centrally is noticed. The plantar fascia should be palpated for defects (rupture) or masses (fibromatosis). Examination of the tendoachilles may reveal tightness.

Clinical course is variable but about 80% of patients state that symptoms settle in about 12 months. The natural history is one of resolution with time and therefore conservative methods must be tried before invasive methods.

Investigations

X-ray of the foot may show a spur in 50% of patients. This spur is not usually the cause of symptoms. Spurs are usually within the muscles superior to the fascia and are not ossification of the fascia origin. X-rays are also useful in ruling out calcaneal stress fractures or other bony lesions. "Fluffy periosteitis" may suggest sponyloarthropathy.

Bone scans are useful for differentiating plantar fasciitis from stress fractures when plain radiographs are normal.

Ultrasonography is not regularly used. It can show an increase in the thickness of the plantar fascia from a normal of 2–4 mm. There may also be local or diffuse echogenicity at the calcaneal insertion.

MRI of the foot shows oedema of calcaneal insertion thick central cord, thickness of the plantar fascia, increased signal intensity in adjacent subcutaneous tissue and calcaneus at the plantar fascia insertion site.

Blood investigations are recommended in patients with an atypical picture or bilateral disease and includes serology to rule out inflammatory arthropathy and other pathologies with CRP and ESR may be indicated if an infection is suspected.

Treatment

There are a variety of treatment modalities suggested for plantar fasciitis. However, there are very few standardised studies to prove the efficacy of many of these. Over 90% patients are able to control their symptoms by conservative means.

Physical therapy

Physical therapy, in the form of stretching, cycling and running in a pool, has been recommended for the management of plantar fasciitis. The stretching exercises improve the elasticity of the fascia and increase its load to failure, therefore increasing the threshold to injury.

There are studies suggesting that stretching + silicon rubber cup gave relief in over 90% of patients.

Plantar fascia massage by rolling increasingly harder balls under the foot has been suggested in a few studies.

Footwear

Footwear modification has been advocated in conjunction with activity modification. The principles are to support the arch, prevent pronation and unload the plantar fascia. Padded shoes also help minimise absorption of shock.

Night splint

Night splint with 5° of dorsiflexion and extended footplate is recommended to be worn at night. Splinting is recommended for a 3-month period and then weaned.

Fascial taping
Useful in diagnosis and provides immediate relief in acute painful stage. Modified low dye taping is a simple method with two components – a horizontal around the heel substitutes for the plantar fascia and a circumferential component supports the midfoot.

Steroid injections
This should be kept for refractory cases. The injection should be deep to the plantar fascia to avoid atrophy of the heel fat pad. Ultrasound guidance can improve the accuracy of the injection

The complication of steroid injections is delayed rupture of plantar fascia. Most of these patients have initial relief of pain but then develop delayed problems such as longitudinal arch strain, stress fractures and hammer toe deformity. Fat pad atrophy and haematoma are other complications of injection.

NSAIDs
Non-steroid anti-inflammatory agents are regularly prescribed and provide pain relief but there are no randomised studies to confirm their efficacy.

Iontophoresis
Iontophoresis of dexamethasone, Phonophoresis, magnetic insoles, ultrasonography and laser therapy have very little evidence to support their use.

Orthotic devices
See the chapter on Orthotics.

Shock wave therapy
This has been used in plantar fasciitis as it has been noted as being capable of inhibiting pain receptors and stimulating healing of soft tissue. There have been many studies in the recent literature with conflicting results.

Surgery
This should be considered only for a small select group of patients who have had pain for over 6–12 months. The options are open/closed plantar fascia release with or without calcaneal spur excision and nerve decompression. Fifty per cent of lateral fibres should be left intact. Most studies showed satisfactory results in over 75% of patients, although there were complications like injury to the posterior tibial nerve, flattening of the arch and calcaneal fracture.

Plantar fascia rupture

Suspected in patients with acute onset of pain in the heel with or without trauma.

Predisposing conditions
- Steroid injections
- Acute hyperextension of foot – wedging of foot in pothole

Clinical features
- Ecchymosis
- Tenderness
- Palpable defect in proximal plantar fascia

Treatment
- Footwear alteration
- Taping
- Casting in refractory cases

Achilles tendinopathy

See the chapter on Calf pain.

Retrocalcaneal bursitis

Retrocalcaneal bursa lies between the Achilles tendon and the superior tuberosity of the calcaneum. Excessive pressure may result in inflammation of this bursa. Frequently this bursitis is associated with an enlarged and prominent superolateral portion of the calcaneus (known as "Haglund's deformity"). Other pathologies which can occur in combination with retrocalcalneal bursitis include Achilles tendon tendinopathy and calcification.

Clinical features
- Pain and tenderness in the retrocalcaneal region
  —dull ache
  —made worse on activity
  —"start up" pain
- Swelling
- There may be features of Achilles tendinopathy

Investigation
- Plain radiograph (can exclude other conditions)
- USS
- MRI

Treatment
Non-operative
- NSAIDs
- U-shaped pads
- Physical therapy
- Activity and shoe wear modification
- Steroid injection (best performed with image guidance, i.e. ultrasound in order to avoid the tendon). Some clinicians immobilise following injection to reduce risk of Achilles tendon rupture.

Operative
- Those that do not respond to non-operative measures are candidates for surgical excision of the bursa and the bony prominence if present.

Peroneal tendinopathy

Seen in patients with a history of inversion ankle injuries. Also occurs with use of footwear with high medial arch without lateral balancing.

Clinical features

Tenderness along the course of the muscle and tendon from fibula, posterior to lateral malleolus, below peroneal tubercle of calcaneum, under cuboid and sole of foot to first metatarsal base in peroneus longus pathology. Tenderness is seen above peroneal tubercle to fifth metatarsal in brevis tendinopathy.

Treatment principles

- Oedema control and immobilisation.
- Lower medial arch and balance lateral border in footwear.

Heel pad atrophy

Is frequently seen in the elderly as well as those with peripheral neuropathy rheumatoid arthritis, steroid use and pes cavus. Hard-soled shoes, obesity and prolonged standing aggravate this condition. Patients complain of pain which is diffuse around the heel with poor localisation.

Treatment includes heel elevation, containment of heel pad and use of insole material.

Stress fractures of calcaneum

Presents with insidious onset of pain about the heel. Follows impact-type activities, e.g. running, marching, and in diabetic patients as Charcot's neuropathy without history of trauma. Vague aching sensation that increases in crescendo fashion with activity and improves on rest. On examination, pain on side-to-side compression (heel squeeze test) of the heel is noted. X-ray may show area of sclerosis from superior portion of calcaneus directed obliquely and inferiorly. Bone scan or MRI may be required to confirm if X-ray is normal.

Treatment is usually rest in a walking cast or brace. If there is no improvement after 3–4 months of immobilisation, surgery in the form of internal fixation will need to be undertaken.

Tibialis posterior dysfunction

Commonly under-diagnosed cause of posterior heel pain. Degenerative tears occur in area of relative hypovascularity.

Pathophysiology

Following rupture, talonavicular joint and subtalar joint collapse. Hindfoot goes into valgus. There is midfoot pronation and forefoot abduction.

Clinical features

- Early – painful swelling of posteromedial border of ankle and fatigue.
- Later – aching along medial longitudinal arch.
- Advanced – lateral side pain due to impingement between lateral border foot and fibula.

On examination

- Tenderness behind medial malleolus or between medial malleolus and navicular.
- "Too many toes" sign when viewed from behind.
- Single heel rise test – either not possible on affected side or foot fails to invert or logitudinal arch fails to rise.

Investigation

X-ray

- standing AP foot
  —Talus is plantar flexed and there is increased angle between the long axis of the talus and calcaneus.
- standing lateral view foot
  —There is increased angle between the long axis of the talus and calcaneus.

Ultrasound

MRI

Treatment

Mild disease can be treated by orthosis with a medial heel wedge or total contact orthosis to allow relative immobilisation while continuing work.

Surgical treatment ranges from tenosynovectomy in the early stages to FDL transfer and calcaneal ostetomy in more advanced stages. In advanced cases with flattening of the foot and fixed deformities, subtalar fusion or triple arthrodesis is indicated.

Sever's disease

See the chapter on Paediatric – osteochondrosis.

Flexor hallucis longus tendinopathy

This is quite a common condition among dancers, gymnasts, trampolinists and cricketers (bowlers).

Clinical features

- Can follow ankle trauma
- Pain behind medial malleolus
- Crepitus
- Tenderness over the tendon
- Pain worse with passive dorisflexion of the hallux

Investigations

- Includes USS or MRI

Treatment

- Treatment is by use of rest, physical therapy, NSAIDs and orthosis. Surgery for those who do not respond to non-operative measures.

It is important to mention that heel pain may be also be due to referred/radicular pain, as well as systemic disease such as infection, inflammatory and neoplasm. These should be excluded when faced with athletes suffering from heel pain.

Further reading

Coughlin MJ, Mann RA. *Surgery of the Foot and Ankle*, 7th edn. Mosby, 1999; 861–79.

Rodstein B, Oh-Park M. Hindfoot pain and Plantar fasciitis. *Physical Medicine and Rehabilitation* 2001; **15**(3): 477–87.

Stephens MM, Walker G. Heel pain: an overview of its aetiology and management. *Foot & Ankle Surgery* 1997; **3**: 51–60.

Stroud C. Heel pain, plantar fasciitis and tarsal tunnel syndrome. *Current Opinion in Orthopaedics* 2002; **13**: 89–92.

Williams SK, Brage M. Heel pain – plantar fasciitis and Achilles enthesopathy. *Clin Sports Med* 2004; **23**: 123–44.

Imaging of sports injuries – plain radiograph (plain X-ray)

AA Narvani

Plain radiography is technically simple, cheap and widely available. In many sports injuries, this should be the first imaging investigation obtained. Even a "normal" plain radiograph can be very helpful by excluding or reducing the likelihood of many conditions. It must, however, be performed competently while paying careful attention to the exposure and positioning. Usually, two perpendicular views are adequate although more specialised views may be required to detect specific injuries.

Plain radiography is particularly helpful in the following situations:

Fractures

- In addition to having a very high sensitivity to detecting the majority of fractures, plain radiography also provides information on the anatomy, displacement and characteristics of many fractures.
- On occasions, subtle fractures may not initially be seen on plain radiography (however, a follow-up radiograph at about 2 weeks post injury will usually show resorption of the fractured bone and increased density at margins secondary to callus production). In such cases, if a fracture is strongly suspected clinically, other imaging modalities such as bone scan, CT and MRI may be required (see chapters on Imaging of sports injuries – bone scan, CT and MRI).

- With stress fractures, plain radiograph may illustrate periosteal new bone formation, callus and a visible fracture line. It may, however, take several weeks before X-ray signs become positive, and in over 50% of athletes with stress fractures, the initial radiographs can be normal. Therefore, again if there is strong clinical suspicion, other imaging modalities should be utilised (see chapter on Stress fractures in sports).

Dislocations/subluxations

- Plain X-ray will be able to diagnose the vast majorities of dislocation and subluxation.
- In subtle cases, further imaging with other modalities such as CT may be required (CT and MRI will also demonstrate other associated injuries as well).

Avulsion injuries

- These are usually secondary to a powerful muscular contraction.
- Plain X-ray can detect acute avulsion injuries.
- Chronic injuries may mimic other pathologies (such as neoplasm) with plain radiographs, therefore other imaging investigations may be required.

Other pathologies

- Plain films may also demonstrate other pathologies which are not related to injuries and cause chronic symptoms. These include:
  —Neoplastic lesions
  —Metabolic bone disease
  —Infection

A plain radiograph may also be performed in combination with intra-articular injection of contrast (plain film arthrography). Although replaced by CT arthrography and MRI (±arthrogram) in many centres, plain radiography with contrast can be useful in evaluating shoulder pathologies (rotator cuff tears, labral injuries, loose bodies, synovitis and capsulitis) and wrist injuries (triangular fibrocartilage complex (TFCC) and ligament tears).

Further reading

Sanders TG, Fults-Ganey K. Imaging techniques. In: JC DeLee, D Drez, MD Miller (Eds) *Orthopaedic Sports Medicine, Principles and Practice*, 2nd edn. Saunders, 2002: 557–614.

Tung GA, Brody JM. Contemporary imaging of athletic injuries. *Clinics in Sports Medicine* 1997; **16**(3): 393–417.

Imaging of sports injuries – ultrasound (USS)

AA Narvani

Ultrasonography is a very valuable diagnostic tool in the management of soft tissue injuries. It is safe as there is no involvement of ionising radiation, yet relatively cheap and readily accessible. It permits dynamic imaging as well as real-time image-guided interventional procedures. It is, however, very operator dependent.

Imaging with ultrasound involves transmission of high-frequency (3–15 MHz), inaudible sound waves from a probe, through a coupling device gel (which is applied topically to the area of interest). These sound waves are directed into the body, and travel through the different layers, i.e. skin, subcutaneous fat, muscle and bone. The velocity and wavelength with which the waves travel through each layer is dependent on the density of the substance of that layer. At a junction between one layer and another layer, at the interfaces, a proportion of the waves are reflected back to the probe. The probe then acts as a receiver, detecting these reflected waves and creating an ultrasound image from them. The greater the difference between the density of the two structures, the greater proportion of the waves that are reflected at interface of the two structures. This is why it is important to use gel between the probe and the skin, as without gel the large difference between the densities of the probe and the air pocket would imply that almost all the waves are reflected back and none will go through the body.

Ultrasonography can be particularly helpful for the assessment of the following structures:

Muscle

Muscle tears

- These are well demonstrated by ultrasound.
- There is disorganisation of the normal architecture of the muscle.
- There may be muscle-end retraction.
- There may also be an associated haematoma (see below).

Muscle haematoma

- Acute muscle haematomas will appear as bright, hyperechoic region.

Myositis ossificans

- USS can be used to diagnose this condition early by demonstrating calcifications within the muscle at 7–10 days post injury.

Muscle hernias

- Because USS is a dynamic investigation, it can be very useful in detecting pathologies which will only become apparent with muscle contraction such as muscle hernias and chronic scars.

Tendons

- Normal tendons will appear as regular tightly packed, longitudinally orientated bundles which are bright (echogenic) compared with the surrounding muscles.
- The following tendon abnormalities can be detected with USS:
  —Tendinopathies, with features such as:
    —loss of normal structure
    —blurring
    —thickening
    —cystic degeneration
    —calcification
    —peritendinous oedema
    —paratenonitis or synovitis
    —neovascularisation of the tendon's substance
    —there may be an associated tear (see below)
  —Tears
    —Can be partial or full thickness.
    —A partial thickness tear will appear as a dark area within the tendon without involving the full thickness of the tendon.
    —A full thickness tear will appear as a dark band extending from one surface to the other surface of the tendon. As the size of the tear increases, this dark band will become thicker, eventually appearing as a dark, hypoechoic gap with massive tears.

Ligaments

- USS can be a very useful diagnostic tool for the assessment of joint ligaments as it would be able to detect oedema, thickening or absence of the ligament.
- Furthermore, as it is a dynamic investigation, the ligaments may be examined under stress.

Bursa

- Bursitis may be diagnosed by USS, if there is fluid distension of a known bursa. This would appear as a dark hypochoic area.

Soft tissue swellings

- USS can aid in establishing a diagnosis with soft tissue masses by providing information on dimensions and morphological characteristics of the swelling such as:
  —surface contour and definition
  —internal structure/contents
  —relationship to the surrounding structure
- The accuracy of percutaneous core needle biopsy (when indicated) may also be increased by using USS to guide the biopsy of these soft tissue swellings.

Interventional procedures

Image guidance with USS may be used in the following procedures:

- Injection of local anaesthetic and corticosteroids
- Dry needling procedures
- Autotransfusion
- Biopsy
  —Percutaneous fine needle aspiration
  —Percutaneous core needle biopsy

Further reading

Colquhoun K, Alam A, Wilson D. Basic science: ultrasound. *Current Orthopaedics* 2005; **19**: 27–33.

Gibbon WM, Long G. Imaging of athletic injuries. *Current Orthopaedics* 2000; **14**: 424–34.

Sanders TG, Fults-Ganey K. Imaging techniques. In: JC DeLee, D Drez, MD Miller (Eds) *Orthopaedic Sports Medicine, Principles and Practice*, 2nd edn. Saunders, 2002: 557–614.

Tung GA, Brody JM. Contemporary imaging of athletic injuries. *Clinics in Sports Medicine* 1997; **16**(3): 393–417.

Imaging of sports injuries – isotope bone scan

AA Narvani

Isotope bone scans provide physiological and function information on osteoblastic activity. The investigation involves injection of a radioactive substance "coupled" to another substance that has affinity for sites of osteoblastic activity. Once taken up by these sites, the radioactive substance decays and emits gamma rays which can be detected by a camera. This would then permit construction of a skeleton functional image highlighting areas with increased osteoblastic activities or bone turnover. Other factors, including blood flow and quantity of mineralised bone, also influence the accumulation of the radioactive substance at particular sites.

Single-photon emission computerised tomography (SPECT) is a bone scan tomographic investigation that involves rotating the gamma camera 360° around the athlete. This permits a multiple projection evaluation resulting in more accurate localisation of the area of the increased uptake.

Isotope bone scans can be particularly helpful in the following situations:

Fractures

Stress fractures

- Isotope bone scanning can be of great use in the diagnosis of stress fractures (sensitivities approaching 100% have been reported) as conventional radiographs are relatively insensitive (initial plain radiography may be normal in over 50% of athletes with stress fractures).

- Owing to the increased blood flow and osteoblastic activity, there is increased radioactive substance uptake at the site of the stress fracture. This will show up as an intense focal area of increased uptake.
- As the stress fracture undergoes healing, this area of increased uptake can become less intense and more diffuse.

Occult fractures

- These are subtle fractures that may not be initially seen with plain radiographs.
- Acute fractures will result in increased radiotracer localisation at the area of the injury, showing up as an intense focal area of increased uptake.
- Similarly to stress fractures, as healing progresses, the area of increased uptake loses its intensity.
- The vast majority of fractures are detected by bone scans taken at 24–48 hours following trauma; however, in more senior athletes and those who suffer from osteoporosis, it may take up to 72 hours post injury before a bone scan becomes positive.

Assessment of union

- Isotope bone scanning may also be used to detect non-union as well as indicating the type of non-union present (atrophic versus hypertrophic).

Spondylolysis

- This condition is thought to represent a stress fracture caused by repetitive hyperextension loading of weakened or defective pars interarticularis.
- SPECT scan is a useful investigation as plain radiographs may not be able to detect the subtle cases.
- Furthermore, SPECT scan would allow the clinician to distinguish between those lesions that have healed from those that have not yet healed. This information can be of great importance since athletes with unhealed lesions generally require prolonged absence from sports so that the lesion can undergo complete healing.

Paediatric injuries

- A bone scan can be used to diagnose epiphyseal plate injuries as well as monitoring the effect of the injury on the growth potential (premature closure of the physis results in decreased uptake).
- An isotope bone scan can also be helpful in the diagnosis of apophyseal avulsion injuries, as these may be difficult to detect with plain radiographs.

Infections

- Although not very specific, isotope bone scans are reported to have a sensitivity of over 95% for detecting osteomyelitis in some studies.

- This accuracy is improved by using labelled leukocytes as these accumulate at the site of the infection.

Tumours

- Isotope bone scans are widely used for detection of osseous metastasis in those with known malignancies.
- Primary bone tumours may result in "hot lesion" on bone scan; however, they have limitations as assessment of the tumour extent is complicated by reactive hyperaemia.
- Myelomas may not be detected by isotope bone scan.
- Most benign bone tumours (with the exception of osteoid osteomas) do not accumulate radioactive tracers; therefore, isotope bone scans should not be the investigation of choice.

Other pathologies

Osteitis pubis

- This condition is a cause of groin pain in athletes. Plain radiograph appearances may be subtle, whereas an isotope bone scan can demonstrate increased uptake over the pubic tubercle.

"Shin splints"

- Isotope bone scan can diagnose this condition by demonstrating superficial uptake along the medial tibial shaft.

Anterior knee pain

- Bone scan can give an indication of the extent of patella overloading in assessment of athletes with anterior knee pain.

Complex regional pain syndrome (reflex sympathetic dystrophy)

- This occurs as a result of autonomic dysfunction secondary to injury.
- Isotope bone scan may detect this by demonstrating increased uptake.

Further reading

Calleja M, Alam A, Wilson D, Bradley K. Basic science: nuclear medicine in skeletal imaging. *Current Orthopaedics* 2005; **19**: 34–9.

Gibbon WM, Long G. Imaging of athletic injuries. *Current Orthopaedics* 2000; **14**: 424–34.

Sanders TG, Fults-Ganey K. Imaging techniques. In: JC DeLee, D Drez, MD Miller (Eds) *Orthopaedic Sports Medicine, Principles and Practice*, 2nd edn. Saunders, 2002: 557–614.

Tung GA, Brody JM. Contemporary imaging of athletic injuries. *Clinics in Sports Medicine* 1997; **16**(3): 393–417.

Imaging of sports injuries – magnetic resonance imaging (MRI)

AA Narvani

Magnetic resonance imaging (MRI) is a wonderful imaging tool. It has had a massive impact on the management of sports injuries since being introduced on a large scale into clinical practice in the 1980s. It allows imaging of a wide range of structures including cartilage, tendons, ligaments, bone and muscle (yet does not involve X-ray radiation) and in most cases is non-invasive.

Mechanism

Although the detailed physics of MRI is complicated and beyond the scope of this chapter, a brief understanding of its mechanism is helpful. MR imaging involves placing the subject in a magnetic field. The hydrogen atoms, in different body tissues, align in this magnetic field. Then, a radiofrequency (RF) pulse is applied to the tissues, which causes the hydrogen atoms in those tissues to alter their original alignment relative to the external magnetic field. Following this radiofrequency pulse, the hydrogen atoms "dephase" and return to their original relaxed state. As they do so, they release energy (echo). This emitted energy is detected by the MRI machine and is converted into images. The time it takes for hydrogen atoms to diphase is called the T2 time and the time taken to return to a relaxed state (and release energy) is called the T1 time.

Dephasing occurs before release of energy, therefore T2 time is always shorter than T1 time. Different tissues and tissue states – e.g bone, muscle, fat, cartilage, oedema, tendon – have different T1 and T2 times. This is due to the fact that relaxation of the hydrogen atoms is dependent on size and bindings of the molecules that contain the hydrogen atom.

The emitted energy (echo signal) is dependent on several factors. This signal would be high if one allows the majority of the hydrogen atoms to diphase, e.g if one starts listening relatively late, therefore giving time for the hydrogen atoms to diphase. If the machine starts listening very early, for a short period of time, the hydrogen atoms may not have "dephased" and therefore the signal would be low. The technical term for when the machine starts listening is called "time to echo" (TE) and is something that can be altered and set on the MRI machine. Therefore, if time to echo is set to be shorter than T2 time of that tissue, then that tissue would not have a high signal on the MR images.

The echo signal's intensity is also dependent on whether or not the majority of the hydrogen atoms have returned to their relaxed state before another radiofrequency pulse is applied. Therefore, if the repeated radiofrequency pulse is applied before the hydrogen atoms return to their relaxed state, they would not be very excitable with the next pulse and therefore the next echo signal would not be strong. Again, how quickly the next radiofrequency pulse arrives is something that could be set on the MRI machine. The technical term for this is "time to repetition" (TR). Therefore, if the time to repetition is set to be shorter than the T1 time of the image tissue, then that tissue would not be presented by a high signal on the MR image.

It can now be appreciated how, by altering the TE and TR parameters on the MRI machine, we can tune it to detect different tissue or pathologies of those tissues. This tuning is performed by having different MRI "weighted" sequences.

T1 weighted sequences

- TE is set at a short time (shorter than 60 ms)
- TR is set at a short time (shorter than 1000 ms)
- Good for demonstrating anatomy
- Fat would be a high signal or bright
- Fluid (oedema) is a low signal or dark
- Can be useful to detect meniscal pathology

T2 weighted sequences

- TE is set at a long time (longer than 60 ms)
- TR is set at a long time (longer than 1000 ms)
- Good for demonstrating pathology
- Fluid (oedema) is bright
- Fat is also a high signal and therefore bright

Proton density (PD)

- TE is set at a short time (shorter than 60 ms)
- TR is set at a long time (longer than 1000 ms)
- Very good for assessment of meniscus

MRI can be used to visualise a wide variety of tissues and their pathologies in different body parts. These include the following.

Bone

Fractures

- Stress fractures
- Occult fractures

Bone bruise

- Best detected on STIR or fat-suppressed T2 sequences.

Ligament

- MRI can be very useful
- T1 sequence good for anatomical detail
- T2 sequence good for detecting ligament pathology

Muscle

Tears

- Intermediate signal on T1
- High signal on T2
- STIR and fat-suppressed T2 sequences are particularly useful as they would permit a distinction to be made between fluid collection or haemorrhage from muscle fat.

Haematoma

- Intensity and appearance dependent on the stage of haematoma.

Other muscular pathologies that could be detected by MRI include:

- Myositis ossificans
- Tumours
- Pyomyositis

Tendon

Tendinopathy

- Acute
  —Intermediate signal intensity on T1 and T2
  —Tendon thickening
- Chronic
  —Thinning and attenuation of the tendon

Tears

- Complete
  —High signal on T2 involving the full thickness of the tendon extending from one surface to another.
  —There may be retraction of the tendon.
- Partial
  —High signal on T2 involving part of the tendon rather than the full thickness.

Cartilage

Articular cartilage

- Useful sequences for relieving surface abnormalities include proton density and fast spin echo.

Menisci

- Preferred sequences include T1, proton density and gradient echo T2.
- Tears may be seen as an intra-substance signal that extends either to superior or inferior surface.

Labrum

- Pathologies of both glenoid and acetabular labrum can be detected by MRI. Accuracy improves when combined with arthrogram.

Further reading

Gibbon WM, Long G. Imaging of athletic injuries. *Current Orthopaedics* 2000; **14**: 424–34.

McKie S, Brittenden J. Basic science: MRI. *Current Orthopaedics* 2005; **19**: 13–19.

Sanders TG, Fults-Ganey K. Imaging techniques. In: JC DeLee, D Drez, MD Miller (Eds) *Orthopaedic Sports Medicine, Principles and Practice*, 2nd edn. Saunders, 2002: 557 614.

Tung GA, Brody JM. Contemporary imaging of athletic injuries. *Clinics in Sports Medicine* 1997; **16**(3): 393–417.

Imaging of sports injuries – computed tomography (CT)

AA Narvani

Since its introduction in early 1970s, computed tomography (CT) has proved to be a very valuable imaging tool. Like plain radiography, CT involves application of X-ray radiation to the body with different body tissues absorbing this radiation at different amounts. However, unlike plain radiography, CT provides three-dimensional information, free of superimposing tissues, thus resulting in much higher contrast resolution.

CT involves transmission of radiation from an X-ray tube which rotates around the patient. This radiation is then received by a ring of radiation detectors which are located around the body. The information received by the detectors is then converted to final images with a computer. With a *spiral* CT, as well as the X-ray tube rotating continuously, the patient is also moved through the X-ray beam. As a result, greater anatomical regions are imaged during a single breath hold, reducing the time taken for the scan and the artefacts caused by movement.

CT provides detailed images of bone. This makes it an ideal choice on investigation for evaluating complicated fractures including those that involve articular surfaces. This evaluation of complex fractures is further enhanced by software packages that produce 3D images. CT can also be a very useful aid in diagnosing of "occult" and stress fractures.

CT can be used in the following injuries:

Head injuries (see the chapter on Head injuries)

CT is a vital tool for evaluation of athletes with serious head injuries, revolutionising management since introduction. It can detect:

- Skull fractures
- Intracranial haemorrhage
  —Epidural
  —Subdural
  —Intracerebral
  —Subarachnoid
- Cerebral contusions
  —This is "bruising" of brain parenchyma.
- Diffuse axonal injury
  —Caused by rotational forces resulting in shearing of multiple axons.
  —Initial CT may not show any major abnormalities other than petechial haemorrhages.

Cervical spine (see the chapters on Cervical spine injuries)

CT indicated when:

- plain radiography fails to show all of cervical spine in those athletes with cervical spine injuries.
- fracture or subluxation is seen on plain X-ray, and further evaluation is required.

Thoracolumbar spine injuries (see the chapter on Thoracolumbar injuries)

CT commonly used to provide anatomical detail of fractures including determination of osseous fragment location in relation to central canal.

Shoulder injuries

- Dislocations ± fractures
  —Subtle Hill–Sachs, Bankart's lesions may not be detected on plain radiography, but can be seen on CT images. Accuracy for detecting labrum lesions may be increased if CT is performed following intra-articular injection of contrast (CT arthrography).
- Proximal humerus fractures
  —By providing anatomical detail, CT can be a vital tool for planning the management of the more complex proximal humerus fractures.
- Scapula fractures
  —Undisplaced fractures may be difficult to see on a plain X-ray whereas CT is accurate in detecting them. Furthermore, CT will reveal the associated surrounding structure injuries.

Chest injuries (see the chapter on Chest injuries)

CT can be an extremely valuable tool in management of chest injuries revealing the kind, location and extent of the chest injury.

Abdominal injuries (see the chapter on Abdominal injuries)

CT is an important adjunct when evaluating athletes with abdominal trauma. It supplies information about:

- Injuries to intra-abdominal organs including retroperitoneal structures.
- Haemoperitoneum and its source.
- Retroperitoneal haematoma and its source.

Pelvic injuries

As well as revealing associated abdominal, pelvic organ and vascular injuries, CT provides vital information when evaluating pelvic and acetabular fractures.

Knee injuries

CT is particularly useful when evaluating tibia plateau fractures.

Acknowledgements

We would like to thank Dr B Langroudi for his comments on this and other chapters on imaging.

Further reading

Barron D. Basic science: computed tomography. *Current Orthopaedics* 2005; **19**: 20–6.
Gibbon WM, Long G. Imaging of athletic injuries. *Current Orthopaedics* 2000; **14**: 424–34.
Sanders TG, Fults-Ganey K. Imaging techniques. In: JC DeLee, D Drez, MD Miller (Eds) *Orthopaedic Sports Medicine, Principles and Practice*, 2nd edn. Saunders, 2002: 557–614.
Tung GA, Brody JM. Contemporary imaging of athletic injuries. *Clinics in Sports Medicine* 1997; **16**(3): 393–417.

Infection and sport

A Kamvari

On the whole, regular moderate exercise is believed to enhance immunity and decrease susceptibility to infections, such as the common cold and also some forms of cancer, whereas sudden intense exercise and over-training appears to have a deleterious effect on the immune response and may be a limiting factor in athletic performance.

An overall view of this situation has been graphically described by Nieman's "J-curve", which is emphasised as being descriptive rather than quantitative (see Nieman 1994).

Exercise – immune interactions

Effects of exercise on the physical barriers to infection

Cooling and drying of the respiratory mucosa causes an increased exposure of the bronchi to viral and carcinogenic particles in the air during exercise, due to a switch in nose-to-mouth breathing and also turbulent and high respiratory flow rates. This in turn reduces cilial motility, which increases mucus viscosity in the bronchi, and thus reduces clearance of the contaminated particles, which can increase the susceptibility of the athlete to viral respiratory infections and certain cancers.

Effects of exercise on the biologic immune defences

Cellular changes

- Leukocyte subpopulations: "leukocytosis of exercise" is one of the earliest and most consistent observations of the exercise-induced immune response in the blood.

- Natural Killer (NK) cells and Lymphokine-activated Killer (LAK) cells increase their activity as well as their concentration in the blood.
- Phagocytic cells increase in numbers during exercise.

Humoral changes

- B Cell Function is not well studied but immunoglobulins (IgA, IgM, IgG) are all depressed during, and two hours post, exercise, but this is a transient change and their concentrations recover after 2 hours.
- Cytokines. Exercise increases production of IL-1, which has a direct cytotoxic effect. It also increases the production of IL-2, IL-6 and tumour necrosis factor (TNF) in plasma.

On the whole, using experimental and epidemiological data, and taking other factors that influence athletes' susceptibility to infection (e.g. pathogen exposure, diet, psychological influences and environmental stresses) into consideration, it has been shown that excessive and stressful exercise weakens resistance to infections and renders athletes more susceptible to frequent and persistent colds, sore throats and influenza-like illnesses. Moderate exercise and training, however, seem to increase immune functions, especially amongst the older age groups.

Upper Respiratory Tract Infections (URTIs) in athletes

These are a spectrum of illnesses, which include infectious rhinitis (common cold), pharingitis and sinusitis.

Epidemiology

The average adult population has two to four colds per year, mostly during the winter months.

Aetiology

- Viral: Most URTIs are caused by viruses, transmitted by secretion, contaminated hands or direct droplet transmission through hand contact with the eyes or nose.
  Infectious rhinitis – mostly caused by rhinoviruses.
  Pharyngitis – mostly caused by rhinovirus, coronavirus, parainfluenza virus or respiratory syncytial virus. Other viral agents include herpes simplex and coxsackievirus and adenovirus. Epstein–Barr virus and cytomegalovirus can also cause pharyngitis, but they also cause other severe systemic symptoms including fatigue, lymphadenopathy, splenomegaly and fever.
- Bacterial: Beta haemolytic Group A streptococcus, chlamydia pneumoniae.

Symptoms and signs

Mild chills and fatigue followed by clear rhinorrhea, congestion, scratchy sore throat, cough, congestion and headache are the most common symptoms.

Patients with bacterial sinusitis often present with a history of purulent rhinorrhea, unilateral sinus or periorbital pain.

On examination, vital signs are normal, but an occasional low-grade fever may be found. The throat often appears erythematous with exudates and, occasionally,

petechiae. Anterior cervical nodes may be swollen and tender. Tenderness over the sinus regions may be present.

Investigations and treatment

Diagnosis of URTIs are usually clinical and do not require further investigation and testing.

Occasionally, if bacterial causes are suspected, throat swabs and cultures may be done to isolate the organisms responsible.

If chronic bacterial sinusitis is suspected a percutaneous sinus aspiration and culture can also be done, but this is usually an impractical procedure for routine diagnostic testing. Imaging with CT and plain radiography can be done if recurrent or chronic sinusitis occurs, which can find mucosal thickening, sinus opacification and altered fluid levels in the sinuses.

Symptoms of viral URTIs usually improve within 5 to 7 days and abate within 10 to 14 days spontaneously, with no treatment.

Vitamin C and zinc supplements have been found to decrease the period and extent of morbidity.

Oral decongestants and antihistamines, paracetamol and ibuprofen can all be used symptomatically.

Antibiotics are only given if bacterial causes are suspected or isolated.

The antibiotic of choice for group A streptococcus infections is Penicillin V, but amoxicillin may also be substituted.

Return to sport

The conventional guidance is that athletes should refrain from exercising in the presence of systemic symptoms that include fever, severe myalgia or lethargy, and tachycardia at rest or severe respiratory symptoms that include wheezing, shortness of breath and deep cough.

Infectious mononucleosis

Epidemiology

Mainly affects adolescents and young adults in developed countries and young children in developing countries.

Aetiology

Infectious mononucleosis is mostly due to Epstein–Barr virus (EBV), less commonly cytomegalovirus (CMV).

Symptoms and signs

Classically presenting symptoms include fever and sore throat, some patients may present with a maculopapular rash, fatigue and left-sided abdominal discomfort due to splenomegaly. There may also be neurological symptoms ranging from encephalitis to a peripheral neuropathy.

On examination, tonsillar hypertrophy with exudates and also generalised lymphadenopathy may be found. Jaundice and haematological abnormalities (thrombocytopenia or haemolytic anaemia) may also be found.

Investigations and treatment

Blood tests generally show an increase in white blood cell count of 10,000 to 20,000/mm^3 with increased atypical lymphocytes.

Serological tests for EBV and CMV IgM and IgG can provide direct evidence of acute or prior infection.

A positive heterophile antibody (Monospot) test is diagnostic.

Infectious mononucleosis is generally self-limiting, and symptoms usually last from 2–6 weeks.

Treatment is therefore mainly symptomatic, and rest.

Corticosteroids are not usually recommended unless there is airway compromise, when the drugs can significantly reduce tonsillar hypertrophy.

Complications

Splenic rupture – up to 40% of traumatic splenic ruptures have occurred in athletes who have been found to have infectious mononucleosis. Most splenic ruptures occur in patients with splenomegaly, but it can happen to patients who do not have an enlarged spleen. Non-traumatic splenic rupture usually occurs between weeks 2 and 4 with an incidence of 1 in 1000.

Persistent fatigue – in a few patients fatigue and lethargy can continue for an indefinite period of time after the rest of the symptoms have been resolved.

Airway obstruction – this can occur if there is severe tonsillar hypertrophy.

Return to sport

Even though total bed-rest is unnecessary, athletes should generally be restricted from training and competing for 3 to 4 weeks.

Athletes returning to contact sports such as rugby or wrestling should refrain from doing so until the resolution of splenic enlargement.

Further reading

Howe WB. Preventing infectious disease in sports. *The Physician and Sports Medicine* 2003; **31**(2).

Nieman DC. Exercise, infection and immunity. *International Journal of Sports Medicine* 1994; **15**(Suppl 3): S131–41.

O'Kane JW. Upper respiratory infection. *The Physician and Sports Medicine* 2000; **30**(9).

Shepard RJ. Exercise, immunity, and susceptibility to infection – a J-shaped relationship. *The Physician and Sports Medicine* 1999; **27**(6).

Knee – acute injuries

P Thomas

The different anatomical structures will be discussed separately, although injuries involving more than one structure can also exist.

Anterior cruciate ligament

This is an intracapsular structure, attached proximately at the posterolateral femur and distally on the tibial spine. The anterior cruciate ligament (ACL) resists anterior displacement of the tibia on the femur. Also, as the knee extends it rotates the tibia externally assisting to "drive" the tibia under the femur.

The usual mechanism of injury includes, in contact sports such as football and rugby, an excessive rotation force on the tibia or a hyperextension of the knee, which usually occurs when a skier falls backwards. Other more complex and multi-directional forces can also lead to an ACL, usually associated with other knee anatomical structure injuries.

Swelling, caused by an acute haemarthrosis is present in almost all patients. Many athletes describe an audible "pop" at the time of the injury. The knee is also painful.

On examination there is effusion present into the knee joint. Seventy-five to 80% of all acute haemarthosis in the knee joint following trauma are usually associated with an anterior cruciate ligament rupture. The tenderness is diffused or present posterolaterally in cases of lateral meniscus tears and posterior capsular damage or medially if there is an associated medial meniscus tear.

The anterior draw test may be negative due to muscle spasm, however the Lachman's test is always positive with a soft or no "end point". In experienced hands, the pivot shift test is also positive.

X-rays may be entirely normal or may demonstrate an avulsion of the tibial spine, more often seen in the young athlete, or Segond's fracture may be present, which is usually associated with an ACL rupture.

Management consists of:

Conservative

- 4–6 weeks' rehabilitation programme to absorb the effusion, restore painless range of movement of the knee joint, regain full muscle strength and proprioception such as side-stepping exercises and "figure of 8" running.
- After this, the patient may be able to return to his sport or will carry on to surgical reconstruction of the ACL, in particular if the knee is unstable on returning to sport or even in daily activities. The individual should be discouraged to continue sport with frequent episodes of instability. Recurrent instability may damage the menisci and the articular cartilage, leading to degeneration and osteoarthritis.
- Derotation braces are still controversial. They may help with stability in some sports such as skiing, tennis or squash.

Surgery

- The decision for a surgical reconstruction will be based on whether the patient is young, with recurrent instability, the level of sporting activity and the personality of that patient.
- During surgery, an autograft from hamstrings, patella tendon or quadriceps is the popular choice among surgeons and will be placed arthroscopically into the knee joint. Allografts and synthetic ligament materials are also used worldwide.
- A prolonged rehabilitation programme is undertaken to allow the patient to return to competitive sport between 6 months to 1 year. In the hands of an experienced surgeon the success rate following surgery approaches 90%.

- The long-term risk of osteoarthritis is unclear, although many publications have suggested that in knees where the ACL is reconstructed then the stability is restored and this reduces the risk of further articular cartilage damage and menisci tearings, therefore reducing the probability of degenerative disease and osteoarthritis. Certainly, a reconstruction of the ACL allows continued sports participation with all its benefits.

Chronic anterior cruciate ligament deficient knee

Symptoms include: giving way, recurrent swelling, pain and locking. The diagnostic tests such as anterior draw test, Lachman's, pivot shift and menisci tests are more obviously positive than the acute rupture of the anterior cruciate ligament. Degenerative disease with crepitus and compartmental pain on movement may be present. An effusion may or may not be present. Arthroscopic surgery may be indicated for the torn menisci and chondroplasty could be performed for frail articular cartilage. A reconstruction is indicated when instability is present with daily activities. The rehabilitation programme is similar as for the acute anterior cruciate ligament reconstruction.

Posterior cruciate ligament

The posterior cruciate ligament (PCL) is an intra-articular but extrasynovial structure, whose course runs from the posterior of the tibia upwards and forwards where it becomes wide at the attachment in the medial femoral condyle.

The function of the PCL is to resist the femur slide over the tibia and also to resist hyperextension of the knee joint.

Mechanism of the injury usually is either a direct blow to the anterior tibia when the knee is flexed or severe hyperextension of the knee joint.

The athlete presents with pain or the feeling of "giving way" when he runs downhill or downstairs. Later on, he will complain of pain at the patellofemoral joint because the patella articular cartilage is damaged as the femur slides forward on the tibia. An avulsion of the tibia attachment is common in the young athlete.

On clinical examination, an increased recurvatum, posterior sag of the tibia and a positive posterior draw test may be observed.

In patients with posterior cruciate ligament tibial avulsions, primary surgical repair will produce excellent results.

Conservative management is successful in most of the patients, achieving full range of movement of the knee joint, strong quadriceps, flexible hamstrings and gradual return to sport with some alterations in training.

Surgical reconstruction is reserved for patients with multiple ligament injuries, or in the few cases of an isolated rupture with continuous functional instability, despite conservative management.

Medial collateral ligament

This represents the most common ligament injury of the knee joint.

The mechanism of injury includes a direct valgus force applied to the knee or a force that increases the external tibial rotation.

Three degrees of injury are recognized:

First degree

- There is pain locally, there is no swelling and valgus stress at 30° of flexion is negative (no medial side opening).

Second degree

- Pain is present locally, there is some swelling and valgus stress at 30° of knee flexion will be positive but with an end point.

Third degree

- Pain is present locally, there is swelling, valgus stress at 30° of knee flexion is positive with no end point and it is usually associated with other ligamentous injury of the knee joint.

The management of the medial collateral ligament injuries is largely conservative. The patient is able to return to his or her sporting activities when there is minimal tenderness at the ligament site, the valgus stress test is pain free, there is full range of movement of the knee joint, and the patient can run and change direction without any pain.

Recovery takes place between 2 weeks to 3 months.

Pellegrini–Stieda disease

This is associated with heterotopic ossification which develops at the disrupted femoral attachment origin of the medial collateral ligament. Symptoms and clinical findings include increased pain, severe localized tenderness and restriction because of discomfort in both flexion and extension of the knee joint. X-rays will reveal the pathology but usually 3–4 weeks later on from the injury. Management includes active mobilization, local infiltration with a corticosteroid agent, aspiration under ultrasound scan guidance and on occasions surgical excision if the ossification is too large.

Lateral collateral ligament, posterolateral corner

The mechanism of injury includes a direct varus force applied to the knee joint or it is a part of a more complex pattern, with damage at the posterolateral corner of the joint. In the majority of cases, surgical management as part of the early exploration of the posterolateral corner complex of the knee is mandatory. Surgical reconstruction in chronic cases is indicated.

Meniscus

The medial meniscus is less mobile compared with the lateral one since the middle third is attached to the joint capsule and the deep layer of the medial collateral ligament. The meniscus is a load-bearing structure which functions as a “shock absorber”. The wedge shape reduces the anatomical disparity between femur and tibial surfaces, therefore contributing to joint stability. It also contributes to the nutrition of the articular cartilage.

A total menisectomy will lead to alteration of the load and stability of the knee joint compartment, leading to degeneration and osteoarthritis. All surgical treatments are aiming to preserve as much meniscus as possible following a tear (repair or partial menisectomy).

The patient will complain of localized joint pain, locking and giving way. On occasions a small amount of swelling can be present. A true locking of the knee represents a loss of the last few degrees of knee extension and is usually associated with a "bucket handle" tear of the meniscus, which is displaced into the knee joint. Associated meniscal cysts may be present, usually at the lateral side of the knee joint.

Clinical tests of McMurray and Apley's compressive tests will both be positive. MRI scans are highly diagnostic and have replaced arthrography.

The management of suspected meniscal tears may involve a period of conservative treatment with rest from activities and physiotherapy. Persisting symptoms beyond 3–4 weeks will lead to arthroscopic surgery where partial menisectomy or repair of the tear with sutures will be performed.

Management of a locked knee will involve arthroscopic surgery and depending on the time of the presentation, repair or excision of the torn peripheral meniscus will be attempted.

A lateral meniscal cyst may be treated by arthroscopic means but, in cases of recurrence, removal by open surgery may need to be considered.

Patellofemoral dislocation

This usually occurs with a sudden internal femoral rotation on the fixed tibia. The patella dislocates laterally and may spontaneously reduce.

Predisponding factors may include:

- increased femoral antiversion
- valgus knee, high patella (patella alta)
- tight patella retinaculum
- shallow femoral groove
- underdeveloped lateral femoral condyle
- overpronated feet
- weak vastus medialis
- wide Q angle.

The diagnosis is easily made if the patella is still dislocated. In cases where the dislocation is reduced the clinical examination may reveal the presence of a haemarthrosis, tender medial patella retinaculum, painful contractions of the quadriceps and a positive Apprehension test.

Management includes the immediate reduction of the dislocation and aspiration of any haemarthrosis. A period of immobilization in a cast or a brace, usually in extension, for a period of 3 weeks is recommended. Then exercises for flexion and gradual range of movement of the knee joint are commenced. This is followed by rehabilitation and strengthening of the vastus medialis. Return to sport will be encouraged when the quadriceps are strong, proprioception is present and the knee is symptom free. A sleeve-type brace is worn when returning to sport, providing additional proprioceptive feedback, reducing the risk of a further dislocation. The presence of recurrent instability will lead to a decision of surgical management.

Other knee injuries

Fractures

- By definition intra-articular, and in most cases will lead to a decision of open reduction and internal fixation.

Osteochondral fractures

- They are commonly associated with patellofemoral instability, they simulate a meniscus injury with pain and locking. Arthroscopic surgery is the treatment of choice.

Ruptures of the extensor mechanism of the knee

- In most of the cases the patella tendon can rupture, less often this injury can occur on the quadriceps tendon in an older athlete. The diagnosis is made by the inability to straight leg raise and the treatment consists of an acute direct surgical repair.

Further reading

Fowler PJ *et al.* Isolated PCL injuries in athletes. *Am J Sports Med* 1987; **15**: 553–7.

Hardin GT *et al.* Meniscal tears: diagnosis, evaluation and treatment. *Orthop Rev* 1992; **26**: 1311–17.

Johnson RJ *et al.* Current concepts review: the treatment of injuries of the ACL. *J Bone Joint Surg* 1992; **74A**: 140–51.

Knee – overuse injuries

P Thomas

Iliotibial band friction syndrome

The iliotibial band is a tendon within the fascia lata inserting into the Gerdy's tuberle on the anterior lateral aspect of the tibia. The iliotibial band drops posteriorly behind the lateral femoral epicondyle during knee flexion, then snaps forward over the epicondyle during the extension phase. This syndrome is the result of the inflammation of the distal iliotibial band and the bursa, which lies underneath it and over the lateral femoral condyle.

Predisponding factors will include: genu varus, excessive feet pronation, any leg length discrepancy, a prominent Greater Trochanter of the upper femur and training errors, e.g. a single run over excessive distance or increasing the running mileage too quickly, excessive hill running.

The pain at first is present going down stairs or downhill. Later on, continuous pain will be present, restricting all running or even daily activities. Tenderness is present 2–3 cm above the lateral joint line at the lateral femoral epicondyle with the knee flexed at 30°. Palpable crepitus may also be present. Ober's test is positive.

The management at first will include rest, ice and anti-inflammatories. Physiotherapy will include localized treatments, stretching of the hip abductors and flexors. Foot orthotics are recommended for any biomechanical discrepancies. At the site of friction, injection of corticosteroid could also be attempted. In persistent cases surgery, with division of the iliotibial band 3 cm above the knee joint at the anteriolateral femoral condyle, may be offered.

Popliteus tendinitis

This is a less common condition than the iliotibial band friction syndrome, however the same predisponding factors could be associated with this condition.

Athletes experience pain which may be reproduced by resisted knee flexion with the tibia held in external rotation.

The management will include rest, ice and compression, anti-inflammatories and localized soft tissue treatments, electrotherapy modalities and stretching of the knee flexors. In more resistant cases the site can be injected with a corticosteroid agent.

Pes anserinus bursitis

At the insertion of the hamstrings at the anterior medial aspect of the tibia there is a bursa present that can become inflamed and cause localized discomfort. The athlete's complaint will concentrate in localized burning and tenderness. The condition is associated with repeated hamstring injuries or even tight hamstrings. The management includes rest, ice and compression, hamstring stretching, anti-inflammatories, orthotics for overpronated feet and local infiltrations using a corticosteroid.

Further reading

Taunton JE, Clement DB, Smart GW, McNicol KL. Non-surgical management of overuse knee injurics in runners. *Can J Sports Sci* 1987; **12**(1): 11–18.

Knee – anterior knee pain

P Thomas

Patellofemoral joint-related pain

Females are affected more compared to males. It is usually seen in adolescence as chondromalacia patellae and in the fourth to fifth decades of life. The predominant symptom is pain anteriorly aggravated by climbing stairs, walking on hills and after a prolonged sitting down position. Crepitus may be present too. Clinical examination reveals irritability of the patellofemoral joint. Biomechanical factors associated with the condition include a wide Q angle, which is above 15° in males and 18° in females, high hypermobile and small patella, shallow intercondylar notch, genu valgus or pronated feet. X-ray assessment includes "skyline" view: lateral tilt of the patella, shallow intercondylar notch and other patella pathology may be detected.

The management of patellofemoral joint pain will focus on:

(1) Quadriceps rehabilitation in particular programmes for the vastus medialis, as in a normal knee there is a tendency of lateral shift of the patella on the femur, which is avoided by the vastis medialis muscle contraction.
(2) McConnell regime involving taping of the patella so it can track correctly when the quadriceps muscle contracts.
(3) Correction of the biomechanics such as pronated feet.
(4) Operative treatment will include a surgical lateral release of the retinaculum, chondroplasty, medial ligament of the patella reinforcement and surgery associated with the effects of osteoarthritis.

Patellar tendinopathy (jumper's knee)

Biomechanical studies have suggested that the greatest tensile forces on the patella tendon during running or jumping occur at the landing phase.

There is a gradual onset of pain at the lower pole of the patella and tenderness locally on palpation. Swelling and crepitus can also be noticed. An ultrasound scan and an MRI scan will reveal defects within the tendon and confirm the diagnosis.

Histology suggests a degeneration of the tendon instead of any inflammatory features. The management of the acute phase will include rest and ice applications. Thermal support could be worn when the acute phase has settled. Attention to orthotics and taping of the patella could also assist to avoid a recurrence. Physiotherapy modalities will concentrate on the quadriceps, the hip extensor and foot plantarflexors strengthening programmes. Recovery will depend on the presence and size of defects and can take from 6–8 weeks and up to 12 months. Recent treatments include under ultrasound scan, guidance dry needling of the defects and autotransfusion of the patient's blood. Surgery will be attempted when the conservative management has failed. Rehabilitation following surgery can last up to 6 months before returning to sports.

Synovial plica

Plicae are the remnants of the septa present in the embryonic knee.

The medial patellar plica runs from the medial suprapatellar pouch to the infrapatellar fat pad. It may impinge of the patellofemoral joint and the medial femoral condyle on flexion following an injury, which will convert the plica thick and tight.

The athlete will complain of aching pain at the front of the knee on flexion, worse in the morning.

The treatment will include rest, ice application, modification of the activities and local infiltration of corticosteroid. However, if symptoms persist, then arthroscopic excision of the plica is recommended.

Fat pad syndrome

Repetitive injury with the knee joint in extension or multiple surgeries may lead to the infrapatellar fat pad proliferation and impingement between the femur and the tibia, usually on extension.

In the most severe cases, the progressive scarring and fibrosis of the fat pad may lead to functional shortening of the patella tendon, which will track down the patella and block the knee flexion (patella baja).

Conservative management is usually effective, including rest, localised soft tissue treatments and awareness of repetitive knee extensions. If conservative management fails then arthroscopic excision of the fat pad will be indicated.

Other causes of anterior knee pain

These include:

- Osgood–Schlatter's disease
- Sinding–Larsen–Johanssen disease
- Trauma:
  —Anterior medial or lateral meniscus tears
  —Patella fractures
- Patella bipartite
- Pre-patella bursitis
- Referred pain from elsewhere (hip joint).

Further reading

Fox JM, Pizzo W (Eds) *The Patellofemoral Joint.* New York: McGraw-Hill (1993).

Van Kampen A, Haiskes R. The three-dimensional tracking pattern of the human patella. *J Orthop Research* 1990; **8**: 372–82.

Lumbar intervertebral disc herniation

AA Narvani

This common condition was first described in the 1930s by Mixter and Bar. Its incidence is reported to be 2.0 and 1.2 per 1000 persons per year for men and women respectively. It more commonly occurs between the ages of 30 and 50 years. Over 95% of symptomatic disc herniations occur at L5-S1 or L4-L5 levels.

Pathology

Intervertebral disc is made out of a central nucleus pulposus and a surrounding annulus fibrosus. The central nucleus pulposus is mainly gelatinous in nature, whereas annulus fibrosus consist of alternating laminae, which are mixtures of type I and II collagens. Trauma or degeneration can cause fissures to develop within the lamina, which can in turn lead to herniation of the nucleus (herniated nucleus pulposus (HNP)).

Bulging of the nucleus through a weakened but intact annulus is referred to as "protrusion". Disc "prolapse" is when the nucleus has gone through the annulus but not the posterior longitudinal ligament. Disc "extrusion" occurs when the posterior longitudinal ligament is penetrated as well by the nucleus. Separation of herniated fragment from the disc allows the loose fragment to lie free in the canal. This is referred to as disc "sequestration".

The herniation of the disc can cause mechanical pressure on the nerve root. In addition it may also cause symptoms by chemical irritation of the nerve root.

Predisposing factors

Reported risk factors for disc herniation include:

(i) Family history of disc herniation.
(ii) Jobs which expose the spine to vibration.
(iii) Smoking.
(iv) Sports or occupations that involve excessive twisting, lifting or bending.
(v) More likely to have symptoms from herniated disc in the presence of congenital conditions that affect the size of the spine.

Clinical features

The clinical features of disc herniation can be divided into

- Radicular features
- Neurological features
- Back pain

Radicular features

Typically there is leg pain in a root distribution, which usually extends all the way below the knee. It is typically sharp in nature and is made worse by coughing, laughing and sneezing. Usually the leg pain is worse than the back pain. On examination, the straight leg test would be positive. With this test, as the leg is lifted, with the knee in extension the patient's radicular pain is reproduced.

Neurological features

Neurological symptoms are dependent on the nerve root involved. Because the vast majority of discs that are herniated are the L4/L5 and L5/S1 discs, the commonest nerve roots that are affected are L4, L5 and S1 nerve roots. L4/L5 disc herniation can cause L4 and/or L5 features depending on the anatomical position of the herniated disc. Similarly, herniated L5/S1 discs can cause L5 and/or S1 symptoms.

Pressure or irritation of L4 will cause an altered sensation or pins and needles in the L4 distribution area (anterior surface of the leg). There may be a diminished knee reflex. There may be some weaknesses in the quadriceps and adductor muscles.

If the L5 nerve root is affected, the altered sensation would occur in the L5 dermatome (lateral aspect of the lower leg, medial part of the foot and big toe). Extension of the big toe and in more severe cases the whole foot may be weak.

With the S1 nerve root, sensation to the lateral aspect and sole of the foot may be affected. Ankle reflex can be absent and there may be decreased power with plantar flexion of the foot.

Cauda equina syndrome

This is an emergency and occurs when there is pressure on the nerves that supply bowel and bladder. It is caused by a central disc herniation causing compression of the nerve roots of the cauda equina. Features include bowel/bladder dysfunction associated with saddle anaesthesia and a varying degree of sensory or motor function loss in the lower limbs. Rectal assessment may reveal a weak anal tone.

Back pain

Commonly there is associated back pain with the radicular and/or neurological symptoms. This back pain has the characteristics of discogenic low back pain (see the chapter on Back pain – discogenic) and it is made worse on flexion of the spine. Sitting is particularly painful. Coughing, sneezing and straining worsen the pain through increasing the intra-discal pressure.

Investigations

In most patients magnetic resonance imaging is the investigation of choice in diagnosis of the herniated lumbar disc disease. It is non-invasive, does not expose the athlete to any ionizing radiation and has the ability to visualize lumbar discs, spinal canal and the lumbar nerve roots accurately. Myelography and CT scan also have a role when MRI cannot be performed.

Differential diagnosis

Other conditions that may present with similar features include the following:

Intraspinal causes

- Spinal stenosis.
- Infection (osteomylitis or discitis causing nerve root pressure).
- Inflammation (arachnoiditis).
- Neoplasm (benign or malignant lesions causing pressure on the nerve root including neurofibromas, ependydomas and spinal metastatic lesions).
- Referred pain from back pain due to other conditions (see the chapter Back pain – overview).

Extraspinal causes

- Peripheral vascular disease.
- Neoplastic lesions causing compression of lumbosacral plexus and nerves).
- Degenerative disease of hip or knee.
- Gynaecological pathology.
- Peripheral neuropathies secondary to conditions such as diabetes or alcohol abuse.
- Sciatic nerve pathology such as trauma or tumour.
- Herpes zoster.

Treatment

It is important to appreciate that in the vast majority of patients, non-operative treatment results in pain relief in a few days to several months. Furthermore, there does not appear to be any significant differences in long-term outcomes when comparing patients who have had surgery, for radicular symptoms secondary to disc herniation, to those that have been managed non-operatively. Surgery does, however, result in better short-term outcomes.

Indications for surgery include:

(i) Cauda equina syndrome.
(ii) Recent onset or progressing sensory or motor deficit particularly in the presence of type and size of disc that make the spontaneous regression of the symptoms unlikely.
(iii) Intractable radicular pain despite conservative management. With non-operative management longer than 3 months in duration, the chances of improvement decrease significantly; therefore, these athletes are candidates for surgery. Non-operative management may also be abandoned earlier in favour of surgery in those with intolerable, severe radicular symptoms, which are not improved with the attempted conservative route.

Non-operative

This consists of:

- Analgesia
- NSAIDs
- Epidural injections/nerve root blocks
- Low back schools
- Exercise programme

In the first few days of symptoms, rest may be combined with analgesia and NSAIDs. If these measures fail to provide any relief, the athlete may then be a candidate for either epidural injection or nerve root block. An exercise programme, consisting of extension exercises, stretching and muscle strengthening, is started once sufficient pain relief is achieved.

Operative

These include:

- Conventional discectomy
- Microdiscectomy
- Percutaneous procedures such as
  —chemonucleolysis
  —Percutaneous automated nucleotomy (PAN)
  —Manual percutaneous discectomy
  —Laser discectomy

Conventional discectomy is associated with low rates of neurological and minor complications (less than 0.5 and 4.7% respectively), and is reported to provide good to excellent short-term results in 90 to 95% of the patients. This success rate, however, does drop over subsequent years as a result of recurrence or scarring.

Microdiscectomy involves a small incision, avoidance of laminectomy and trauma to facets, and excising only sufficient disc material to relieve compression of the nerve root. It may be performed with the aid of an operating microscope. It is argued that this procedure results in lower risks of complications in healing, less pain in the early post-operative period and earlier return to normal activities.

Chemonucleolysis involves application of enzymes that dissolve the disc. It is associated with risks of allergic reaction or toxicity, and may have a role in a very selective group of patients.

Percutaneous automated discectomy involves evacuation of disc space through a cannula, which is placed in the disc space with an automated probe. This may also be performed manually with a probe. An endoscope may also be used during manual percutaneous discectomy. The efficacy of this procedure remains to be proven. In laser discectomy, various laser systems are utilized to coagulate, shrink, carbonize, vaporize or ablate the nucleus pulposus. There are doubts about the efficacy of this procedure and it is not used on a wide scale.

Return to sport

As with other sports injuries, return to sport is permitted once the athlete is pain free, able to achieve a full range of movement and has regained enough strength to perform their sport-specific activities. In addition, there should be complete neurological recovery, as neurological deficits may predispose the athlete to other injuries. With non-operative management, once pain relief is achieved, this process may take less than 4–6 weeks. Most athletes who have been treated surgically are able to participate at around 8 weeks following surgery.

Further reading

Eismont FJ, Kitchel SH. Thoracolumbar spine in adults. In: JC DeLee, D Drez, MD Miller (Eds) *Orthopaedic Sports Medicine, Principles and Practice*, 2nd edn. Saunders, 2002; 1525–62.

Postachinni F. Management of herniation of the lumbar disc. *J Bone & Joint Surgery (Br)* 1999; **81**-B: 567–76.

Maxillofacial injuries in sport

F Monibi

Trauma to the head and neck can range from fairly superficial cuts and bruises to serious and life-threatening injuries, which can result in neurological complications as well as facial scarring and disfigurement. This chapter aims to summarise the assessment of the head and neck as well as highlighting common injuries and complications.

Assessment

- Secure airway.
- Ensure breathing is adequate.
- Control haemorrhage.
- How was the injury sustained?
- Did the patient lose consciousness?
- Are visual disturbances (flashes, diplopia, blurred vision, pain) present?
- Does the patient have clear-fluid discharge from the nose or ears?
- Is the patient having difficulty opening or closing the mouth?
- Does the patient feel like the teeth come together normally?
- Areas of paraesthesia/anaesthesia?
- Systematic maxillofacial examination:
  —Assess for asymmetry.
  —Check zygomatic complex by looking down from behind the patient.
  —Check for abrasions, swelling, haematoma and lacerations.
  —Inspect open wounds for foreign bodies.
  —Inspect the teeth for mobility, fracture or misalignment. If teeth are avulsed, make sure they are accounted for.
  —Palpate for bony injury, crepitus and steps, especially around orbital rims and zygomatic arches.
  —Eyes: inspect for the presence of exophthalmos or enophthalmos. Visual acuity, abnormality of ocular movements and pupil size, shape and reaction to light, both direct and consensual.
  —Look for intra-oral lacerations, ecchymosis or swelling. Bimanually palpate the mandible, and examine for signs of crepitus or mobility.
  —Place one hand on the anterior maxillary teeth and the other on the nasal bridge. Movement of only the teeth indicates a Le Fort I fracture. Movement at the nasal bridge indicates a Le Fort II or III fracture.
  —Gently manipulate each tooth individually for movement, pain, gingival and intra-oral bleeding, tears or crepitus.
  —Palpate the mandibular condyle by placing a finger in the external auditory miatus while the patient opens and closes the mouth. Pain or lack of movement of the condyle indicates fracture.
  —Perform a thorough cranial nerve examination.

Fractures

Maxillary fractures

Le Fort I fracture is a horizontal maxillary fracture across the inferior aspect of the maxilla and separates the alveolar process and hard palate from the rest of the maxilla.

The fracture extends through the lower third of the septum and includes the floor of the maxillary sinus extending into the palatine bones and pterygoid plates. Clinically, the upper dental arch is mobile and bruising can be observed in the upper labial sulcus.

Le Fort II fracture is a pyramidal fracture extending from the nasal bone extending through the lacrimal bone downward through the zygomatico–maxillary suture continuing posteriorly and laterally through the maxilla.

Le Fort III fracture is a separation of all of the facial bones from the cranial base including fractures of the zygoma, maxilla and nasal bones. The fracture line extends posterio-laterally through ethmoid bones, orbits and pterygo-maxillary suture into the spheno-palatine fossa.

Mandibular fractures

These can occur in multiple locations of the jaw and the condylar neck. Fractures often occur bilaterally at sites away from the site of direct trauma. Common areas of mandibular fracture are where unerupted teeth or long roots may present weak spots. These areas are the angle of the mandible and the area of the lower canine. Para-symphyseal fractures often present with condylar neck fractures and are difficult to see radiographically.

Clinical findings of mandibular fractures include pain on jaw movement, and mis-alignment of the teeth on biting. Mobility of the segments, crepitus and steps can be palpated along the fracture sites.

Intra-oral oedema, haematoma, gingival bleeding or tears may be present. An anterior open bite can occur with bilateral condylar or angle fractures. Trauma to the inferior alveolar nerve may cause paraesthesia and/or anaesthesia of the lower lip and chin.

Frontal bone fractures

Presentation

Usually a result of a blow to the forehead. The anterior and posterior wall of the frontal sinus may be involved.

Orbital floor fracture

Presentation

Orbital floor fracture ("blow-out fracture") can occur on its own or can be accompanied by a medial wall fracture. A teardrop-shaped herniation of the orbital contents into the maxillary sinus is a typical radiographic presentation. The incidence of ocular injury is high, but globe rupture is rare. Usually the globe of the affected eye has dropped and appears lower. The eye movements of the affected eye will be restricted due to the interference with the extra-ocular muscles.

Management

Surgical debridement and repair with autogenous or synthetic graft.

Nasal fractures

Presentation

The immediate result of nasal fracture is usually epistaxis. On examination, the nose may appear flattened or may deviate to one side. Nasal fractures may extend from the nose to the ethmoid bones and can result in damage to the medial canthus, lacrimal apparatus or nasal-frontal duct. They also can result in a dural tear at the cribriform plate.

Zygomatic arch fractures

Presentation

Zygomatico-maxillary complex fractures are usually a result of direct trauma. Fracture lines can involve the zygomatico-temporal, zygomatico-frontal and zygomatico-maxillary components of the zygomatic tripod. Fractures of the zygomatico-maxillary buttress usually extend through the infra-orbital foramen and orbital floor. Concurrent ocular injuries are common.

Alveolar fractures

These can occur in isolation from a direct low-energy force or can result from extension of the fracture line through the alveolar portion of the maxilla or mandible.

Dislocation of the mandible

Presentation

The patient is unable to close their mouth. Although not especially painful the procedure for relocating the mandible will become progressively more difficult as time goes by.

Management

The mandible is relocated by firm downward and backward pressure. This is applied to the external oblique ridges of the mandible, which are located on the buccal surfaces of the lower molar teeth.

Fractured teeth

Presentation

Pain with extreme hot and cold sensitivity. Bleeding from the gingivae and exposed pulps of teeth, often in conjunction with soft tissue injuries.

Management

So long as the patient does not have any other more serious injuries, the patient should be referred to a dentist as soon as possible, who should stabilise the teeth and explore the wounds for tooth and foreign body fragments before suturing takes place. Soft tissue radiographs are very helpful in locating glass and other difficult to see fragments.

Avulsed teeth

Presentation

Teeth can either fracture or be completely avulsed from their sockets and the mouth. This is most common in high-impact sports injuries with a blunt object and usually affects the upper front teeth, particularly in patients with a large overjet.

Management

It is important for the tooth to be *kept*, gently cleaned, without touching the root surface and placed back into the patient's mouth, into the socket, or kept in saline or fresh milk. If the tooth is placed back into the socket care must be taken to place the tooth the right way round. Often the contra-lateral tooth will provide a clue. The patient should be referred to a dentist immediately for follow-up treatment.

Soft tissue injuries

Intra-oral lacerations can be sutured with either 4/0 silk on a curved cutting needle or resorbable materials, which will be resorbed within 7–10 days (e.g. vicryl rapide).

In case of deep lacerations, the connective tissue can be sutured with a longer-lasting resorbable material such as PDS or Vicryl.

Further reading

Echlin P, McKeag DB. Maxillofacial injuries in sport. *Curr Sports Med Rep* 2004; **3**(1): 25–32.

Mourouzis C, Koumoura F. Sports-related maxillofacial fractures: a retrospective study of 125 patients. *Int J Oral Maxillofac Surg* 2005 Sep; **34**(6): 635–8.

Muscle properties relevant to sports and exercise (including fatigue)

B Lynn

Muscle is the tissue whose properties dominate all others when we want to understand exercise and sports performance. The basics of muscle biochemistry, physiology and anatomy are well covered in medical and sports science texts, so this chapter will concentrate on aspects particularly relevant to sports and exercise. Table 1 lists the four key proteins. Myosin and actin interact through crossbridges (the myosin "heads") to slide the myofilaments and produce force. These two proteins form 85% of total muscle protein. Troponin and tropomyosin are the key regulatory proteins that bind calcium, so revealing the myosin-binding site on actin and allowing contraction to proceed. Titin is a structural protein comprising 7% of all muscle protein. Its role is not fully defined, but in genetic trawls for performance-related genes, titin has emerged as a candidate. α-actinen is in the list for the same reason, one form of the gene being much more common in sprinters than in non-sprinters.

Table 1 Muscle proteins.

Protein	Function
Myosin	Contractile protein, thick filaments
Actin	Contractile protein, thin filaments
Troponin	Regulatory protein, calcium binding
Tropomyosin	Interacts with troponin
Titin	Elasticity; filament alignment?
α-Actinen	Actin binding to Z-line

Power – the force–velocity curve

Muscle is an unusual kind of motor. It generates maximum force at zero velocity. As it speeds up, force falls away, with a clear upper limit on contraction speed. Since power is the product of force and velocity, this means that there will be a maximum power at some intermediate velocity since power will clearly be zero both when velocity is zero (isometric contraction) and when force is zero (at maximum velocity). In practice, maximum power occurs at approximately one-third of maximum force, which also corresponds to about 1/3 maximum velocity. This optimum is important, for example, when cycling and is the reason gears can help. These allow us to adjust the force and velocity of limb movement, thus keeping our muscles operating close to the maximum power part of the force–velocity curve under different loads (e.g. varying uphill gradients).

Contraction and length changes: concentric, eccentric, isometric

Typically, a muscle is activated, generates force, and shortens. Such contractions are termed *concentric*. Sometimes the muscle contracts against a matching force, with no external shortening. This is an *isometric* contraction. Finally, muscle may be stretched by an opposing force during activation. This may seem wasteful, but in fact muscles acting as "brakes" play an important part in locomotion (e.g. on heel strike the ankle flexors contract while being stretched in order to limit ankle extension). Such contractions are called *eccentric* (meaning "away from centre", not crazy!). In the previous section it was stated that during isometric contraction muscle force was at a maximum. However, this is not strictly true. It is true for muscle shortening. However, during eccentric contractions higher forces can be developed. This is due to the ability of crossbridges between myosin and actin to support higher passive loads than can be created during shortening. Interestingly, these additional forces do not need any extra ATP (adenosine triphosphate) splitting, so eccentric contractions are metabolically very efficient. However, there is a small price to be paid as eccentric contractions cause microdamage leading to diffuse onset muscle soreness (DOMS).

Fibre types

Muscle contains three different types of fibre with different inherent speeds and hence power production (Table 2). Slow (type I) fibres predominate in postural muscles where prolonged contraction is the main requirement. These fibres have relatively slow kinetics, but lower basal energy requirements. The other two classes have faster kinetics. The fastest of them, the type IIb, are specialised for short, explosive actions (e.g. jumping, throwing) and metabolise almost entirely anaerobically. Different individuals can have very different proportions of the three fibre types, largely through inheritance, but also partly by training (see the chapter on training). Perhaps unsurprisingly, sprinters and other athletes in explosive events have a large proportion of fast fibres while endurance athletes are just the opposite, with rather few fast fibres and lots of slow ones.

Table 2 Fibre types in human skeletal muscle.

Property	Classification		
	Slow	Fast	
	I or S	IIa or FR	IIb or FF
Twitch speed	Slow	Fast	Super fast
Power	Low	Intermediate	High
Energy utilisation	Low	Intermediate	High
Glycolytic capacity	Low	High	High
Oxidative capacity	High	Medium-high	Low
Myoglobin (giving red colour)	High	Intermediate	Low
Myosin heavy chain isoform	MHC-I	MHC-IIA	MHC-IIX
Fatigue resistance	Hard to fatigure	Moderate-high fatigure resistance	Easily fatigued
Prevalence in limb muscle of sprinters	20–40%	60–80%	
Prevalence in limb muscle of endurance athletes	60–90%	10–30%	

Muscle metabolism – different fuels for different durations of exercise

At the level of actin and myosin, the energy for force generation comes from hydrolysing ATP. However, cells do not store ATP, so a continuous re-supply is necessary during contraction. Re-supply comes from metabolism of carbohydrate and fatty acids. The fastest method is rapid breakdown of glucose to lactic acid – the process of glycolysis. However, even this takes several seconds to get going and ATP will last less time than this. In fact, ATP concentration must not be allowed to get low as it has many important control functions in the cell. ATP levels are maintained by having another compound, creatine phosphate (CP, also called phosphocreatine), that does

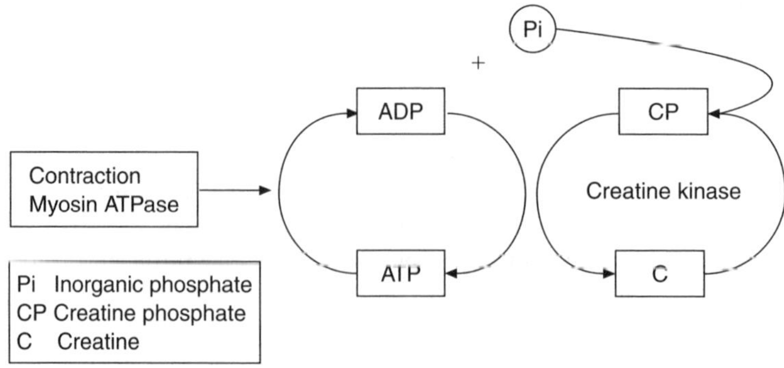

Figure 1 Reactions involved in maintaining ATP levels in the first few seconds of muscle contraction.

act as a short-term store. CP can rapidly phosphorylate ADP back to ATP, an action catalysed by the enzyme creatine kinase. This cycle of reactions is given in Figure 1.

Glycolysis is fast, but subject to two limits. Only carbohydrates can be used, so this supply depends on muscle glycogen. However, the real limit is set by the acidity of the end product, lactic acid. Lactic acid accumulates locally, lowering the muscle pH, and diffuses into the circulation where it is buffered by bicarbonate. However, this in turn pushes up blood carbon dioxide levels. This means that during continuous heavy exercise, e.g. distance running, another energy store must be available after about 30 s and must be supplying the bulk of energy by 2 min. This role is performed by oxidative phosphorylation of glucose. Glucose is broken down by the glycolytic pathway as far as pyruvate, then pyruvate enters the mitochondria. There, via the TCA cycle and the electron transfer chain, large amounts of ATP are generated using oxygen as an additional reactant and generating carbon dioxide and water as waste products.

Oxidative phosphorylation of carbohydrate can provide enough energy for high levels of activity, but cannot generate ATP as fast as pure glycolysis. So, typically, exercise levels for durations of 2 min or more are well below the peak levels that can be maintained for 1 min or less. For very long duration exercise, exceeding about 1 hour, carbohydrate stores start to be used up. Muscle glycogen will be mostly gone and only limited amounts of glucose can be removed from the blood if blood sugar is to remain at a high enough level for normal brain function. Some glucose is available from the breakdown of liver glycogen, and thanks to glucose synthesis in the liver from lactate and other sources. However, this is not enough to support high levels of exercise.

The fuel for long-term exercise is fat. The body has massive stores of fat (too massive in many of us!), enough to keep us running for days. However, it can only be converted into ATP relatively slowly, although training can increase this rate (see the chapter on training). Fats (triglycerides) are broken down to fatty acids and glycerol. The relatively small amounts of glycerol can be metabolised as carbohydrate. The larger amounts of fatty acids need to undergo beta-oxidation ending up with acetyl-CoA. Acetyl-CoA is the fuel for the TCA cycle, so enters the mitochondria and undergoes breakdown to CO_2 and water, yielding lots of ATP in the process.

The way muscle fuel sources change with time is summarised in Figure 2.

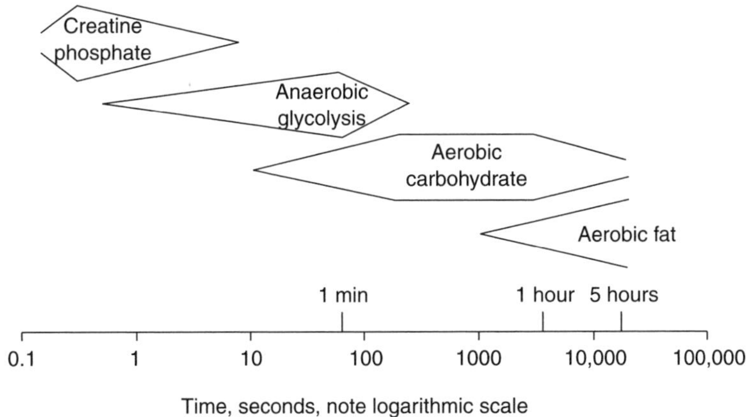

Figure 2 Succession of fuels used during exercise of different duration.

The sequence of fuel use has some clear implications for sports performance. Firstly, it is clearly essential for endurance athletes (events lasting more than 60–90 minutes) to maximise carbohydrate availability. So "carbohydrate loading", e.g. having some big pasta meals in the 72 hours before an event, is useful. Also, drinking carbohydrate-containing fluids during an endurance event can contribute significantly to performance duration.

It might appear from the above that if one is exercising to reduce body fat, it is necessary to do so for more than an hour continuously to burn significant amounts of fat. This is not the case. We may burn little fat during the actual exercise if doing this in 20–30 min bursts. However, we are reducing overall energy stores, and in replacing these fat will be used. In fact, the relation between physical activity and weight control is complex and probably an important aspect is that physical activity improves appetite control, helping to balance energy intake and energy expenditure.

Motor control

Although the properties of muscle tissue itself are crucial, several aspects of performance in sport and exercise depend importantly on the way this tissue is controlled. The motor unit comprises the currency of motor control. This consists of a single alpha motor neurone plus all the muscle fibres to which it connects. A single motoneurone action potential will excite every one of these fibres, so the motor unit is the smallest control element available to the nervous system. A motor unit may consist of just ten fibres in muscles specialised for fine control (e.g. extra-ocular muscles), but is typically 1000–3000 in the large limb muscles. All the fibres in a single motor unit are of the same type (S, FR or FF).

The link between motor nerve fibres and muscle is the motor end plate. In sport and exercise situations this appears to perform reliably as a one-to-one path for excitation. However, there are some fatigue situations where a degree of neuromuscular block may occur.

The motoneurones themselves are the final path for central nervous system motor control signals. Voluntary contractions involve motor cortex and the pyramidal (corticospinal) tract. Involuntary reflex control involves mainly inputs from muscle and joint proprioceptors and from the vestibular system, crucial for maintaining basic postural stability. There is also important protective feedback from high threshold nociceptors in muscles and joints that limit muscle force (for example during eccentric contractions). Locomotion is largely involuntary, involving automatic circuits at brainstem and spinal levels.

Motor learning is an important part of all sports and exercise training. A key structure here is the cerebellum, but basal ganglia and cerebral cortex undoubtedly are also involved. Finally, a key issue in motor performance is motivation and "psyching oneself up". Here cortical and limbic circuits must be crucial.

Fatigue

Muscular fatigue is often the limiting factor in sports and exercise performance. So establishing the basis of this phenomenon has occupied much research. Apparently excessive fatigue is a problem about which health professionals are often consulted. This section will cover central and peripheral mechanisms of fatigue directly related to exercise. The more generalised phenomenon of chronic fatigue will not be addressed. Aspects of chronic fatigue are seen in unexplained underperformance syndrome (UUS) and are discussed in the chapter on UUS.

Fatigued muscles show characteristic falls in peak force and in speed of contraction. Power, the product of these two, is profoundly reduced. The time course of individual twitch contractions is also prolonged due to a slowing of relaxation. The causes of these changes are multiple and will first be considered for different durations of exercise. But one aspect of fatigue is worth pointing out. It is never due to ATP depletion. ATP never drops below 70% of the resting level. Clearly ATP levels must remain high as it is essential for many functions in the cell and for the maintenance of cell integrity.

For maximal efforts up to 1 hour or so the principal factor in fatigue appears to be accumulation of end products from muscle contraction, notably inorganic phosphate ions. Accumulation of phosphate, one of the products of ATP splitting during cross-bridge cycling, will directly inhibit further ATP splitting. In addition, there is evidence that accumulation of phosphate also interferes with excitation–contraction coupling, reducing calcium release during excitation (Westerblad and Allen 2002).

For endurance exercise, accumulation of phosphate and other ions appears to be less important. Here the problem is running out of glycogen. Supplies of glycogen and glucose are limited. Parallel carbohydrate metabolism is also needed for lipids to enter the TCA cycle and be oxidised. Thus, as mentioned earlier, athletes pre-load with carbohydrate before endurance events and drink carbohydrate fluids during them.

We recover quickly from the immediate fatigue following exercise, but only up to a point. After strong exercise there is a lingering fatigue for several days. During this phase, maximum muscle contractions are possible but require more effort. Electrical stimulation experiments show that muscles respond normally to high frequency (>50 Hz) stimulation, but have reduced force generation at lower frequency. Hence the term "low frequency fatigue" for this phenomenon. This is actually not a very good term as it implies that low frequency stimulation produces the fatigue, which of course is not the case: maximal high frequency stimulation is the usual trigger. Westerblad and Allen propose that we use the term "delayed low-frequency recovery" (DLR) instead. The mechanism of DLR may be micro-trauma leading to interference with excitation–contraction coupling. If this is the case, then it is similar to the muscle weakness seen following eccentric contraction (part of the diffuse onset muscle soreness, DOMS, phenomenon).

Central fatigue

It is well recognised that during a fatiguing voluntary contraction if you shout encouragement to the competitor there is usually an increase in force. This phenomenon can be studied more precisely using the twitch interpolation technique where a maximal shock is applied to the muscle motor nerve during a voluntary contraction. Such experiments show that voluntary activation often fails to evoke a maximum contraction, and this is more often true in fatigue. A more subtle aspect of changing motor control in fatigue is that the motor unit firing frequency falls, but usually only by enough to allow for the fall in tetanic fusion frequency caused by the slowing of relaxation time in a fatigued muscle. The causes of these changes in motor control during fatigue are not well understood, but presumably depend in large part on feedback from sensory receptors in the muscle.

In summary

- Muscles produce most power at approximately one-third of their maximum force production.
- Contractions may be concentric, isometric or eccentric (force production during muscle lengthening).
- There are three quite distinct fibre types in skeletal muscle: slow twitch fibres (I or S), fast, fatigue-resistant fibres (IIa or FR) and fast fatiguing fibres (IIb or FF).
- Different fuels are used for exercise of different durations: anaerobic glycolysis for up to 2 min; oxidation of carbohydrate as the main fuel from about 2 min; additional oxidation of fats for exercise exceeding around 1 hour.
- Motoneurones form the final path for neural motor control and a single motoneurone can innervate up to 3000 muscle fibres, all of the same fibre class.
- Fatigue is a complex phenomenon involving both muscle factors (slower contraction of lesser force caused largely by accumulation of inorganic phosphate), lack of carbohydrate fuel for prolonged exercise, and reduction in neural drive.

Further reading

Spurway NC. In: RJ Maughan (Ed) *Basic and Applied Sciences for Sports Medicine.* Oxford: Butterworth Heinemann, 1999; Chapter 1.

Westerblad H, Allen DG. Recent advances in the understanding of skeletal muscle fatigue. *Current Opinion in Rheumatology* 2002; **14**: 648–52.

Nerve injury – overview of peripheral nerve injuries

O Haddo

Morphology

Peripheral nerve trunk

Made up of highly organised fascicles and blood vessels, surrounded by thick connective tissue (epineurium).

Fascicle

Made up of several axons surrounded by perineurium.

Axon

A protoplasmic extension of the neuron.

It may be myelinated (one axon to one Schwann cell, surrounded by endoneurium) or unmyelinated (one Schwann cell to several axons, no endoneurium).

Schwann cells
These are glial cell responsible for myelination.

Myelin
Made up of 70% lipid and 30% protein.

It affects speed of action potential conduction. It is interrupted at regular intervals by Nodes of Ranvier.

Blood supply
Intrinsic – complex plexus within the connective tissue.
Extrinsic – longitudinal vessels on the surface of the nerve and running along its course.

Conduction
Afferent – From sensory receptors to central nervous system (CNS). Receptors found in skin and muscles (somatic) or in viscera (visceral)
Efferent – From CNS to periphery. To skin, muscles and joints (somatic) and autonomic (sympathetic and parasympathetic)

Pathology of nerve injury

Wallerian degeneration
This refers to the degeneration of myelin and fragmentation of the axon, distal to the injury site. The Schwann cells undergo proliferation and play a role in the clearance of debris and in the regeneration process.

A similar process occurs at the proximal stump, but only up to the next Node of Ranvier.

Regeneration
After some time, the proximal axon sprouts buds that work their way through the proliferation of Schwann cells and, in the absence of obstruction at the injury site, enter the endoneural tube of the distal end of the nerve. Regeneration occurs at a rate of 1 mm/day. In the presence of discontinuity, these buds clump together to form a neuroma.

Classification

Seddon (1943)
Neurapraxia – this refers to a reversible conduction block with selective focal demyelination. This is not a degenerative lesion.
Axonotmesis – this refers to injury to the axon and myelin, but with an intact epineurium. This is a degenerative lesion.
Neurotmesis – this is also a degenerative lesion and refers to complete loss of continuity of a nerve fibre.

Sunderland (1951)
1st degree – conduction block as with neurapraxia.
2nd–4th degrees – refer to worsening degrees of axonal damage.
5th degree – complete anatomical disruption to the nerve.

However, distinguishing between the various stages can be very difficult initially and may only be possible with nerve exploration or after a long time from the injury.

A useful classification is to divide nerve injuries into *non-degenerative* and *degenerative* lesions. This concept was brought to light by Thomas and Holdorff in 1993:

Focal conduction block
Transient – ischaemic, other.
Persistent – demyelinating.

Axonal degeneration
With preservation of basal laminal sheaths.
With partial section of a nerve.
With complete transection.

Clinical features

In the assessment of patients with nerve lesions, the mechanism of injury and the energy involved is an important factor in determining the extent of nerve lesion.

Neuropathic pain has implications on the type of lesion. In general terms, pain is present in partial nerve lesions, but absent with complete lesions.

Examination should include assessment of sensation in the distribution of the affected nerve, to include light touch and pinpoint sensation as well as two-point discrimination. Muscle power assessment is in accordance with the MRC grade.

Sympathetic dysfunction usually presents as warm and dry skin, secondary to loss of vascular tone and sweat secretion.

Tinel's sign is indicative of the presence of bare axons, which are easily stimulated by the tapping action over the nerve. It can be used to identify the level of injury, but also nerve regeneration as it progresses distally with time.

Allodynia refers to the experience of severe pain with normal stimulus. This occurs in cases of pre-ganglionic nerve injuries, where nerve activities within the dorsal root ganglion persist.

In situations of severe trauma associated with nerve injury, patients are treated with ATLS protocol, taking into consideration other injuries including cardiorespiratory, skeletal and vascular.

Investigations

Electrophysiological studies can provide important evidence on the type and site of nerve lesion. They can also act as prognostic indicators.

Repeat studies can be useful in assessing amount of recovery.

Other investigations include plain radiographs, magnetic resonance imaging and angiograms for assessment of associated injuries.

Non-operative management

In the case of suspected focal conduction block (neurapraxia), the doctor may choose to adopt conservative measures. These include careful observation for signs of recovery and regular physiotherapy to maintain a passive range of movement of the affected joints.

This is an acceptable option, as the prognosis for recovery with neurapraxia is very good. It is important, however, to keep a close eye on the patient, with careful documentation of their existing neurology.

If there are no signs of recovery within the initial weeks (maximum 6 weeks), or if there is any doubt as to the type of nerve injury sustained, then surgical exploration is recommended, as per the indications below.

Nerve exploration

This is highly skilled surgery and requires specialised expertise and equipment.

The aims of surgery on nerves are:

(1) to establish diagnosis
(2) to remove cause of compression, whether external or internal
(3) to repair or graft a severed nerve

The indications for surgery include the presence of nerve lesion with:

(1) open wounds
(2) surgery or injection
(3) high energy injuries
(4) associated arterial injury
(5) closed fracture requiring urgent reduction and internal fixation
(6) worsening symptoms
(7) failure to progress within expected time
(8) persistent neuropathic pain
(9) severe traction injury

Surgery is, however, only one step in the management of patients with peripheral nerve injuries. A multidisciplinary approach is required, with the aim of achieving pain-free, adequate functional recovery, in order to allow reintegration into work and society. This process requires a lot of time and hence the need for specialised units to deal with such injuries.

Further reading

Birch R, Bonney G, Wynn Parry CB. *Surgical Disorders of the Peripheral Nerves.* New York: Churchill Livingstone, 1998.

Nerve entrapment syndromes – upper limb

P Thomas

Suprascapular nerve entrapment

The suprascapular nerve supplies sensation to the posterior aspect of the shoulder and acromioclavicular joint. It innervates the supraspinatus and infraspinatus muscles. It is a repetitive injury with stretching of the infraspinatus branch, as seen in volleyball players, producing wasting of the infraspinatus muscle. EMG and nerve conduction studies will confirm diagnosis.

Management will consist of rest and also corticosteroid injection at the suprascapular notch. If conservative management fails then surgical treatment is indicated.

Median nerve entrapment

Anterior interosseous syndrome

It occurs after strenuous repetitive elbow exercises. The nerve can be compressed by the pronator teres or flexor digitorum superficialis. The nerve does not carry any sensory branch so the changes are only motor related. Weakness of the flexor pollicis longus and index finger profundus will result in weakness of the interphalangeal joint of the thumb and distal phalangeal joint of the index finger. The athlete is unable to make a circle using his thumb and index finger together.

The management consists of rest and splinting of the extremity. If this fails then surgical decompression of the nerve will follow.

Carpal tunnel syndrome

It affects sports with repetitive flexion and extension of the wrist.

Anatomically the carpal tunnel accommodates the medial nerve, the finger flexors in one sheath and flexor pollicis longus in a separate sheath. Irritation of the synovial sheath covering the tendons can produce swelling and oedema, which increases the pressure on the medial nerve.

The discomfort is described as "pins and needles" which wakes the individual in the middle of the night and he or she has to shake the hand to find relief. Tinnel's test and Phalen's test are usually positive.

Treatment consists of splinting in slight extension for up to 1 month. The tunnel can be injected with a corticosteroid substance. If conservative management fails then surgical decompression will follow.

Ulnar nerve entrapment

Ulnar tunnel syndrome

The deep branch of the ulnar nerve itself can be compressed at the ulnar canal or at the hamate carpal bone region (racquet sports, golf, cricket, baseball and hockey).

Symptoms could be only motor, sensory or mixed. Numbness of the little finger, inability to hold a piece of paper between thumb and index finger (Froment's sign) are common clinical features. Management consists of splinting, anti-inflammatories and rest. If this fails after a period of six months then surgical decompression is recommended.

Cyclist's palsy

Leaning on the handlebars for extended periods of time can lead to swelling in the hypothenar area. Padded gloves, varying riding positions, soft padded protection of the handlebars will assist with recovery.

Bowler's thumb

It represents compression of the ulnar digital nerve of the thumb whilst gripping the ball. Numbness, tingling or pain is present at the medial aspect at the base of the thumb. The management consists of rest, anti-inflammatories, cryotherapy, splinting and corticosteroid injection.

Radial nerve entrapment

Distal posterior interosseous nerve entrapment

It occurs in gymnasts with repetitive wrist dorsiflexion that may compress the nerve as it is entering dorsally to the wrist capsule. Symptoms consist of deep dull ache with forceful wrist extension. A different diagnosis is carpal instability. Treatment consists of activity modification, rest and splinting.

Superficial radial nerve entrapment

The nerve can be compressed at the wrist between the extensor carpus radialis longus and branchioradialis with repetitive pronation and supination as in throwing and rowing sports. It also can occur if gloves are strapped too tight. A burning type of pain in many cases is present during the night and there may be sensory changes over the dorsal radial aspect of the wrist and hand affecting the dorsal thumb and index fingers. Tinnel's test is positive but Finkelstein's test is negative. Treatment will consist of rest, anti-inflammatories, splinting and modification of the sport activities.

Further reading

Lichtman DM (Ed) *The Wrist and Its Disorders*. Philadelphia: WB Saunders, 1988.
Nicholas JA *et al.* (Ed) *The Upper Extremity in Sports Medicine.* Mosby, 1990.

Nerve entrapment syndromes – lower limb

O Haddo

The term "entrapment neuropathy" applies to compression or tethering of nerves within their normal course, as they pass through an area of anatomical susceptibility. In fact this term may be seen as an extension of compression neuropathies.

Certain factors can lead to focal nerve lesion and the onset of symptoms in entrapment neuropathy. These factors may be internal or external or a combination. External factors include pressure onto a vulnerable area. Internal factors may be intraneural (e.g. intraneural lipoma or intraneural changes arising from conditions such as alcoholism or diabetes) or extraneural (e.g. tumours or malunion post fractures).

Pathology

It is thought that pressure on a nerve causes ischaemia, leading to oedema. This, in return, leads to further increase in pressure.

The pressure effect causes demyelination, and eventually axonal loss (large axons are preferentially affected).

This leads to a decrease in the velocity of nerve action potential through areas of compression.

Fibroblasts invade into the oedema, laying down collagen and causing connective tissue thickening.

Meralgia paraesthetica

This relates to the entrapment of the lateral cutaneous nerve of the thigh on its course underneath the inguinal ligament.

This condition is rare, with symptoms of pain and paraesthesia on the lateral aspect of the thigh, worsened by prolonged standing, walking and running and relieved by rest. Examination may show tenderness over the inguinal ligament and altered sensation in the distribution of the nerve.

Treatment of persistent symptoms is surgical decompression.

Pudendal nerve entrapment

The pudendal nerve is formed from the 2nd, 3rd and 4th sacral nerves. In its course, it passes between the ischial spine and sacrotuberous ligament, which is the site of possible entrapment.

This condition can be seen in cyclists, especially over long distances, but it may also present without an obvious precipitating factor.

The symptom is that of pain on the affected side of the perineum. Digital rectal examination may show tenderness.

Treatment is either in the form of injection under imaging (usually computer tomography) or by surgical decompression.

The piriformis syndrome

The sciatic nerve exits the pelvis through the greater sciatic foramen, passing deep to the piriformis muscle. In situations of piriformis hypertrophy or excessive muscular activity, the sciatic nerve is at risk of entrapment.

This condition presents with pain, paraesthesia and weakness in the sciatic nerve distribution. Electrophysiological studies can confirm the clinical picture.

Treatment is by surgical division of the piriformis muscle.

The common peroneal nerve

The common peroneal nerve is at risk in its course around the fibula neck.

Pressure on the nerve may occur from a ganglion or other lesions and from entrapment by the arch of the peroneus longus muscle. In the case of athletes, trauma to or around the knee is the main cause for lesions of the common peroneal nerve.

The symptoms include pain and paraesthesia on the lateral aspect of the lower leg. There is also associated weakness in ankle dorsiflexion, big toe dorsiflexion and foot eversion.

In a case of persistence of symptoms, long after the injury to the knee has settled down, surgical exploration and decompression offer good results.

Tarsal tunnel syndrome

The tibial nerve passes posterior to the medial malleolus beneath the medial retinaculum.

A sporting injury to the ankle, soft tissue or fractures, may cause compression of this nerve at this site. This leads to pain and loss of sensation over the first web space or in the sole of the foot.

Surgical decompression relieves symptoms.

Plantar digital nerve entrapment

This is more common in women, usually involving the third web space. The primary symptom is pain in this region and radiating into the toe, which is made more severe by walking. Examination shows tenderness on the plantar aspect of the third web space, or tenderness on compression of all the metatarsals by hand.

The pathology is thought to involve microtrauma against the transverse metatarsal ligament, causing formation of a neuroma.

Injection with steroid may be helpful; otherwise excision of neuroma is required.

Discussion

It is important to emphasise that these syndromes are rare, but they should certainly be considered as part of the differential diagnosis. History and examination are absolutely necessary to give an idea of the possible diagnosis. Electrophysiological studies can be helpful in establishing the diagnosis, as well as pinpointing the site of nerve entrapment.

Non-surgical treatments are available for these conditions. Surgery must not be taken lightly as it is associated with various risks, including persistence of symptoms.

Further reading

Birch R, Bonney G, Wynn Parry CB. *Surgical Disorders of the Peripheral Nerves*. New York: Churchill Livingstone, 1998.

Orthoses in sport

JL Livingstone

Functional foot orthoses are an effective treatment for sports-induced injuries of the lower limb and there is evidence to support the use of orthoses in prophylaxis of injuries that may occur in both professional and amateur athletes.

Clinicians are faced with a wide range of options in terms of orthosis when prescribing treatment modalities for patients.

The choice of device prescribed should depend on careful examination of the patient and discussion of the type of sport and footwear the patient wishes to pursue.

Orthotics

Foot orthotics are insoles that can

(1) Accommodate a deformity or lesion of the foot.
(2) Provide control to the movement of the foot and lower limb.
(3) They can be prefabricated.
(4) They can be custom made to a prescription of a cast of the patient's foot.

The function of the lower limb in sport

In sporting activity the functional mechanics of the lower limb and foot act in a triplanar motion, sagital, transverse as well as frontal.

Posting of an orthosis in one plane of motion has effects due to the structure and function of the subtalar joint (STJ) and mid tarsal joint (MTJ) on the other two planes of motion.

A patient's gait will depend on their sporting activity, the more cutting (sudden changes in direction) involved in a sport the more lateral or medial instability (frontal plane motion) may need to be controlled.

There are inherent differences between walking and running. Walking is a dual support activity, whilst when running only one foot is in contact with the ground at any one point.

Sporting activity can include walking, running and cutting such as in football (soccer) or may predominantly be unidirectional running such as in a marathon; the type of orthosis required will vary accordingly.

The function of the foot is to act as a spring to allow energy transfer to occur through the contact phase of the gait cycle. An orthosis should facilitate effective movement from heel strike through to toe off by allowing for correct alignment of the osseous structure and function of the muscular, ligamentous and fascial systems in the lower limb.

At heel strike the foot should contact the ground in a supinated or varus position. Pronation of the foot and internal rotation of the tibia occurs to shock absorb from heel strike though to mid stance.

Mid stance through to toe off, supination of the sub-talar joint creates a more rigid lever for propulsion.

Dorsiflexion of the first metatarsal phangeal joint instigates the windlass mechanism, a tightening of the plantar aponeurosis, which raises the medial longitudinal arch.

Static assessment of a patient can reveal

- Forefoot to rearfoot alignment.
- Range of motion.
- Limb length measurement.

The static assessment, however, does not necessarily reveal how a person will act in a dynamic situation. Careful assessment of an athlete's gait should always be undertaken before intervention.

The use of slow-motion video analysis allows gait pathology to be highlighted but also allows gait to be viewed in multiple directions simultaneously.

A pressure plate or in-shoe pressure systems show the force and pressure loading of the foot in walking or running.

Sagital plane progression, or rather the ability of force or pressure to travel unimpeded through the foot from heel strike to toe off is often assessed through the use of video and pressure-measuring systems.

Failure of the first metatarsal phalangeal joint (1st MPJ) to hinge at heel lift results in a decrease in loading over the metatarsal head and increased pressure loading over the phalanx, functional hallux limitus. It occurs if the full range of motion is observed in the 1st MPJ when the patient is non-weight bearing but fails to occur upon weight bearing.

Condition treated

Orthoses can address

- Limb length discrepancies that occur in up to 90% of the population (see Bluestone and D'Marco, 1985).
- Prolonged STJ pronation.
- Lateral instability.
- Sagital plane blockage.

Orthoses provide effective and essentially complication-free treatment to a number of lower limb pathologies that occur in sporting activity.

Common conditions in which orthoses are used in the management of the sporting patient include:

Back pain remains one of the more controversial subjects in the context of effective treatment by use of orthoses. Physiotherapists, osteopaths, chiropractors and podiatrists alike embrace the supposition of asymmetry leading to muscular imbalance in the lower back resulting in continual mechanical back pain. Orthoses can increase sagital plane progression by addressing ankle equinus or failure of the first ray to function effectively. Heel raises can compensate for a limb length discrepancy or an ankle equinus, varus posting will limit sub talar joint pronation. Allowing the 1st MPJ to plantarflex in relation to the foot promotes the function of the windlass mechanism and hence facilitates sagital plane progression.

Hip pain has many aetiologies, including trochanteric bursitis and piriformis syndrome. Addressing imbalances in symmetry of gait as well as limiting excessive pronation can be useful in treating hip pain. Excessive pronation of the STJ leads to internal rotation of the tibia placing a strain on both piriformis and the medial structures of the hip, and this can be prevented with orthoses incorporating a rearfoot varus post or medial skive alteration to the cast.

Knee pain has probably attracted the most interest in the efficacy of orthoses in its treatment. Careful diagnosis should be carried out before conservative care is undertaken but orthoses can be effective in treating a range of knee pathology from Patella Femoral disorders through to mild osteoarthritic changes within the knee joint itself. Sagital plane function as well as pronation and supination should be considered.

Lateral ankle instability either as a result of a ligamentous ruptures or strains, commonly to the anterior talo-fibular ligament, or from peroneal subluxation or tendonitis can be addressed effectively acutely with the use of a laterally wedged device. Long-term injuries require more careful consideration of the underlying function of the patient. Excessive pronation of the STJ leads to failure of peroneus longus to function effectively and can lead to lateral symptoms but also failure of the 1st MPJ to function leading to sagital plane pathology.

Achilles tendinosis and plantar fasciitis both should be treated aggressively with physical therapy modalities such as stretches, icing and electrotherapies. The use of orthoses is beneficial in addressing underlying structural pathology but also in providing increased shock absorption. Lateral forefoot or valgus wedging can be used to reduce tension in the plantar aponeurosis, as well as increasing 1st MPJ function allowing the windlass mechanism to function more effectively.

Tibialis posterior tendonitis occurs from overpronation or direct trauma and a medially-posted orthosis will help by allowing healing to occur and can be used to prevent recurrence.

***Metatarsalgia* can occur due to**

- Pressure overloading of the metatarsal heads.
- Strain to the metatarsal phalangeal joint ligamentous structure.
- Stress fractures.

In an overpronated or hypermobile foot the first ray can become ineffective leading to overloading of the second or third metatarsal head. The devices used should address underlying mechanics such as pronation but adaptations such as Morton's extensions (to increase first ray weight bearing) or metatarsal pads (to reduce pressure over the metatarsal heads) can be utilised; a reverse Morton's extension is padding placed under toes 2–5 to cause more plantar flexion of the 1st MPJ.

First metatarsal phalangeal joint (1st MPJ) pathology may be:

- Sesamoiditis.
- Osteoarthritis (hallux limitus/rigidus).
- Hallux valgus.

The 1st MPJ is designed to hinge at heel lift allowing the windlass mechanism to function and raise the medial longitudinal arch. Orthoses prevent failure of this mechanism to occur due to overpronation or can be designed specifically to increase the function of this mechanism. Placing a pad anterior to the 1st MPJ with a cut-out beneath the metatarsal head results in a plantarflexion of the metatarsal in relation to the phalanx (known as a Functional Hallux Limitus pad or Kinetic Wedge). A dancer's pad is padding under the medial arch and second metatarsal head to offload the metatarsal head and is especially useful in sesamoiditis. A Morton's extension pad under the 1st MPJ can be used in hallux limitus or rigidus.

Orthotic prescription

Orthoses restrict or promote motion; if muscular weakness or restriction is not addressed they will only function to a limited effect. The orthosis is a functional device not a crutch; alteration in the patient's motion will require time, and exercises and stretches as part of a rehabilitation programme are also required.

Footwear may need to be adapted or changed to accommodate the devices and like all new shoes a wearing-in process may be required. Orthoses should not be prescribed or changed drastically just before a sporting event, such as an important game, marathon or tournament.

Orthotics may be used to treat an acute or chronic injury. In acute injuries, prefabricated devices can often be modified to provide a quick and effective treatment that allows the athlete to return to sporting activity whilst protecting the traumatised area.

Professional athletes, by pushing their bodies to more extremes will, as a consequence, also wear and use their device more. A child may outgrow the device quickly or indeed as their body grows their mechanics change requiring different prescription.

Acute injury may only require provision of temporary devices, whereas for correction of underlying biomechanical pathology the patient may expect to wear orthoses for the rest of their sporting life.

Initial discussion with the patient should also include whether orthoses will be required for use when not doing their sporting activity.

Orthoses, like footwear, will wear in time; they may need replacement and can be a life-long commitment. Many orthotic laboratories provide insurance programmes to cover the cost of refurbishment or replacement but not practitioner fees and patient time. To this end, both the patient and the practitioner should consider cost, both initial and long term, at the initial stage of deciding on intervention.

The type of sporting activity undertaken is an important consideration when prescribing orthoses. The use of different footwear that will be worn for different activities should also be considered.

It is possible that the patient will require more than one device to accommodate different training and sporting practices or indeed different footwear.

Orthoses can be used to treat tri-planar pathology, such as excessive or prolonged pronation or supination of the sub-talar joint through the gait cycle or to deal with specific pathology, such as an inversion strain.

Footwear can also dictate the type of device in terms of function; if the patient requires additional shock absorption the orthosis can be used to provide this in a shoe that would not normally provide a decrease in force.

Footwear should always be fitted around the orthosis and the foot. Previously-used footwear, whether they be custom-made football boots, a favoured trainer size and style may no longer be comfortable when used in conjunction with a device designed to change the function of the foot or lower limb.

Manufacture of orthoses

Orthoses can be manufactured from a cast taken of the patient's foot or can be a prefabricated device. Various casting techniques exist for the manufacture of custom-made functional devices (see Figure 1).

(1) Sub-talar joint (STJ) neutral cast. The STJ is held in the neutral position and a plaster of paris impression is taken. This is the most favoured method used by podiatrists.
(2) Weight-bearing cast.
(3) Semi-weight-bearing casts.
(4) In-shoe casts.

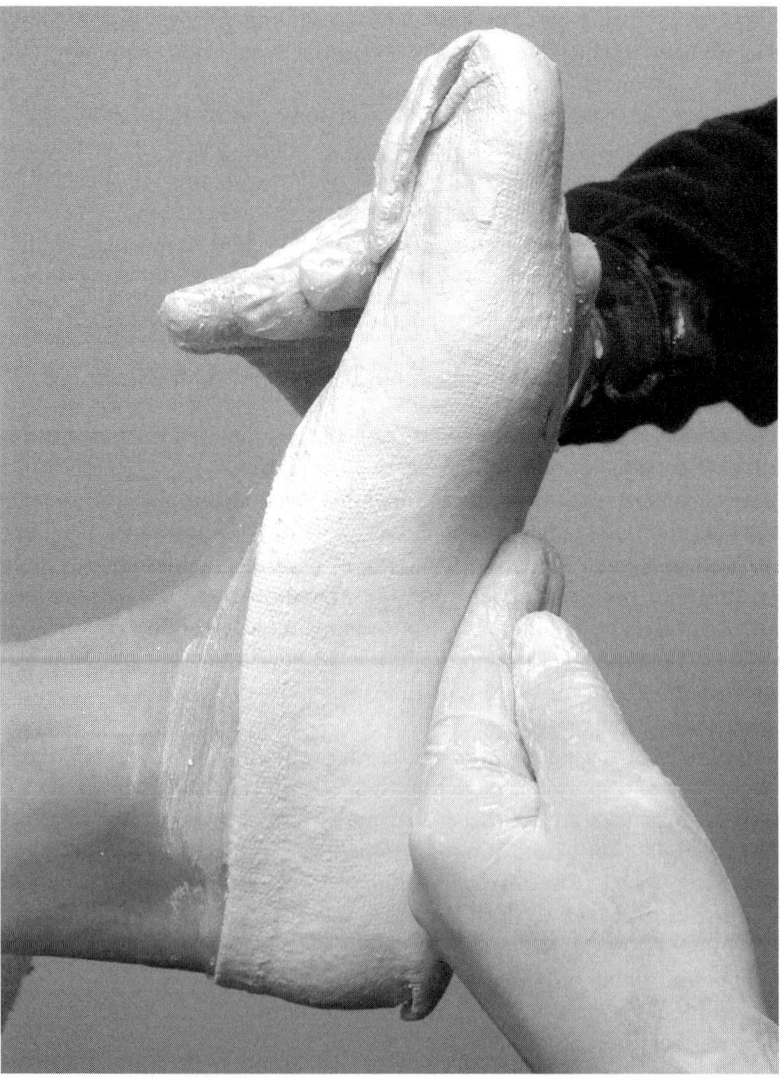

Figure 1 Orthosis casting technique.

The choice of shell material requirements depends on:

(1) How rigid a device should be.
(2) How comfortable it will feel on initial usage.
(3) How much shock-absorbing quality is required.

The more rigid the device the more control of motion that can be exerted in relation to frontal plane mechanics. A rigid device is often not tolerated by the athlete as the foot and leg undergo multiple changes in direction and speed during sporting activity.

Semi-rigid materials such as

- ethylene vinyl acetate
- polypropylene
- carbon fibre

are commonly used to provide control whilst allowing for the flexibility required in sport.

The softer the shell material, the less the longevity of the device. One solution is to provide a reasonably rigid shell material and use a top cover of a softer material. Leather has been used but combinations of leather; open or closed cell rubber or neoprene top covers can be used to increase shock absorption (see Figure 2).

Heel cup depth is an important consideration. The deeper the heel cup the more rearfoot control can be exerted both on the medial and lateral column. In a UCBL (University of California Biomechanics Laboratory) device (see Figure 3), limitation of rearfoot motion is achieved through a deep heel cup. This would not be suitable for the vast majority of sporting activity, as some rearfoot motion should be allowed for changes of direction. In a shallow depth heel cup the patient will find it easier to accommodate the device into shoes. Heel cup depth also affects its width, the deeper the heel cup the wider the device.

Additions and modifications can be used to provide:

(1) comfort
(2) offload pressure
(3) increase the function of a device

Metatarsal pads or bars can be used to offload pressure on metatarsal heads as well as causing toes to plantar flex.

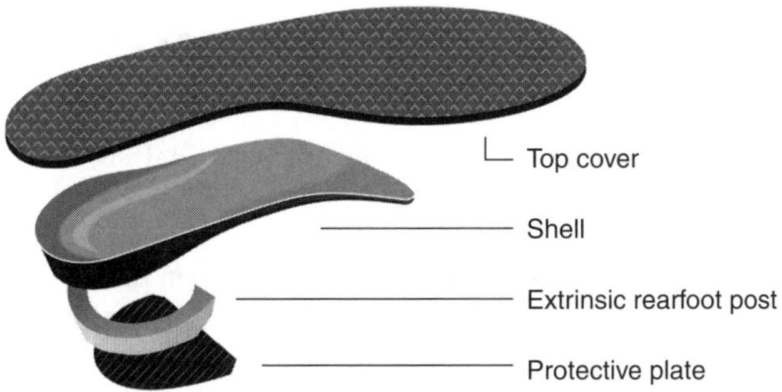

Figure 2 Anatomy of orthosis.

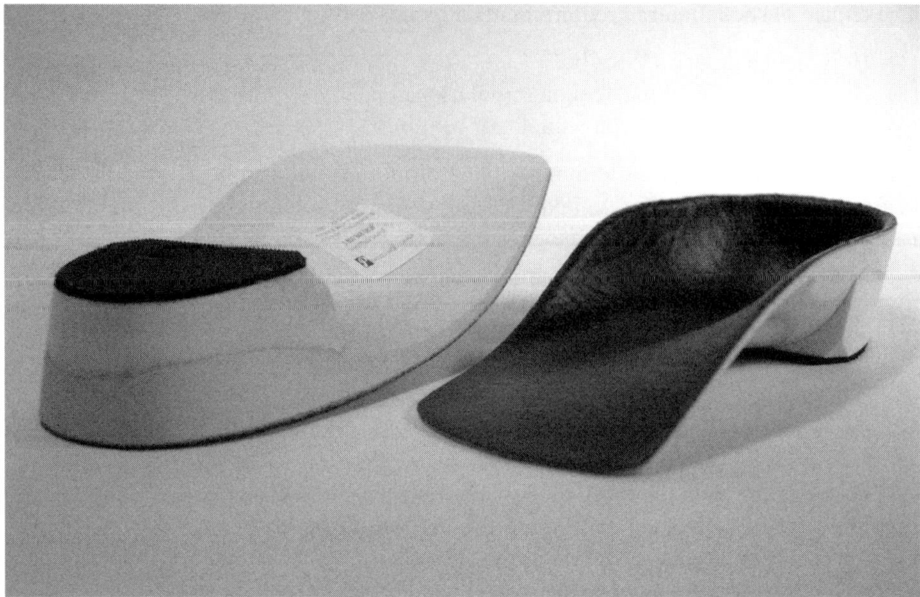

Figure 3 Picture of UCBL orthosis.

Specific pads can be incorporated into a device to offload a lesion such as a corn.

Modifications can be used to increase first-ray function: these commonly include first metatarsal or ray cut-outs to the shell or a plantar facial groove built into a shell.

A cuboid pad will stabilise the calcaneo-cuboid joint, which also ultimately will result in an increase function of the 1st MPJ.

A Morton extension (a pad extending under the 1st MPJ) is used to limit 1st MPJ motion, which is especially useful in arthritis of the 1st MPJ.

A reverse Morton extension extends under the second to fifth metatarsals to toes and results in increased 1st MPJ function.

Troubleshooting orthoses

Whilst an orthotic is very effective at treating sporting injury, problems with their use and prescription do occur.

On issue, the patient should be assessed with the device both non-weight bearing and weight bearing for fit as well as to check accurate location of modifications and additions.

Gait analysis, both slow-motion video and pressure analysis, can also be used to assess the function of the device.

Orthoses should be comfortable; an athlete cannot be expected to perform at their best if they are constantly thinking about a lump or bump in their shoe.

Heel cup depth is vitally important to the function of any orthosis, too narrow and the foot does not sit inside the device, leading to a lack of control and function.

If the orthosis limits too much motion of the lower leg, it can result in torsional forces that lead to muscular pain or indeed irritation of anatomical bursae.

Mechanical back pain can occur as a natural aspect of any change in function that occurs in the treatment of sports injuries.

Reduction in the use of the device initially should resolve the pain, allowing its use to be increased over time.

Stretching and exercises also play an important role in prevention of muscular pain when first wearing orthoses.

Iliotibial band syndrome can occur due to over-correction of pronation or restriction of motion of the foot.

Trochanteric bursitis (lateral hip pain) or pes anserinus bursitis (anterior medial knee pain), where inflammation occurs, can be due to the orthosis trying to cause motion that has not previously been commonplace in an athlete's gait.

Casting the foot inaccurately or an incorrect prescription can lead to blisters and callosity, the device not functioning appropriately or pain.

Common sites for blisters and callosity are under the 1st MPJ, the medial arch or the lateral aspect of the heel. First-MPJ or medial arch blisters can occur from the device failing to allow the first ray to plantar flex, or if the orthotic shell is too long. A first-ray cut out should resolve this issue.

Conclusion

Orthoses are effective, in this author's opinion, in treating a wide range of muscular skeletal disorders of the lower limb that occur acutely or are chronic in the sporting patient. The use of orthoses should be combined with rehabilitation programmes to maximise their benefit and effect. Careful assessment of the patient's underlying mechanical function should be undertaken before prescription is considered. Discussion with the patient regarding their compliance and footwear should be undertaken for successful treatment outcomes to occur.

Acknowledgement

The author would like to thank Paris Orthotics for their kind support in supplying the illustrations used.

Further reading

Bluestone SM, D'Marco JC. Limb length discrepancy, identification, clinical significance and management. *JAPMA* 1985; **75**(4): 200–6.

Nigg BM, Nurse MA *et al.* Shoe inserts and orthosis for sporty and physical activities. *Med & Science in Sport & Exercise* 1999; **31**(7): 421–8.

Osteoarthritis and sport

AA Narvani

The benefits of exercise to health are numerous and well documented. As well as providing entertainment, enjoyment and satisfaction, sporting activity is associated with improved physiological well-being and reduced incidence of osteoporosis and cardiovascular diseases. Furthermore, sport provides a profession for many athletes.

Osteoarthritis (OA) is the commonest disease of the joints and is reported to affect up to 25% of the people over the age of 55 in western societies. As well as having the potential to impose a great amount of suffering for the individual patients, it is a huge burden to the society. It is also a growing problem because it is associated with ageing and people are living longer.

The impact of osteoarthritis is so great, that the question "is sporting activity associated with osteoarthritis?" is one that all sports clinicians will have to answer at some stage of their career.

This chapter will highlight some of the difficulties with answering this question, and aims to provide some ammunition for sports clinicians when they are advising athletes on sports participation and the risks of OA.

Difficulties with studies on sports and OA

The influence of sporting activities on the development of OA is complex because of the following reasons:

(i) Sports covers a huge range of activities, which range from walking to activities that subject joints to tremendous forces, such as American football.
(ii) How is OA diagnosed, e.g. by clinical or radiological assessment?
(iii) Is any influence of sporting activity on the development of OA a direct influence or as a result of an injury that occurred as a consequence of the sport?
(iv) If sport is linked with OA, does this association outweigh the numerous positive influences of sports in physiological and psychological well-being?

The link

Studies that have investigated the link between OA and sports suggest that the risks of joint degeneration is dependent on two important factors:

- joint abnormalities or history of joint injury
- type/level of sporting activity

Joint abnormality or history of joint injury

The presence of joint abnormality or a history of joint injuries is the most crucial risk factor for developing OA. There are a significant number of studies that suggest that all those joints that are unstable, mal-aligned, incongruent, dysplastic, have damaged cartilage, have sustained ligamentous and meniscus damage (knees) or have abnormal proprioception are at increased risk of developing OA. Those athletes with muscle weakness and neurological deficits are also at higher risks of developing degenerative joint changes. It appears that in the presence of such abnormalities and injuries, participation in even low-impact sporting activity leads to increased risks for developing degenerative changes. This is thought to be due to sporting activity preventing optimal healing of the injured joint and causing further damage. It has been suggested that continued joint loading in the immediate period following joint injury may interfere with chondrocyte restoration of their matrix. Similarly, incongruency of the joint caused by different mechanisms leads to amplified shear forces on some parts of the cartilage and therefore increases the risks of developing degenerative changes.

Level of impact and torsional loading

In normal joints, those that have none of the above-mentioned abnormalities and which are not injured, the level of impact and torsional loading becomes a very important factor. There are a number of studies that have shown that, in normal joints, although repetitive running may lead to altered articular cartilage composition and osteophyte formation, it does not lead to joint degeneration (see Buckwalter and Martin 2004). Sporting activities that involve intense impact and torsional activities on the other hand, appear to result in increased risks of OA. These sports include American football, rugby, singles tennis, squash, soccer and basketball. The mechanism for this increased risk of OA in high-impact and torsional-loading sports in apparently normal joints may be the presence of unrecognised joint injury and damage.

Therefore, essentially, the athletes can be divided into four groups:

(i) Athletes with joint abnormalities/injuries who participate in sports that subject the joint to minimal or low impact and torsional loading.
(ii) Athletes with joint abnormalities/injuries who participate in sports that subject the joint to relatively high impact and torsional loading.
(iii) Athletes with no joint abnormalities/injuries who participate in sports that subject the joint to minimal or low impact and torsional loading.
(iv) Athletes with no joint abnormalities/injuries who participate in sports that subject the joint to relatively high impact and torsional loading.

Table 1 summarises the risk of OA in these four groups of athletes.

Summary

The association between sports and OA is difficult to study, nevertheless there appears to be a definite link between sports and OA in abnormal or injured joints.

Table 1 Risk of osteoarthritis in different type of activities.

	Low impact/torsional loading	High impact/torsional loading
Normal joint/no injury	Does not usually lead to increased risk of OA	Increased risk of OA
Abnormal joint/injury	Increased risk of OA	Increased risk of OA

Participation in sports that involve high impact or torsional loading of the joint, even in the absence of joint abnormality or injury, is also shown to increase the risk of OA. Although this possible deleterious influence of sport may not outweigh the many benefits of exercise in most individuals, it is necessary to

(i) minimise impact and torsional loading in athletes (particularly in the presence of joint abnormalities or injury),
(ii) reduce the risk of joint injury,
(iii) address correctable abnormalities.

As well as all sport injuries prevention measures (see the chapter on the prevention of sports injuries), actions that may be taken to achieve the above aims include the change of training programmes, utilisation of special shoes that minimise impact, strengthening of the muscles and even changing the sport of some athletes.

Further reading

Buckwalter JA, Martin JA. Sports and osteoarthritis. *Current Opinion in Rheumatology* 2004; **16**(5): 634–9.

Conaghan PG. Update on osteoarthritis part 1: current concepts and the relation to exercise. *The British Journal of Sports Medicine* 2002; **36**(5): 330–1.

Lievense AM, Bierma-Zeinstra SMA, Verhagen AP, Bernsen RMD, Verhaar JAN, Koes BW. Influence of sporting activities on the development of osteoarthritis of the hip: a systemic review. *Arthritis & Rheumatism* 2003; **49**(2): 228–36.

Osteoarthritis – treatment

AA Narvani

Osteoarthritis (OA) is a multifactorial disease process that is thought to occur as a result of imbalance between degeneration and repair of the articular cartilage. It is an extremely common condition with a huge impact both on the individuals affected and on society as a whole. The aim of this chapter is to highlight briefly the different treatment modalities available, with some examples of where they are utilised. The pathology and clinical features of OA are not discussed here.

Non-pharmacological therapy

Physical therapy

Physical therapy can have a substantial role and is utilised frequently in particular for osteoarthritis of the knee. The aims here are to:

- control pain and inflammation
  —cold/heat therapy
  —ultrasound/diathermy/microwave/shortwave/laser (role of all yet to be proven)

—TENS (transcutaneous electrical neuromuscular stimulation) (further studies required to establish role)

- to improve *range of motion* (see the chapter on Physiotherapy – rehabilitation)
- to improve *muscle strength* (see the chapter on Physiotherapy – rehabilitation). This can be of vital importance as weak lower limb muscles (as seen in many with OA of the knee) results in the reduced ability of these muscles to attenuate potentially injurious impact loading).
- to improve muscle *coordination and balance*

Types of exercise that can be used include:

- isolated isometric, isokinetic and isotonic exercises
- combined exercise programmes
- water exercise (reduces the loading forces on the knee)
- walking
- cycling (further studies are required)

Activity modification

As well as increasing the risks of developing OA, sporting activities that involve intense impact and torsional activities can also enhance the rate of progression of OA (see the chapter on osteoarthritis and sport). Therefore activity modification, including avoidance of sports that involve intense impact and torsional activities, can be very important.

Load modification

The means by which load modification could be achieved include:

- *weight loss*
- *foot orthoses* (controversial)
  —the aim of lateral wedge insoles is to reduce the force on the medial compartment of a varus knee by altering foot biomechanics
  —they may also offer some shock absorption
  —whether or not these are of any benefit is yet to be proven
- *knee orthoses*
  —can aid those with severe deformities and instability
- *walking aids*
  —can be offered to those with knee and hip OA
  —not popular in those who like to pursue sporting activities
- *patella taping* (controversial)
  —may reduce patella–femoral joint loading in those with OA of this joint
  —role yet to be established

Topical modalities

These can be used for the knee as it is quite a "superficial joint". They include:

- *NSAIDs* (many question the efficacy of the topical NSAIDs)
- *Capsaicin*
  —proposed to work by reducing inflammation and attenuating pain pathways.
  —role not established yet

Oral pharmacological agents

- *Non-opioid analgesics*
  —Paracetamol
    —relatively cheap and safe
    —first line agent in many
- *NSAIDs*
  —well-known side effects (including GI ulceration and bleeding, renal, respiratory dysfunction)
  —selective COX-2 inhibitors are associated with reduced risk of GI toxicity; however, there are fears of increased risk of myocardial infarction and stroke with long-term use (see Krishnan *et al.* 2005). Further studies are required.
- *Narcotics*
  —effective analgesics but associated with significant side effects and dependency
- *Glucosamine and chondroitin*
  —constituent components of the hyaline cartilage
  —proposed mechanisms of action include enhanced production of cartilaginous matrix, attenuation of proteolytic activities, and anti-inflammatory action
  —further studies are required on their efficacy
  —so far, studies have shown these to be relatively safe

Intra-articular agents

- *Corticosteroids*
  —commonly used
  —benefits tend to be short lived
  —may have a role in acute flare
  —reports of repeated injection resulting in enhanced cartilage degradation
  —should not be used in the presence of infection
- *Visco-supplementation*
  —hyaluron and hylan derivatives
  —used for knee OA
  —hyaluronic acid is a component of synovial fluid which contributes to its visco-elastic properties
  —most common preparations involve one injection per week for about 4 weeks
  —further research is required on the degree of benefit

Surgical interventions

Arthroscopic debridement

Although arthroscopies of many joints, including shoulder, hip, ankle, elbow and wrist are becoming common practice, the most frequent joint where it is used as a treatment modality for OA is the knee joint. The role of arthroscopic debridement in the treatment of OA, even in knees, remains controversial. Those who benefit most appear to be the ones who also have meniscal tears, unstable chondral flaps and those with less deformity. Arthroscopic debridement could also be by laser and thermal chondroplasty to aid stimulation of fibrocartilage formation, the efficacy of all of which is not established yet.

Abrasion arthroplasty

- The damaged cartilage surface is abraded to bleeding bone.
- The aim is for the bleeding to cause nourishment of the damaged area and formation of fibrocartilage from primitive blood cells.
- Efficacy yet to be proven.

Drilling/microfracture

- Have been used in the treatment of osteochondral defects (OCDs) of the knee and ankle.
- Involves penetration of the subchondral bone by different techniques: drilling or stabbing with an awl for microfracture.
- Aim is to facilitate repair process and formation of fibrocartilage.
- Role in management of OA yet to be shown.

Mosaicplasty

- Also used mainly for osteochondral defects of knee and ankle.
- Involves transplantation of small circular autografts, in a mosaic pattern, into the osteochondral defects.
- The small circular autografts are harvested from a non-weight-bearing region.

Autologous chondrocyte implantation

- A number of studies have been performed on their use for OCDs of knee and ankle.
- It is a two-stage surgical procedure which involves harvesting healthy cartilage cells from a non-weight-bearing area. The condrocytes are sent to a laboratory for culture in order to generate a large number of cells which are then implanted into the defect by different techniques.
- Further research is required.

Osteotomy

- Popular in treatment of uni-compartment OA of the knee
  —Aim is to shift the weight-bearing line from the diseased compartment to the normal compartment and therefore shift the load to the unaffected compartment.
  —Various techniques are available, details of which are beyond the scope of this chapter.
- Osteotomy for hip OA may be suitable for those with relatively early stage OA.

Arthroplasty

Total joint replacement

- Well established for hip and knee with extremely good outcomes.
- Prosthesis also available for other joints including shoulder, elbow, ankle, fingers and 1st MTPJ.

Unicompartmental joint replacement

- Unicompartmental knee replacement has become very popular in recent years for unicompartmental OA. Offers a quick recovery; however appropriate patient selection is of vital importance.

Resurfacing

- Resurfacing arthroplasty of the hip has undergone a resurgence of interest in recent years. Its advantages include:
  —it preserves more bone than standard hip replacement
  —the physiological-sized head enhances stability and range of movement. This makes it ideal for those who intend to pursue different sporting activities (see Narvani *et al.* 2006).

Excision

- Joints where excision arthroplasty as a treatment of OA can be used include the first metatarsal phalangeal joint and the first carpo-metacarpal joint.
- Hip excision arthroplasty (girdlestone) may be indicated in those with severe symptoms in whom other surgical procedures cannot be carried out.

Arthrodesis

- Ankles, subtalar, wrists and toes are common joints where arthrodesis is considered for advanced OA.
- Hip and knee arthrodesis may be considered in a selective population of young, active patients (manual labourers, etc.) with severe OA who are poor candidates for joint replacement (where joint replacement may lead to early failure) and in whom other types of surgeries are contraindicated. It also may have a place in those with a prior joint infection.
- Shoulder arthrodesis can be offered to those with severe symptomatic shoulder OA who are not suited for shoulder replacement.

Further reading

Krishnan SP, Skinner JA, Wilson D. Novel treatments for early osteoarthritis of the knee. *Current Orthopaedics* 2005; **19**: 407–14.

Narvani AA, Tsiridis E, Nwaboku HCI, Bajekal RA. Sporting activity following Birmingham Hip Resurfacing. *International Journal of Sports Medicine* 2006; **27**: 507–9.

Vad V, Hong HM, Zazzali M, Agi N, Basrai D. Exercise recommendations in athletes with early osteoarthritis of the knee. *Sport Med* 2002; **32**(11): 729–39.

Paediatrics – sports medicine

P Thomas

Physical activity during childhood is necessary for normal growth and development. This can be achieved by free play or game activities. The participation of growing children in organized sports activities with set regimes of training has been criticized as it may place an impact on the physiological and psychological growth of the child. However, modern lifestyles and cultures have reduced the traditional "free play" routine and there is a trend for children to obtain physical activity only through organized sports programmes. There is a variability in the physical growth in children of the same chronological age. For example, a group of 14 year olds may contain children with biological ages from 11–17 years. Therefore, there is a mixture of children in any age group with differences in height, weight and even skill development.

Girls are taller than boys and may have greater muscular strength between 11–14 years, due to the earlier onset of a growth spurt. There is no reason to separate the sexes for sporting activity up to 14 years old when strength, height and weight will begin to favour the growing boys.

The maximum aerobic power of a child is nearly the same as an adult; however, the anaerobic power is lower until the age of 14–16 years old. Children have a higher maximum heart rate at rest and exercise compared with adults. The systolic arterial blood pressure is relatively low at rest and exercise. The breathing pattern is shallow with a result of lower absorption of oxygen from the inspired air.

Children are vulnerable to environmental temperature extremes as the sweating mechanism is not fully developed until the adolescence growth spurt. Heat injury may cause a permanent damage to the thermal regulatory system and may cause long-term heat intolerance. Children, in particular those with low fat insulation, lose heat quicker during immersion in cold water.

Psychological maturation in sport must be adjusted to the child's age. In the first 7 years, motor learning will provide the foundations for later acquaintance of skills necessary for sporting performance. In this period, free play will allow the child to practise skills such as running, jumping, swinging and climbing, and therefore the child will improve balance, coordination, proprioception (position sense). After 5–6 years old, children can organize themselves into groups and play more complex games and seek adult approval for their performance and compare it to their peers. A child becomes aware of rewards, self-esteem, achieving goals and gaining the admiration of others. Formal games with rules are appropriate after the age of 8–9 years old. Careful encouragement in effort rather than outcome will avoid the risk of developing the stereotype of the children feeling a failure at the end of a performance.

The most obvious anatomical difference present in a child is the cartilaginous growth plate. The growth plate is vulnerable during vigorous sport. Often the same proportional forces that will cause a rupture of ligaments in adults may cause growth plate injuries instead in the immature skeleton. In addition, very intense strength training in children may cause growth plate damage and deformity. Epidemiological studies suggest that child injury rates are at about 3 per 100 children per year. The injury rate in children below 12 years old is very low; however, there is a sharp increase at the age of 14 in boys and this continues with age in contrast to girls, where the injury rate appears to peak at about 15 years of age. The most common single injury is a sprained ankle joint. Collisions in rugby and football account for more than half of all child injuries.

Prevention of injuries will include the careful application and modification of sport regulations, equipment design for size and skill, protective equipment and footwear, appropriate sports selection for the individual child and experienced coaching staff with a knowledge of child development and sport routines.

Further reading

Micheli CS (Ed) *Paediatric and Adolescent Sports Medicine.* Boston, MA: Little Brown, 1984.

Paediatrics – sports injuries

P Thomas

Head and cervical spine

Head and neck injuries are extremely rare in children below 11 years old; however, there is a dramatic increase in the 15–18 year old group, including most of the fatalities and permanent spinal cord injuries. Children younger than 10 years old have a relative high incidence of atlantoaxial type of damage while the older children may suffer a subaxial injury.

At the field site, the medical team is responsible for determining the status of the neurovascular system and also for providing safe transport to the nearby hospital. A cervical spine collar should always be worn during any transfer to hospital.

Particular care should be taken when children with Down's Syndrome take part in sporting activities. Down's Syndrome is associated with an increased atlantoaxial instability. In children where lateral flexion/extension X-rays show an abnormal odontoid or excursion of more than 4–4.5 mm then advice should be provided to restrict these children from certain sports.

Pre-participation screening must assess the range and symmetry of cervical spine movement. The Klippel–Feil syndrome with two or more cervical vertebrae that are fused will reduce the range of the cervical spine movement and increase the risk of injury. In these children, radiological assessment must follow.

Thoracic and lumbar spine

Acute injuries and fractures at the thoracolumbar spine in children are very rare but they follow a similar pattern to those occurring in the adult population.

There is a distinct difference between children and adults when overuse stresses apply over the spine. In children the stress primarily concentrates at the posterior elements of the vertebrae at the pars intrarticularis, facets and pedicles. In contrast, in adults the overuse stress is applied anteriorly with progressive degeneration of the intervertebral discs before the posterior vertebrae elements are involved.

Although there is a genetic predisposition in the occurrence of spondylolysis, it seems these injuries are, in effect, stress fractures. The early diagnosis of this condition is essential to prevent a complete fracture and a non-union that may follow. In a young athlete with a history of repetitive extension activities and the presence of pain with extension of the spine, in particular on single leg extension testing, then spondylolysis must be suspected. A bone scan and CT scan can confirm the diagnosis before the fracture occurs. The treatment before fracture will include rest from sport, antilordotic braces and, recently, the intravenous injection of parmidronate biphosphonates has been introduced to achieve an early resolution. When a non-union develops then surgery will be considered.

Disc herniation may occur in children. Young people with short pedicles and narrow neuroforamina have an increased risk of suffering a disc hernia during sports. An MRI scan can confirm the diagnosis. Conservative management is successful in most cases with relative rest, physiotherapy protocols of exercises and, on occasions, supportive bracing.

Shoulder

Young athletes practising in swimming and throwing sports may suffer from repetitive stresses which can result in a subsequent tightening of posterior structures of the glenohumeral joint, increased mobility of the scapulothoracic region, anterior subluxation of the glenohumeral joint with symptoms simulating anterior instability and rotator cuff impingement. Rotator cuff tears are rare in young athletes.

A multiaxial instability of the shoulder can be demonstrated in some young athletes. Clinical testing of the shoulder in different directions may confirm a combination of more than one direction of instability. Management will include strengthening and balance programmes for the major muscles around the shoulder since surgery is rarely if ever required.

Elbow

A fall on the hand with the elbow bent can lead to a supracondular fracture of the elbow. The humerus fractures above the condyles and the distal fragment with the forearm rotates and is pushed backwards in most cases. An urgent reduction under anaesthesia is required. A displaced fracture can cause an associated injury to the brachial artery or the radial and medial nerves. Even after reduction in some patients, when the elbow is flexed the swelling may cause reduced circulation of the forearm and pulses in the periphery may be absent. Early correction of the elbow in a more extended position will assist in restoring the circulation distally.

Racket sports or those sports that involve fast striking of a ball, e.g. cricket or baseball, with repetition can cause a number of pathological events around the elbow – a condition known in American literature as the "little leaguer's elbow" (see chapter on Elbow – throwing injuries). Typically it will include a range of traction injuries at the medial epicondyle, an impaction injury on the lateral aspect of the elbow, osteochondritis dissecans, loose bodies and premature arrest of the medial physis. Both CT and MRI scans will be diagnostic. The treatment consists of arthroscopic multiple drilling of the osteochondral defects and removal of the loose bodies. This will be followed by a lengthy rehabilitation programme and absence from sport. Finally, when the medial epicondyle physis is fused, in many of these cases the symptoms will resolve.

Wrist and hand

The young gymnast who practises floor work, the repetitive impaction and dorsiflexion of the wrist can be responsible for a premature closure of the distal radius physis and, later on, the development of a Madelung-type situation with positive ulna variance and distortion of the distal radioulnar articulation.

A fall onto the outstretched hand can cause a distal forearm fracture. The location of the fracture will depend on the age of the child: very young children will fracture the forearm at the junction of the diaphysis to metaphysis; near puberty the same injury could cause a fracture through the radial physis (the Salter–Harris classification with types from 1–5 will be used). Later on, in the young athlete after puberty, the same mechanism of injury will cause either a fracture of the radial metaphysis and ulna or a scaphoid.

Hip and pelvis

The most common group of injuries occurring in the young athlete are an apophyseal avulsion of a muscle group which inserts into the pelvis or proximal femur. These groups are as follows:

- Anterior superior iliac spine and sartorius muscle
- Anterior inferior iliac spine and rectus femoris
- Iliac crest and abductors and lateral abdominis
- Ischial tuberosity and hamstrings
- Lesser trochanter of femur and iliopsoas

The above injuries are commonly seen in mid-adolescence, coinciding with periods of relative rapid growth. The majority are treated by conservative means; however, large avulsions at the ischium may be treated by a surgical reduction and fixation, or, if they are diagnosed later on when non-union has already occurred, then excision of the non-united fragment will relieve the irritation of the sciatic nerve.

Field sports practising on hard surfaces could cause osteitis pubis pain in young athletes. X-rays and bone scans will assist with the diagnosis. Conservative management is usually successful. In young athletes after puberty, intravenous injections of parmitronate biphosphonates have been recently used to promote an early recovery.

A displacement at the femoral physis level or slipped upper femoral epiphysis (SUFE) may occur without any major trauma. Many of these young athletes are obese or sexually underdeveloped and usually there is an endocrine imbalance in their medical background. This condition is seen between the ages of 9–16 years old. The symptom presented in many cases is pain at the lateral thigh and knee joint instead of any hip discomfort. Later on, when the displacement has progressed, then the patient will limp, the leg becomes obviously shorter and rotates externally. Anteroposterior X-rays and "frog view", including both hips, will confirm the diagnosis. The patient must be provided with crutches to non-weight bear and be immediately referred to an orthopaedic surgeon.

Young athletes involved in contact sports may suffer from thigh contusions. The immediate treatment consists of rest, ice and the use of crutches. If a haematoma developes then severe pain will appear. Myositis ossificans is a recognized complication that can occur following attempts of rapid rehabilitation and return to sport after injury. In cases of a haematoma collection visible on an ultrasound scan then an attempt to aspirate it under ultrasound scan, guidance could be considered. In cases where myositis ossificans has developed, then gentle therapy is required to maintain isometric strength and a range of movement of both hip and knee joints until the bone-mass will eventually reunite with the femur below, a process that can take between 6–12 months to complete.

Knee

Fractures and physeal injuries are commonly present in the middle to late adolescence. Salter–Harris types of fracture at the distal femur should be accurately reduced because of the high risk of growth arrest and angular deformity. The same principals should be observed in any proximal tibial physeal fractures which are also common in adolescence. Patella fractures must be distinguished from patella bipartite which is apparent at the superior and lateral aspect of the patella. X-rays of both knees will assist diagnosis.

The incidence of anterior cruciate ligament ruptures has increased in recent years. Similar to the adult, a haemarthrosis is usually present. An avulsion fracture of the tibial spine can usually be seen in young athletes, arthroscopy can determine any displacement and, in such cases, reduction followed by internal fixation will follow. Anterior cruciate ligament disruption in young patients has a poor overall prognosis and some form of reconstruction surgery is recommended in most cases. Before puberty, the accepted routine following an anterior cruciate ligament rupture is careful rehabilitation and protection of the knee until skeletal maturity when surgery will be planned. However, if symptoms of instability and meniscal tears exist, then surgery that must avoid any physeal damage may be considered to provide stability.

Isolated meniscal tears are rare in children and may be associated with anterior cruciate ligament damage. Many of these tears are in the periphery of the meniscus and respond much better to arthroscopic repair compared to the adult population.

Acute chondral and osteochondral injuries will produce a haemarthrosis. If the fragment is large then reduction and internal fixation is indicated.

In acute dislocation of the patella, after reduction, a period of immobilization with the knee in extension will follow. Progressive rehabilitation will provide satisfactory results. An avulsion of the tibial tubercle, which is not displaced, can be treated with immobilization with the knee in extension. However, if the fragment is displaced or involves the articular surface of the tibia then an open reduction and internal fixation will be indicated. The patellofemoral pain, which usually develops at the time of the growth spurt, is usually associated with a tight iliotibial band and a weak function of the vastus medialis. This imbalance will result in a maltracking of the patella and may lead to changes of the patella articular cartilage and functional pain. In the majority of all patients a physiotherapy programme with stretching of the lateral structures and strengthening of the vastus medialis will achieve satisfactory results. In addition, orthotics will address malalignments of the leg and foot and may assist further with the recovery. In the few cases where after 6 months the pain persists because the lateral retinaculum of the patella is tight then arthroscopic lateral release may improve the patella tracking combined with physiotherapy regimes.

Ankle and foot

The ligament attachments of the ankle joint are subphyseal so most ankle injuries involve the physis. Therefore, a sprain of the ankle joint that in adults can cause anterior tibiofibula ligament (ATFL) damage; in contrast, in children it can cause a physeal injury of the fibula, presented with direct pain over the physis, which carries a good prognosis of healing. There are specific ankle fracture patterns that can occur in the juvenile athlete, such as the juvenile Tillaux fracture, which is a Salter–Harris type 3 injury of the partially fused physis of the distal tibia, and also the Triplane fracture, which is a combination of Salter–Harris types 2 and 3 injuries at the distal tibial physis. Awareness of these injuries will lead to X-rays and CT scans to confirm the diagnosis because surgical reduction will be necessary in many of these injuries. Pain at the accessory navicular region can be seen in young athletes. This is caused by the repetitive action of the posterior tibialis tendon attached at the navicular bone. A below-the-knee plaster-cast worn for between 4–6 weeks will allow healing. Appropriate padding inside the footwear to protect the prominent navicular will assist in reducing the irritation in this area of the foot. If conservative management has failed then resection of the accessory navicular bone may need to be considered.

Stress fractures of the distal tibia, calcaneum and tarsal bones may occur in young athletes. A stress fracture of the navicular bone is difficult to diagnose. A bone scan and CT scan may confirm the diagnosis. Immobilization for 8–12 weeks non-weight bearing is necessary to allow healing. The non-union rate is high and surgery with an open approach and bone grafting will be necessary in these situations.

Tarsal coalitions are caused by fibrous cartilaginous or bony bars between the tarsal bones. They are seen between the calcaneum and navicular bones or calcaneum and talar bones. There is a strong family history and they are often seen bilaterally. Although they are present from birth, they start to cause symptoms in adolescence with sport and physical activity. They are associated with a rigid flat foot so it is always important for the examining physician to be aware that a painful flat foot in adolescence may be associated with the presence of tarsal coalitions. Peroneal muscle spasm can also be observed. The foot can be investigated with special weight-bearing X-rays but in most cases CT scans can be diagnostic. In mild cases, a plaster-cast between 4–6 weeks followed by a modification of sport activities will improve symptoms. In severe cases the early surgical excision of the bar is indicated.

Further reading

Salter R, Harris WR. Injuries involving the epiphyseal plate. *J Bone and Joint Surgery* 1963; **45**: 587–622.

Paediatrics – osteochondrosis (osteochondritis)

P Thomas

Osteochondrosis are self-limiting idiopathic disorders of the development of the primary or secondary ossification centres. They represent the most common group of overuse injuries during childhood.

Osgood–Schlatter disease

The repetitive traction by the patellar tendon applied to the tibial tuberosity will cause a partial avulsion of the secondary ossification centre followed by a repetitive cycle of healing and bone accumulation. It represents the most common complaint in young athletes less than 16 years old; it is more frequently observed in boys but also is seen in young girls at around 12 years of age.

The pain is severe at the end or after activity and clinical examination reveals a tender enlargement of the tibial tubercle. At first presentation X-rays are not necessary; however, if the symptoms have failed to subside, or in those athletes who present after the age that ossification and fusion of the tibia tuberosity is expected, then radiological examination is indicated.

The treatment will begin with appropriate counselling and explanation of the condition to the athlete and his or her parents. Programmes to strengthen the quadriceps, balance regimes between quadriceps and hamstring, concentric contractions followed by eccentric exercises and progressive loading will allow the young athlete to return to sport activities. Ice applications after activity will relieve symptoms in most cases. Corticosteroid injections are not indicated and anti-inflammatory treatments are not useful. In the severe case of an avulsion then a complete rest between 3–4 weeks from running is necessary. Plaster-casts or rigid braces are not always necessary in severe cases.

Sinding–Larsen–Johansson's disease

The patellar tendon applies repetitive traction at its attachment at the inferior pole of the patella. In some cases a separate ossicle from the inferior patella may be developed. Prognosis and management are similar to the Osgood–Schlatter disease.

Sever's disease

This is a traction apophysitis of the heel in young athletes between 8–16 years old. The repetitive plantar flexion and impact on the unfused calcaneum apophysis may cause inflammation and microfractures.

The pain usually appears at the end of training and the young patient may limp or walk on the toes. Findings include tenderness over the calcaneum apophysis, gastrocnemeus muscle tightness reducing the ankle dorsiflexion, which in normal circumstances is expected to be at around 15° with the knee straight.

Attention is focused on the footwear, including well-fitted shoes with a firm heel counter and orthotic correction in malalignments. In some cases, a heel raise may be added. Other treatments include strengthening exercises for the foot dorsiflexors, stretching of the tight gastrocnemeus, activity modification and in severe cases even dorsiflexion night splints.

X-rays are not necessary in first presentation. They will usually show fragmentation and sclerotic changes of the apophysis. If the treatment fails to alleviate symptoms then X-rays will be necessary to distinguish between Sever's and other pathologies, such as neoplasm or Brodie's abscess (chronic infection).

Navicular bone apophysitis

This condition presents in adolescence located at the medial and inferior aspect of the navicular bone, usually affecting the accessory navicular bone.

Kohler's disease

This condition presents in young athletes between 4–7 years old affecting the navicular bone, which on X-rays appear sclerotic.

A walking cast for 6 weeks followed by orthotic support will assist with recovery.

Freiberg's condition

This usually affects the epiphysis of the second and sometimes third metatarsal heads. Symptoms usually appear in children older than 12 years of age but sometimes they present in adult life when the degenerative changes of the metatarsophalangeal joint will develop.

X-rays will confirm deformity and fragmentation of the epiphysis with an often flat metatarsal head.

If the diagnosis was made before the closure of the growth plate then deformity may be reduced by modification of physical activity to exclude running and jumping. In addition metatarsal neck supports and wearing shoes without a heel will assist in off-loading the metatarsal heads. In later stages of the condition, in adult life, surgical procedures will be considered in painful situations.

Osteochondritis dissecans

The cause for this disease is unclear, although in some cases repetitive trauma may be associated with this condition.

The history is typically of a male between 10–16 years old with the most common site affected being the medial femoral condyle of the knee joint. The other anatomical sites where the condition could be found include the talar bone, the capitellum at the elbow, the first metatarsal head, and even the head of the femur. At first, the presented complaint is pain after activity but in later stages of the disease where there is a separation of the fragment, then effusion and locking may occur.

X-rays can demonstrate a demarcated area or irregular ossification. An MRI scan can predict the probability of the fragment separation. An increased uptake on bone scan suggests healing and incorporation of the fragment.

Treatment in early stages will include modification of sport activity to prevent separation of the fragment. Arthroscopic drilling can revascularize and stabilize the fragments. If the fragment is loose then early reduction and internal fixation is indicated.

Scheuermann's disease

This condition affects the growth plates of the spine with irregular growth where increased compression forces could lead to secondary angular deformity and kyphosis.

The young athlete presents with pain during and after activity where X-rays will confirm irregularity of the vertebrae body with progressive anterior wedging.

It is usually present during the last years of skeletal growth, so early diagnosis will reduce activity of repetitive flexion of the spine. Physiotherapy programmes will minimize the tightness of the fascia and will strengthen the abdominal muscles. In addition, braces to reduce thoracic kyphosis and decrease lumbar lordosis can be provided, when there is anterior vertebra wedging of more than 5° or the disease affects two or more vertebrae.

Further reading

Michels IJ. Overuse injuries in children's sports: the growth factor. *Orthopaedic Clinics of North America* 1983; **14**: 337–60.

Physiotherapy – general principles

T Betts

The aim of the following chapters is to provide an outline of the general principles of sports injury management. It is intended to be a brief introduction to aspects of acute injury treatment, rehabilitation management and on-field and team physiotherapy.

Initially a description of injury treatment and healing will be given, followed by a description of acute treatments and rehabilitation of muscles. These chapters are not intended to be a definitive guide to injury treatment or a recipe of diagnostic-specific treatments. Instead it is hoped that they provide a stimulus to understanding the goals and main beliefs that guide physiotherapists in sports.

The gradual progressive/stepwise treatment of the injured tissue/limb is based upon the healing status of the injury, acute to sub-acute to chronic, from early tissue damage through to full natural healing. Initially the therapist should determine the appropriate focus for treatment. Following models of clinical reasoning, the therapist can match the treatment to the stage of healing assessed. A working model is suggested below (Figures 1 and 2) which sketches out the differences in healing time of injured tissues. A mental model similar to that suggested can help the therapist plan treatment progressions. The therapist should always ensure that the subjective signs follow the expected treatment phase.

Phase 1 early > control inflammation
Protect injured tissues
Phase 2 Intermediate > initiate loading of injured tissue
Phase 3 Late > progress load and movement
Phase 4 Advanced > sports specific
Return to athletics activities

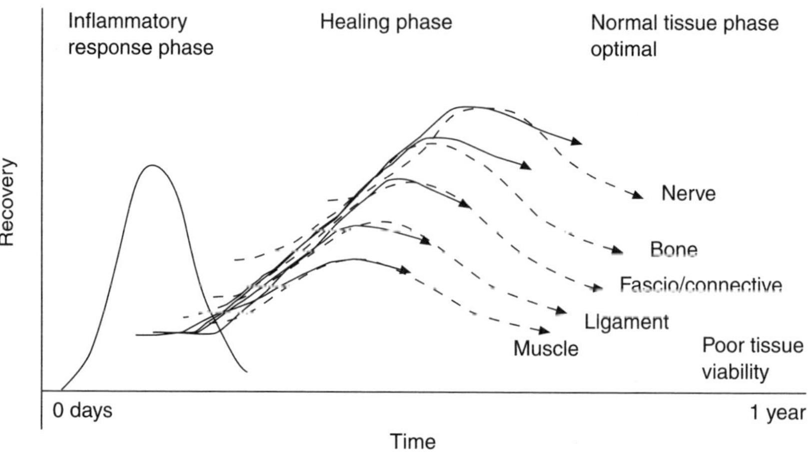

Figure 1 A schematic representation of phases of healing, after tissue injury.

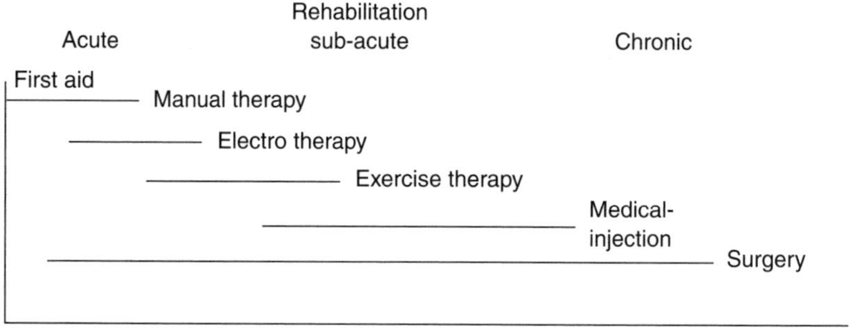

Figure 2 Treatment management approaches from acute to chronic healing.

Treatment should also include:

- Continual r eassessment at each phase
- Goal-directed therapy – incremental – short-term, long-term, daily, weekly, monthly
- Psychological and social support

Measurable (quantifiable) assessment tools

- Motion – goniometre
- Strengthen – oxford scale/dynometer/isokinetic
- Balance – Balance Error Scoring System (BESS) – sway, timing
- Tissue integrity – investigations, stress testing
- Endurance – holding and repetitions
- Functional – SAQ drills – jump and hop tests, throwing and catching

Pre-conditioning programmes

Prior to any sports it is essential that the athlete is physically prepared for the specific sport and is generally conditioned to tolerate the loads of sporting activities. It has been suggested that athletes of all sports should have pre-conditioning programmes that involve specific exercise to optimize physical performance and prevent injuries. Here are a few examples of pre-conditioning exercises specific to joints/body areas based upon promoting joint stabilization.

Aim

Injury prevention, for first-phase rehabilitation and early injury recovery.

Principles

- Low effort
- Low load
- Avoid impact and torsion
- Selective muscle control
- Reduce conscious inhibition of mass movement/muscle actions patterns

Examples

Foot

- Lumbrical strengthening of forefoot
- Medial arch muscle strengthening
- Balance/proprioception exercises

Knee

- Inner range/static quads
- Selective VMO control
- Balance/proprioception

Hip

- Inner range gluteals (isometric)
- Hip abductors – lateral supporters
- Balance/proprioception

Lumbar spine

- Core stabilization training – deep abdominals/deep lumbar muscles/gluteal muscles (pilates)
- flexibility training (yoga)
- postural education (Alexandra technique)

Preconditioning exercise principles

Correct muscle action

- EMG bio-feedback
  —EMS stimulation
  —Palpation

Correct movement control

- Visualization/imaging
- Mirror
- Guidance (move) tactile

The principles of treatment to muscle injury

Grade I
- Initial rest and pain/swelling control methods
- Early motion and early muscle activity
- Progressive return to sports within 1–3 weeks

Grade II
- Initial rest and pain/swelling control methods
- Protection and rest from early motion
- Progressive muscle exercises – isometric/eccentric/concentric/isokinetic
- Progressive return to sports within 3–9 weeks

Grade III
- Initial rest and pain/swelling control methods – surgery?
- Complete immobilization and protection/rest from early motion
- Progressive muscle exercises, initial very low effort/resistance – isometric/eccentric/concentric.
- Progressive return to sports within 12–36 weeks (3 months–9 months)

The principles of treatment to ligament injury

Grade I
- Initial rest and pain/swelling control methods
- Early motion and early ligament stress activity
- Progressive return to sports within 1–3 weeks

Grade II
- Initial rest and pain/swelling control methods
- Protection and rest from early motion
- Progressive ligament stress activities
- Progressive protective muscle exercises – isometric/eccentric/concentric/isokinetic
- Progressive balance and proprioceptive retraining exercises
- Progressive return to sports within 6–9 weeks

Grade III
- Initial rest and pain/swelling control methods – surgery?
- Complete immobilization and protection/rest from early motion
- Progressive ligament stress activities – exercises
- Progressive protective muscle – exercises – isometric/eccentric/concentric/isokinetic. Initially very low effort and resistance muscle training/strengthening.
- Progressive balance and proprioceptive retraining exercise
- Progressive return to sports within 12–54 weeks (3 months–12 months)

Further reading

Kibler WB *et al.* Shoulder rehabilitation strategies, guidelines, and practice. *Orth Clin N Am* 2001; **32**: 527–38.

Magee DJ. *Orthopaedic Physical Assessment.* WB Saunders, 1987; 266–314.

Maitland GD, Corrigan B. *Muscular, Skeletal and Sports Injuries.* Elsevier Health Sciences, 1994.

Physiotherapy – acute injury management

T Betts

To treat an injury immediately after it has occurred, the therapist should follow the principle of **PRICE:**

Protection
Rest
Ice
Compression
Elevation

These principles prevent the initial injury from escalating into a more severe condition by controlling and reducing the extent of the inflammation of the injured tissue and limiting the potential for further trauma caused by moving the tissues too early. They also help provide the physiological environment to achieve optimal repair and healing.

The advice given for "PRICE" is:

Protection

Protect the injured tissue from further damage. This can be achieved with taping, strapping, orthotic supports. For the foot and ankle, air cast supports; for the upper limb, shoulder braces; and for the spine, corsets and/or collars.

Rest

Minimal movement around the injured area is necessary to prevent further damage. The athlete should try to stop any weight-bearing or upper limb movements for 24–72 hours.

Ice

Regular ice packs every 3–4 hours for 10–30 minutes reduces excessive inflammatory tissue flooding the injured tissue site. Ice also helps to reduce pain perception.

Compression

A compression support bandage, such as tubigrip or adjustable neoprene support, helps to keep swelling controlled within the damaged area.

Elevation
The injured limb should be elevated above the heart whenever possible to assist lymphatic damage of inflamed tissues.

Any injury to the body should be treated by the principles of PRICE during the acute phase. Diagnosis is essential to discover the extent of tissue damage (Grades I–III) and the body tissue injured – bone, ligament, muscle, tendon, fascia, nerve, vessels.

The aim is to reduce pain, metabolism, muscle spasm and minimise the inflammatory process. Hard evidence for cry therapy, based on stringent literature review criteria is poor. There are few studies that incorporate rigorous comparisons of treatment deviations and specific protocols based on prospective, randomised blinded studies. However, current guidelines encourage the use of PRICE and practical evidence suggests PRICE encourages the recovery process after injury.

After the acute inflammation stage has been reached, it is important to move onto the next stage of injury management. The next stage is often described as the proliferation/mobilisation phase followed by the remodelling phase. In these phases it is important to begin the gradual process of moving the injured tissue. Initial rest and protection needs to be followed by movements of the tissue to promote the remodelling phase of healing. Mobilisation techniques can be described as:

(1) *Passive* – the limb tissue is moved by an outside force, e.g. including CPM, Maitland.
(2) *Active assisted* – the therapist aids the movements of the limb, which is controlled by the athlete.
(3) *Active* – the athlete is in control of the direction speed and range of movement.

The extent of body tissue damage will dictate the amount of mobilisation allowed. With soft tissue injuries it is imperative that the extent of tissue damage is diagnosed accurately. For example, a classification of soft tissue injuries is:

Grade 1 A minor soft tissue strain or stretch with tissue integrity maintained.
Grade 2 A moderate to substantial tissue damage, partial rupture/tear of soft tissues.
Grade 3 A full rupture of soft tissue fibre between origin and attachment.

Many classifications will sub-divide Grade 2 to give a more precise description of how much tissue tear exists, from 0–100% rupture.

In principle, Grade 1 tears (minor strains) can be managed by early motion/mobilisation after 3–7 days. Movement of a damaged limb in directions that do not cause pain can begin immediately.

For Grade 2 tears, it is important to maintain protection and rest for longer periods of time, 7–14 days or longer if a substantial tear exists. Until the integrity of the tissue damage is restored, movement at this stage can cause further damage, delay healing and lead to long-term dysfunctions.

In Grade 3 ruptures, complete rest and protection is necessary for many weeks or months. Often surgical reconstruction or repair is required to restore tissue integrity and physiological competence.

Having established the extent of the injury, a treatment plan can be developed that dictates the timing and progression of mobilisations to the affected area. The underlying principle is gradual. Progressive movements, which are pain-free (or minimal) throughout the range of motion and that do not overly challenge tissue integrity, should be encouraged. Controlled motion acts as a trigger and guide to the remodelling phase.

Once functional tissue range and/or integrity are restored, strengthening/resistance programmes can begin to provide natural protection to the joints. Stabilisation programmes and sports-specific functional restoration provides the injured tissue with protection in the future prior to the return to sports. Rehabilitation programmes should be guided by physiological principles of tissue injury and repair rates (see Figure 1 in the previous chapter).

The role of electrotherapy in the acute rehabilitation of sports injuries

Ultrasound therapy

Ultrasound is a mechanical vibration, which uses high-frequency acoustic energy to oscillate biological tissues and stimulate healing. This helps accelerate tissue healing by stimulating cellular activity within the inflammatory, proliferation and remodelling phases. Ultrasound stimulates growth factors within macrophages and mast cells (white blood cells) to clear tissue debris accumulated after injury. Ultrasound can be used pulsed and/or continuously. For acute injuries, pulsed ultrasound is recommended, it is non-thermal, and has an analgesic effect. Continuous ultrasound produces heat and is used for chronic injuries. The frequency and intensity of ultrasound is varied according to the stage of the injury, the size of the area of tissue being treated and the type of body tissue.

Interferential stimulation

Interferential stimulation uses low-frequency current produced within tissues, with low skin impedance. This is created by two medium-frequency currents that cross to produce a "beat frequency". The interferential current improves the permeability of muscle and nerve tissue and stimulates the healing process.

Combination therapy

Combination therapy consists of a mixture of interferential stimulation and ultrasound to provide cellular stimulation and tissue fluid flow at lower intensity outputs. Ultrasound can stimulate healing of the ligament while interferential stimulation reduces general capsular swelling.

Pulsed short wave

Pulsed short wave uses magnetic field energy to stimulate cellular activity. Biological research suggests that the process of cellular mitosis is enhanced by the use of pulsed magnetic energy. The transportation of fluid flow across the cell at the surface of the membrane enhances the resolution of inflammatory exudates.

Iontophoresis

Iontophoresis is used to help the penetration of the anti-inflammatory medicine into injured soft tissues or joints. It is the therapeutic process by which pharmacological agents (non-steroidal anti-inflammatories) are transported through the skin into the tissues using electrical currents. This technique can help make the application of the anti-inflammatory medication more effective.

Neuromuscular electrical stimulators

Electrical muscle stimulators work between frequencies of 0 to 50 Hz. Faradic and Russian stimulation currents are two types regularly used. Many companies have produced disease and selective muscle-specific stimulation programmes. The aim is to stimulate weak and atrophied muscles that a patient is unable to activate consciously. In acute injuries or post-surgery, muscle stimulation can maintain muscle activity whilst avoiding placing excessive resistance stress through the joint. In chronic or overuse injuries, muscle stimulators provide a trigger for inhibited and disused muscles.

Electrical biofeedback

Electrical biofeedback uses surface electrodes which are applied to the muscle belly of selective muscles, and the electrical muscle activity is recorded. The information is converted into visual and auditory signals and the patient is able to alter their muscle activity appropriately by volitional control of their muscles. Electromyography is a useful tool to aid with the re-education of pain-inhibited muscles. Because the athlete can see the activity of the muscle being recorded they can adjust and alter the behaviour of the muscle. For muscles that are weak at selective joint ranges or during specific movements the athlete can learn to increase the muscle activity while repeating the affected movements. For muscles that work excessively or inappropriately during selective movements the athlete can learn to reduce the muscle activity.

In chronic overuse injuries, muscles initially inhibited by pain may remain dysfunctional after the pathology has resolved (despite gym exercises). Effective biofeedback training can re-educate muscle-response timing, selective to specific sporting movements, including throwing, catching and bowling for the upper limb and lunging, squatting and jumping for the lower limb.

TENS (Transcutaneous Electrical Nerve Stimulation)

TENS is used to provide pain relief. TENS stimulates biological analgesic systems within the body through the pain gate and opiate systems.

High-frequency stimulation of large diameter nerve fibres reduces the perception of pain by closing the gate to pain fibres at the spinal cord level. The pain gate theory proposes that pain is transmitted via the spinal cord by small diameter a-delta and c fibres. TENS machines set at high frequency (80 to 130 Hz) and high pulse rates (60 to 80 pulses per second) stimulate large diameter nerves in the spinal cord and inhibit the information transmitted to the spinal column by the small diameter pain fibres.

Low-frequency stimulation of nerve fibres helps to release the body's own pain-relieving substances (endorphins or endogenous opioids). Opioids work on the central nervous system to stimulate control of pain transmission and also influence the spinal cord, inhibiting the transmission of messages of tissue damage to the brain. The TENS machine is set at frequencies below 80 Hz with a pulse rate below 4 pulses per second. This can produce a low-intensity muscle twitch; it can be used on acupuncture or trigger points.

Heat

Heat can be used to promote blood flow, provide analgesia, and to relax muscles. It is applied to the damaged tissues only after acute inflammation has resolved (to avoid increasing any exudates). Hot packs and whirlpools provide superficial heating, and deep heating modalities include continuous ultrasound and shortwave diathermy. Superficial heating techniques are useful to encourage the circulation in ligaments and tendons just beneath the skin. Deep heating modalities are useful for fascia and deeper structures.

The role of massage in the acute to chronic rehabilitation of sport injuries

Massage has many proposed benefits, including physiological and psychological. Massage helps to reduce swelling, breaks down scar tissue (adhesions), and improves circulation to facilitate healing. There are many different techniques used in massage and these include kneading, effluage, picking up, pounding, shaking, rolling, hacking, vibrations and myofascial release. These techniques range from movements designed to promote fluid mobility and circulation within arterial, venous and lymphatic vessels, to techniques designed to aid the mechanical breakdown of fibrotic and/or adhered scar formation that could prevent healing.

Massage can

(i) Promote local circulation, to remove inflammatory exudates.
(ii) Provide pain relief. Gentle pressure stimulates pain gating at the spinal cord level.
(iii) Break down scar tissue adhesions, which restrict normal joint movement.
(iv) Promotes correct scar tissue formation in healing soft tissue injuries.
(v) Encourage relaxation.

Further reading

Cyriax J. *Textbook of Orthopaedic Medicine, Edition 11, Diagnosis of Soft Tissue Lesions*. London: Baillière Tindall and Cassell, 1984.

Meeusen R, Lievens P. The use of cryotherapy in sports injuries. *Sports Med* 1986; **3**: 398–414.

Travell JG, Simons DG. *Myofascial Pain and Dysfunction: The Trigger Point Manual*. Lippincott: Williams and Wilkins, 1998.

Physiotherapy – rehabilitation

T Betts

An adequate rehabilitation programme must address muscles, flexibility and proprioception. Following optimisation of the above, then the athlete can progress to sport-specific exercises and then finally return to sport. Attention must also be paid to cardiovascular fitness throughout the rehabilitation programme.

Muscular rehabilitation

The rehabilitation of the musculo-tendon units is of paramount importance to the successful return to sports by athletes. Muscle performance is a composite of strength, power, endurance, balance and coordination, therefore all these factors must be addressed in an appropriate rehabilitation programme.

Muscular strength

All sports-related activities involve a fluid combination of isotonic (which can be concentric or eccentric), isometric and isokinetic exercises. The coordination and modulation of these activities have a very important influence on performance. Most sports activities involve phases of stretch-shortening cycles of muscle work (e.g. overhead throwing, the golf swing, striking a football, jumping and landing upon one leg, and grand plié). It is therefore essential that pre-injury training and post-injury rehabilitation is targeted at all of these aspects of muscle function to reduce injury susceptibility.

Isometric exercise

Isometric exercises involve the static loading contraction of muscle fibres, without the movement of the associated joint. Isometric activities, if at high intensity and prolonged, can have negative effects causing metabolic fatigue and injury. However, isometric muscle contractions also enhance joint stability and are a good measure for testing muscle performance.

Isotonic exercise

With this exercise, there is a constant external resistance, but the movement of the joint is permitted. The two types of isotonic exercise are:

(i) *Concentric*
- muscle shortens as it contracts
- external resistance force is *less* than the internal force generated by the muscle
- required for acceleration
- the most common type of muscle action used to produce force, power and speed during take-off jumping and sprinting.

(ii) *Eccentric*
- muscle lengthens as it contracts
- external force *greater* than the internal force generated by the muscle
- required for deceleration and braking
- sports-related activities that are eccentric include squatting down (urging forward and downhill walking/running)

- Several studies into muscle activities have demonstrated that eccentric loading can lead to injuries of the skeletal muscle system, causing tears, weakness and gross swelling.
- Eccentric loading exercises can also be used to promote tendon repair following overuse injuries and have been demonstrated to aid recovery of function and reduction of pain in the Achilles tendon and elbow joint.

Isokinetic exercise

Isokinetic exercise machines apply variable resistance at pre-determined speeds throughout the joint range. Isokinetic exercises are progressed by altering the speed and resistance of the machine. The athlete should train to restore normal ratios and muscle strength characteristics.

Open and closed chain exercise

With open chain exercise, the distal extent of the extremity is free to move through the space. With closed chain exercise, the distal extent of the extremity is fixed, therefore requiring simultaneous agonist and antagonist muscular contraction and coordination. Furthermore, with closed chain, all the joints that compose the kinetic chain are set in motion. As a result, closed chain exercises are thought to simulate functional activities to a greater degree.

Muscular power

Power is trained by progressive (over)loading of resistance using weights or power cords/tubing.

Muscular endurance

Endurance can be developed with a gradual increase in repetitions and holding times. High repetition at low loads develops the endurance capacity of muscles. The speed of progression is determined by the response of the muscle to the previous exercise. Initially, the athlete should complete enough repetitions to start muscle fatigue. Subjective feelings of tiredness or muscle ache or increasing difficulty maintaining the exercise are signs of fatigue. The repetitions should be counted and the number used as a base line. Gradually the number of repetitions (or time taken to complete the exercise) is increased.

Muscular coordination

Muscular coordination exercises and correction of abnormal muscular patterning form a very important part of an accurate rehabilitation programme. Various methods involving muscular re-education, including biofeedback techniques, stability exercises and Pilates can be utilised.

Flexibility

This is dependent on all the joint structures, including the capsule and ligaments, and the muscular-tendinous unit.

Injuries, and in many occasions their treatment (by immobilisation), can lead to capsular and other soft tissue tightening, with the end result being joint stiffness. Therefore, exercises to prevent this from occurring must be commenced as soon as it is safe to do so. It is beyond the scope of this chapter to discuss the details of each different range of motion exercises, but broadly speaking these could be divided into:

(i) Passive exercises (which also include continuous passive motion)
(ii) Active exercises
(iii) Active assisted exercises

The flexibility of the muscular-skeletal tendon unit is essential for the optimal performance of sporting activities and to reduce injury susceptibility. Enhancing flexibility has been reported to:

(i) maintain mechanical strength throughout the range
(ii) prevent joint contractures and/or muscle imbalance
(iii) maintain adequate range of motion specific to each sport
(iv) reduce injuries caused by rapid stretching
(v) improve performance
(vi) decrease risk of delayed onset muscle soreness

Different types of stretching techniques used include:

Passive (static) flexibility:

- Slowly and passively stretching the muscle to full range, and maintaining this stretched position with continued tension.

Active (dynamic) flexibility:

- Ballistic. Rapid jerking actions at the end of range to force the tissues to stretch.
- Contract relax (CR). Isometrically contracting the stretched muscle, and then relaxing and passively stretching the muscle still further. This action is usually performed by a partner.
- Contract-relax-agonist-contract (CRAC). The same as CR, except that during the final stages of the stretching phase the muscle opposite the stretched muscle is contracted.

Rehabilitation of proprioception

Proprioception/balance exercises are challenged through the axial loading of joints. Axial loading exercises or closed kinetic chain exercises uses body weight against ground reaction forces. Unstable or external perturbation promotes reflex reaction forces/impulses by muscles that stabilise joints. By standing on a wobble board or responding to manual rhythmic pushes in multiple directions, the body learns to correct itself. The theory is that delayed reaction timing leads to instability within joints caused by excessive motion within the neutral zone of the joint motion parameters. Too much motion beyond the neutral zone can over-stretch the elastic-ligament structure that surrounds and protects joints.

Pathological laxity can lead to instability. Inhibition of muscles that stabilise joints caused by acute recurrent inflammation reduces the active response needed to correct excessive and/or unhealthy joint motion. Equipment that challenges motion correction within a small base of support encourages the body to correct alignment to an optimal position. This position alignment is when the limbs and/or trunk are moving the least against the ground reaction force. Severe or gross motion against the ground produces "swaying" when upon a wobble board (or balance machinery). This "swaying" is displayed as the body (trunk or limb) attempts to re-find (retune) the position of minimal motion or maximum energy efficiency. Rapid muscle activity controlled by central nervous processes repositions the joint. Good proprioception (as seen by high-class, elite athletes and dancers) involves minimal body sway movement when challenged by very small bases of support. Poor proprioception (novice athletes, babies) involves large body sway under big bases of support (i.e. both feet on flat ground).

To progress, improve and/or retrain proprioception, the athlete should be progressively advanced from large, stable support bases, to small unstable bases. Finally, the specific sporting context should be replicated to enhance the functional restoration of proprioceptive abilities. For example, footballers can practise proprioceptive exercises using a football while wearing football boots, dancers can practise plié and point work on a wobble board or a safe equivalent balancing surface.

Further reading

Carpenter JE, Blasier RB, Pellizzon GG. The effects of muscle fatigue on shoulder joint position sense. *Am J Sports Med* 1998; **26**: 262–70.

Hesselink MK, Kuipers H, Geurten P, Van Staaten H. Structural muscle damage and muscle strength after incremental number of isometric and forced lengthening contractors. *Muscle and Cell Mobility* 1996; **17**: 335–41.

Swanick CB, Lephart SM, Giannatonio FP, Fu FH. Re-establishing proprioception and neuromuscular control in the injured athlete. *J Sports Rehabilitation* 1997; **6**: 182–206.

Tongue BN, Schwane SA. Effect of intermittent eccentric contractions on symptoms of muscle micro-injury. *Med Sci – Sports Exercise* 1995; **27**: 1378–84.

Physiotherapy – the team physiotherapist

T Betts

The team physiotherapist has many roles and multiple functions within the sports team. These roles can change from one sport to another. However, the chief role within any sport of the therapist is to organise and support the treatment of all the musculo-skeletal injuries of athletes within their team. Together with the medical team they should work to maintain;

(1) the individual assessment and treatment of injured athletes,
(2) the screening and development of fitness profiles for all the athletes pre-season/prior to joining a team,
(3) the organisation of a medical team, which is multi-disciplinary and includes fitness coaches, nutritionists, podiatrists, psychologists, surgeons, general practitioners/team doctors,
(4) organise the correct and safe use of sporting clothing and equipment,
(5) organise and purchase the most modern and evidence-based electrotherapy and general treatment equipment,
(6) develop protocols for on the field work and life-threatening incidents,

(7) develop rehabilitation protocols for common injuries, with monitoring of incidents and recovery rates.

Together with the fitness staff, the coach and the doctors, the physiotherapist should compile a profile of the athletes. There are many different occasions when this can be done and it can depend on the seasonal variations of the sport. For example,

- Pre-season/post season
- Pre-tour/post tour
- Mid season breaks/intervals
- Post intense physically demanding periods of the season/tour
- Regular intervals relating to the yearly calendar

The fitness profile should be as comprehensive as possible. To get a thorough understanding of a fitness and physiological profile of an athlete read the chapter on fitness testing.

The physiotherapist's role within the team is to treat acute injuries and manage long-term injuries. The physiotherapist should have a working knowledge of the current treatment regimes used for a wide variety of the most common injuries treated. Access to the Internet and search engines or sports journals with current research trials is essential to maintain up-to-date treatment methods. The therapist must be able to interact with both the athletes and other medical staff. They should be good communicators who are able to provide information to both the injured athlete and those responsible for other aspects of their health and being. These include the head coach, family members, team physicians and surgeons.

Typically, the treating physiotherapist will have rolling caseloads of injured athletes. However, the beginning of the week may start with preparation of the athletes for training. Treatment may involve manual therapy, massage, electrotherapy and or taping. The physiotherapist may have to organise investigations, physicians/surgical opinion and then gather and communicate the results. This will continue until the weekly match and/or performance. Then the therapist will have to assess the condition of the athlete and report to the medical coaching and management staff on the availability and level of recovery. Between everybody, a decision on who can perform is made and the appropriate injury prevention measures instigated. The team should work together in the week to plan the treatment programme and support the injured athlete socially and psychologically whenever necessary.

In specific sports, the therapist must understand the rules regarding head injuries, bleeding and concussion. The principles of ABC – airways, breathing, circulation – must be adhered to at all times. The therapist should ensure that they are up to date with the latest rules and procedures for resuscitation.

It is essential to have a well-stocked kit bag, which has all the items needed to apply first aid and immediate cooling. A well-stocked kit bag should include the following items:

Kit bag

- Ice pack/spray
- Cold water – sterile
- Taping – multiple lengths: 2 cm, 5 cm, 7 cm (elastic + non-elastic)
- Scissors

- Tape removal appliance
- Vaseline
- Bandages
- Massage oil/cream
- Salts
- Ankle supports (joint supports), toes, elbows, knees, neck and lumbar spine brace
- Cotton wool
- Sterile gloves

A para-medical equipment pack is also essential for the modern-day sports therapist. This should include:

- Radios for communication with medical staff and coaches
- Frac-pac bag
- Gases
- Stretchers
- Stitching/cleaning material

The principles of on-field assessment

Assessment of the injured athlete on the field involves:

- Evaluation of severity of injury – structure/grade
- Risk of assessment for continuing to play
- Application-appropriate immediate treatment
  —Cryotherapy
  —Massage
  —Protection/support
  —Remove from field of play

Actions a therapist should do for the athlete immediately at the site of injury:

(1) Observe (use principles of ABC).
(2) Establish if the athlete is conscious.
(3) Questions – where is your pain?
(4) How did it happen?
(5) What do you feel now?
(6) Did you hear/feel anything when it happened – popping, snapping, tearing sensation?
(7) Assessment – look/feel/move.
(8) Active/passive/resisted/accessory movements.
(9) Can you stand up? (Lower limb injured.)
(10) Can you continue?
(11) Head injury questions – see chapter on Head injury.

Acknowledgement

We would like to thank Mr Gary Lewin for his comments on this chapter.

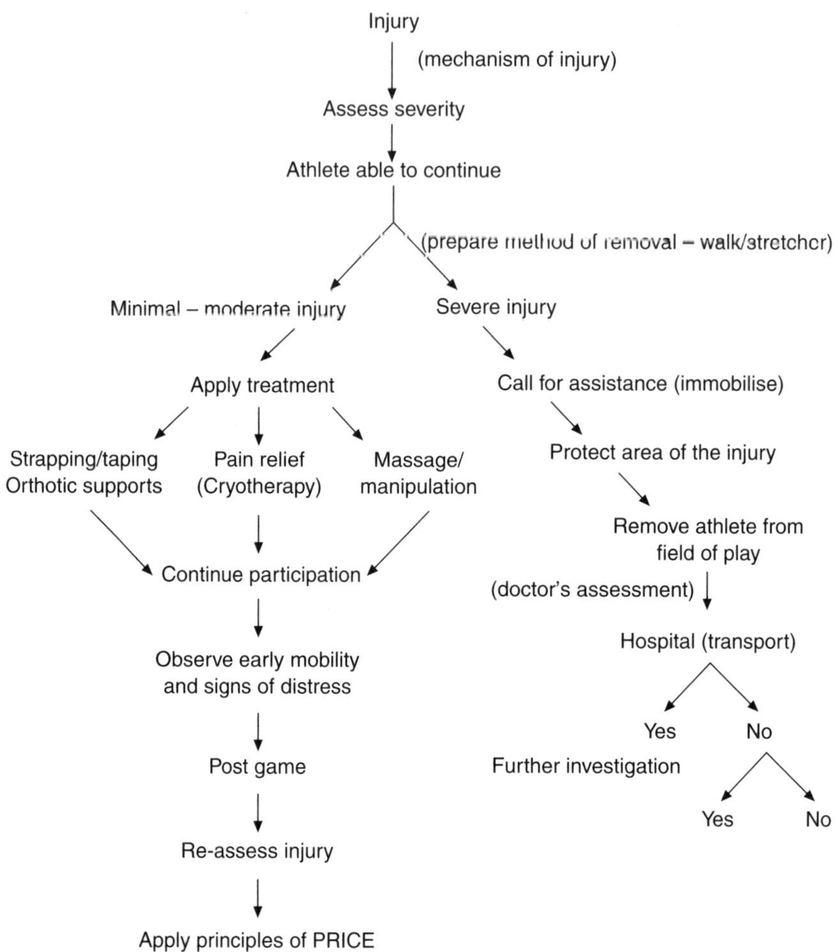

Figure 1 Paradigm for on-field assessment.

Further reading

Corrigan B, Maitland GD. *Musculoskeletal & Sports Injuries*. Edinburgh: Butterworth Heinemann, 1994.

Magee DJ. *Orthopaedic Physical Assessment.* WB Saunders, 1987; 266–314.

Norris CM. *Sports Injuries, Diagnosis and Management*, 2nd edn. Butterworth Heinemann, 1998.

Prevention of sports injuries

AA Narvani

Treating sport injuries can often be complex, difficult, expensive and challenging. Therefore all efforts must be made to prevent these injuries, and all individuals working with athletes, including sports clinicians, must have an understanding of the different injury prevention strategies. All these strategies involve identification of risk factors as well as attempts to minimise the risks and their impact. There are a number of classifications for these strategies in the literature, but one of the most practical ones is presented in Figure 1.

Screening

Screening forms a vital part of any injury prevention strategies. As well as identifying those athletes who are particularly at risk of injury and the specific risk factors, screening permits an assessment of fitness, general health, condition of musculoskeletal

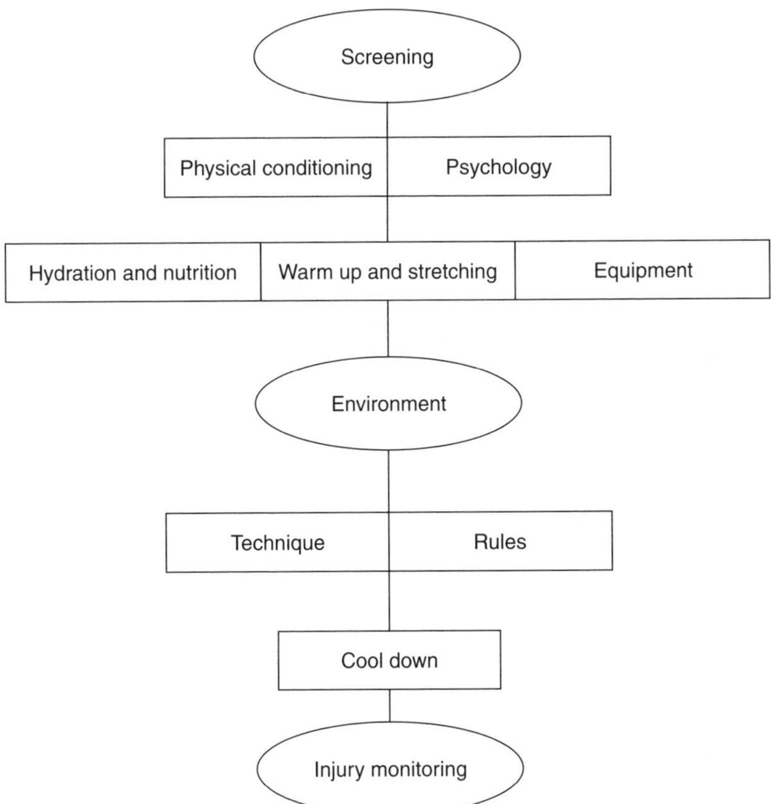

Figure 1 Schemes for injury prevention.

system and efficacy of the rehabilitation programme for existing injuries to be made. A screening programme may consist of:

- health questionnaire
- lifestyle assessment questionnaire
- history
- physical examination
- investigations
- follow-up screening

Physical conditioning

Appropriate physical conditioning and balanced training result in better performance and reduced risk of injury. The training programme must be gradual, allowing the athlete to recover, and implemented in phases (preparation, pre-competition and competition). It must focus on all of the following skills:

- flexibility
- strength
- aerobic capacity
- anaerobic capacity
- stamina
- speed
- coordination and timing
- technique and sports-related skills
- agility
- proprioception

Psychology

See the chapter on Psychology – injuries.

Hydration and nutrition

As well as influencing performance, inadequate hydration may lead to injury by compromising muscle blood flow and function, temperature regulation, cardiovascular response, concentration and therefore technique. It is, therefore, important that the athlete drinks adequate quantities of fluid before, during and after exercise.

Equally, nutrition can also play an important part in injury prevention. Inadequate carbohydrate intake may lead to decreased glycogen stores and increased muscle/protein breakdown in order to compensate for the reduced carbohydrate fuel supply. Insufficient protein intake can also lead to decreased muscle mass and strength, therefore increasing the risk of muscle damage and injury. Iron deficiency may lead to increased lactic acid production and therefore increased risk of muscle damage by compromising oxidative potentials in the muscle. Similarly, inadequate calcium intake can increase the risk of osteoporosis and stress fractures. Supplementation of diet with antioxidants such as vitamins C and E may also reduce the risks of muscle injuries by reducing and minimising the effect of the free radicals produced during exercise.

Warm up and stretching

The proposed benefits of warming up include better oxygen delivery to muscles through increased blood flow and better release of oxygen by haemoglobin, decreased muscle stiffness, increased range of motion (controversial) and better psychological preparation.

The proposed beneficial effects of stretching include:

- increased compliance of the tendon unit
- increased tendon compliance leads to a "higher ability of tendon to absorb energy"
- decreased load transfer across the muscle-tendon unit during "high-intensity stretch-shortening cycles" in sports involving jumping and bouncing activities)
- decreased risk of injury to tendon
- decreased risk of injury to the muscle

The role of stretching in the prevention of injuries does, however, remain very controversial. Although there are a number of studies that have shown the beneficiary effects of stretching, there are also other authors who have not shown any advantages in stretching prior to exercise. It does appear likely that whether stretching has any benefits or not is dependent on the type of exercise and sport performed by the athlete (see Witvrouw *et al.* 2004). Those that pursue sports which involve eccentric contractions and a high intensity of stretch-shortening cycles, such as basketball, football and long jump, require a "compliant" muscle–tendon unit that is capable of storing and releasing excessive amounts of elastic energy. As stretching has been shown to increase the compliance of the muscle–tendon unit, such athletes would benefit from stretching. In contrast, those who take part in sports that do not involve high-intensity "stretch-shortening cycles" such as jogging, cycling and swimming, do not require a highly elastic muscle–tendon unit. In such athletes, there is no requirement for the tendons to act as energy-absorbing structures, and therefore they may not benefit from stretching exercises. Furthermore, making the tendons more compliant in such athletes may result in decreased ability and decreased performance as rapid tension changes and swift joint motion responses would be more difficult.

Equipment

Correct equipment can play a vital role in injury prevention. Along with other gear, equipment includes shoes (see the chapter on sports footwear), rackets, skis, gloves and other items of clothing, all of which should be appropriate and complement the athlete.

The role of protective equipment is to prevent or reduce the risk of injury by decreasing the impact of the force on the body part and spreading this force over a large surface area. It may also provide protection of an injured body part during recovery.

Protective equipment includes:

- helmets
- eye protection
- mouth guards
- shoulder padding
- gloves

- elbow guards
- genital guards
- thigh guards
- knee pads
- shin pads
- ankle braces

Environment

Environmental factors that may lead to an increased risk of injury include:

Weather
- temperature
- rain
- icy conditions
- fog
- snow
- wind

Surface
- uneven surface increases risk of injury
- hard surface may lead to greater force on musculoskeletal system
- inappropriately slippery surface can lead to injuries

Facilities
- availability of first aid equipment
- availability of qualified staff
- appropriate free space around the playing area
- protective padding around the playing field if indicated
- field equipment must be regularly checked to ensure it is in working order

Technique

Poor technique can lead to injury. It is, however, difficult to define what "good" technique is, but it should consist of efficient and comfortable movements with least effort in order to perform the optimal sporting task. Correct technique acquired at an early stage prevents developing bad habits. Poor techniques in jumping, landing, stroke, swing, serve, throw, kick, grip, boxing and posture can all lead to injuries. It is important to emphasise that technique may need to be changed as a result of injury. This is where the role of a biomechanist becomes important in management of sports injuries.

Rules

All rules must take the safety of the athletes into consideration and should ensure maximum protection for the athlete. Equally, it is vital that these are followed by all parties concerned, including the athletes themselves, coaches, managers, medical staff and referees. When rules are not followed heavy punishments must be enforced, especially if the safety of any individual is compromised as a consequence.

Cool-down

It has been suggested that the cool-down reduces risk of injury and optimises performance by:

- allowing a gradual drop in heart rate
- allowing continued oxygen delivery to muscles, therefore restoring them to the condition they were in prior to exercise
- enabling removal of lactic acid and other waste products from muscles
- promoting flexibility
- lowering risk of muscle soreness

Cooling down should include gentle aerobic exercise (jogging) and stretching.

Injury monitoring

Data collection of injuries and circumstances associated with the injuries should be an important part of any sport injury prevention strategy. As important is analysis of these data and implementing changes in order to reduce the risk of the injuries occurring again.

Further reading

Grisogono V. Prevention and prophylaxis. In: B Helal, J King, W Grange (Eds) *Sport Injuries and their Treatment*. Chapman & Hall, 1986; 1–17.

MacKay M, Scanian A, Olsen L, Reid D, Clark M, McKim K, Raina P. Looking for the evidence: a systemic review of prevention strategies addressing sport and recreational injury among children and youth. *J. Science & Medicine Sport* 2004; **7**(1): 58–73.

Witvrouw E, Mahieu N, Danneels L, McNair P. Stretching and injury prevention, an obscure relationship. *Sports Medicine* 2004; **34**(7): 443–9.

Psychology – performance enhancement

P Thomas

Psychology applied to sport can enhance the athlete's performance. Clinical psychology will target and prevent the athlete's individual problems, and will also provide educational programmes that have an impact on the knowledge of the athletes and coaches.

There are many existing prescription programmes that focus on modelling and enhancing performance. One of them, the "self-regulation" Kirschenbann includes five stages:

(1) *Identify the problem.* Change of the routine activities, such as training, eating times and work involvement, setting goals to alter the "problem habit".

(2) *Commitment.* A positive mental action to change and improve.
(3) *Execution.* The athlete systemically monitors his or her performance. The athlete approaches the positive aspects of their performance during the competition, and focuses on routine mistakes and performance problems using cognitive methods to reduce any negative effects.
(4) *Environmental management.* Social support and a secure environment to train and achieve goals or preparation.
(5) *Generalisation.* Relevant habits can be destructive to the athlete's concentration. Cognitive efforts to reduce a compulsive–obsessive style in elite sports preparation and performance.

Sports psychology is applied to the needs of the individual athlete and can create a model suitable for his or her personality and the complexities of the chosen sport. This model will include:

(1) Arousal control: in an effect the correct amount of personal power that is necessary to deliver on the day of the competition.
(2) Cognitive factors: the appropriate learning of skills around an individual sport.
(3) Reduce stress and psychological tension: appropriate steps to be taken to reduce muscle spasm, increase heart rate and breathing rate.
(4) Attention ability: the athlete can focus and perform using external stimuli such as the crowd support or internal routines such as self-focusing with mediating techniques.
(5) Emotions: strategies are employed to reduce anxiety, anger, depression or confusion and they will include "positive chat", music, socialising, reading, etc.
(6) The athlete's own adherence to his or her preparation performance routine and competition rituals.

Team sport

The selection of individual athletes to achieve full potential within a team set-up, with the sharing of common goals with other team mates, can be a challenging task. The best individual athletes will not necessarily be able to fuse into a successful team.

Effective communication systems should be placed between the team players to promote the goal settings.

Cohesiveness into the team ranks being observed by the coaches, team captain and officials within the team, enhances confidence and the trust of the individual players with all members of the team.

The coach has the responsibility to design the tactics for the group and promote the individual's performance, creating a successful working unit. He or she must also ensure that there is equal distribution and appraisal of achievements.

Further reading

Gill DL. *Psychological Dynamics of Sport.* Human Kinetics Publishers, 1986.

Hackford D, Spielberger C (Eds) *Anxiety in Sports – American International Perspective.* New York: Hemisphere, 1989.

Psychology – sports injuries

P Thomas

Psychological factors contributing to sports injury, recurrence management and return to sport are discussed in this chapter.

Psychological predictors in the occurrence of a sport injury

An athlete's personality may influence the risk of an injury. The social support by family, friends, coaching staff, and staff trust in the athlete's ability will reduce the risk of an injury. Other injuries in past life-events will play a role in the occurrence of a sport injury.

The psychological response to injury

Response to an injury generally follows the stages of grief, recovery with denial of the injury at first, with the athlete demonstrating over-optimism, followed by emotional swings of anger and depression, and this is usually the time that the treatment will be questioned. Later on there is a bargaining period, when the athlete accepts and adapts to the injury and questions the guarantees of certain treatments. The final stage is of general acceptance when the athlete resigns to the limitations of the injury, takes part in the treatment protocols and actively accepts the rehabilitation process. Self-motivated and extrovert athletes will usually recover quicker. The history of other injuries and social support are both important for recovery from an injury. Aspects such as timing of the injury in the season, the "illegal" action of a colleague that caused the injury, will produce a negative feeling.

Rehabilitation process

The athlete has to accept positively the physical protocols of treatment so rehabilitation can begin. The psychologist will have to concentrate on motivation techniques, using goal-setting, relaxation, and positive interaction and self-talk, also involving in support other individuals such as the team coach, teammates and friends.

Ready to return to competition

Physical readiness must be accomplished by psychological readiness to avoid anxiety during the return, avoiding bad performance and new injuries. It is based on protection of the confidence levels of the individual athlete who has overcome an injury and feels prepared to return to competition.

Further reading

Bunker LK, Rotella RJ *et al.* (Eds) *Sports Psychology: Psychological Considerations in Maximizing Performance.* New York: Movement, 1985: 273–87.

Williams JM (Ed) *Applied Sports Psychology: Personal Growth in Peak Performance.* Palo Alto: Mayfield, 1986: 343–63.

Pulmonary disorders and exercise

S Parnia

In normal subjects, exercise is rarely limited due to pulmonary causes, as most people maintain a substantial breathing reserve. However, in some cases exercise may be impaired by a number of acute and chronic pulmonary disorders. These include exercise-induced asthma (EIA), vocal cord dysfunction (VCD), exercise-induced anaphylaxis, and exercise-induced urticaria as well as chronic lung disease. The aim of this chapter is to review these conditions and their relationship with exercise.

Acute pulmonary disorders and exercise

Exercise-induced asthma (EIA) or bronchospasm, and vocal cord dysfunction (VCD) are perhaps the two most common and disabling acute pulmonary disorders that may limit exercise in athletes. Other rare pulmonary disorders that may prevent or limit an individual's ability to participate in sports include exercise-induced anaphylaxis and urticaria.

Exercise-induced asthma

Exercise-induced asthma or bronchospasm is a common disorder and is thought to occur in 50% to 80% of asthmatics, as well as up to 40% of patients with allergic rhinitis, and 10% of normal subjects.

Essentially, exercise-induced asthma is airway obstruction that is induced by exercise. Symptoms thus resemble the symptoms of other obstructive lung disorders and may include wheezing, coughing, shortness of breath and, in some cases, chest discomfort. Post-exercise coughing is the commonest symptom, and in many cases wheezing may actually be absent. Although the symptoms of EIA may usually occur 5 to 10 minutes after strenuous exercise, they actually peak 5 to 10 minutes after cessation of exercise and resolve approximately 30 minutes after the exercise has ended. Cold, dry air is more likely to induce EIA and it is thought that the 5-lipoxygenase pathways play a significant role in the pathogenesis of EIA, as does underlying pulmonary eosinophilic inflammation.

Diagnosing EIA can be accomplished by means of exercise testing together with the measurement of obstructive lung function parameters such as FEV_1. Alternatively, some practitioners may perform a methacholine or histamine challenge test.

Prevention and treatment of EIA involves a number of steps. In those people who suffer with chronic asthma, it is important to treat the underlying condition successfully. This involves the identification and avoidance of specific allergens (in the case of allergic asthma), such as house dust mite, together with appropriate pharmacological treatment. Many professional pulmonary bodies such as the British Thoracic Society and The American Thoracic Society have published detailed guidelines on the management of asthma. Routine usage of inhaled corticosteroids improves pre-exercise FEV_1 and reduces the propensity to develop EIA. Additional agents include leukotriene modifiers and long-acting $beta_2$-adrenergic agents. Montelukast (10 mg po daily), a leukotriene receptor antagonist, has been shown to be superior to salmeterol (42 mcg inhaled BID), a long-acting $beta_2$-adrenergic agonist, in preventing EIA in patients with chronic asthma over an 8-week trial.

Athletes may be able to control EIA by performing a period of exercise prior to the actual exercise event. It has been shown that, in some cases, initial exercise is followed by a period of relative refractoriness to EIA if another period of exercise is commenced approximately 1 hour after the first. Thus, the non-pharmacologic options include induction of a relative refractory period prior to the exercise event and controlling the atmospheric conditions such as cold weather. Avoidance of winter sports and choosing to exercise indoors under climate-controlled conditions minimises the occurrence of EIA. Recent studies have also demonstrated that low-sodium diets may improve post-exercise pulmonary function. Hence, dietary intervention may be useful in asthmatics and in those with EIA as well.

As well as following guidelines for the treatment of asthma, pharmacologic options to manage EIA alone include the use of inhaled $beta_2$-adrenergic agonists such as salbutamol (albuterol) or inhaled sodium cromoglycate (cromolyn sodium)15 minutes before exercise. Sodium cromoglycate is not as effective in preventing EIA when compared with $beta_2$-adrenergic agents, which may prevent EIA in up to 90% (the use of sodium cromoglycate may prevent EIA in up to 40%) of patients. Athletes should therefore take the regular daily requirements of these drugs in combination with an extra dose before exercise.

Training goals in the athlete with EIA are no different than for normal subjects and asthmatics should choose their exercise and training activities carefully. It should be remembered that cold, dry air exacerbates asthma and is a major factor in inducing EIA. Activities that do not generate high minute ventilations such as tennis, handball, karate, wrestling and golf are preferred, as are water activities such as swimming, diving and water polo. High minute-ventilation activities such as long-distance running, cycling, basketball and football or those taking place in a cool and dry climate, such as ice hockey and ice skating, are more likely to induce EIA.

Vocal cord dysfunction

Vocal cord dysfunction (VCD) is characterised by inappropriate vocal cord adduction during the respiratory cycle. This condition is more common in young female athletes. Patients may feel that they are unable to get air in and they may also develop wheezing and shortness of breath. Unlike asthma there is a lack of responsiveness to bronchodilators.

Many patients with VCD are thought to suffer with EIA and they may initially be referred with this condition. In order to distinguish between these two conditions, pulmonary function testing as well as exercise testing may be useful. Evidence of upper airway obstruction is often elucidated during an exercise test. In addition, the diagnosis can be made using direct laryngoscopy after the signs of vocal cord dysfunction have been triggered with exercise.

Treatment is effective both for immediate relief and prevention. Panting or coughing may abort an attack and some patients should be advised to attempt to stop an attack using such maneuvers. Additional interventions that may help include administration of a short-acting sedative or inhalation of heliox (a mixture of helium and oxygen), which helps by reducing flow resistance as it is a less dense gas. Other measures include speech therapy consultation to teach diaphragmatic breathing and oral airway relaxation during an attack. Chronic use of sedatives or antidepressants may also be useful in preventing or reducing the incidence of attacks.

Exercise-induced anaphylaxis and urticaria

Rare yet potentially life-threatening disorders to which some individuals are susceptible are anaphylaxis and urticaria, which can occur during exercise. The mast cell is thought to mediate the development of these conditions, as increased levels of histamine, tryptase, and leukotrienes are involved. Exercise-induced urticarial disease may manifest itself with the development of small papules surrounded by an erythematous region. In other instances there may be single larger (10 cm–20 cm) macular erythematous and pruritic lesions. Lesions usually appear on the upper thorax or neck but may spread. Classically they appear in response to exercise, passive warming, and emotional stress. A more dangerous and potentially fatal presentation is when patients present with classic exercise-induced anaphylaxis. As well as urticaria, there may be angioedema together with upper airway obstruction, and hypotension. Symptoms may also include shortness of breath, wheezing, dizziness, loss of consciousness, as well as gastrointestinal symptoms and headache. These symptoms may last 30 minutes to 4 hours after termination of exercise.

The diagnosis of exercise-induced urticaria or anaphylaxis is based primarily on history. A history of atopy is also supportive. For patients suspected of having this condition, an exercise test (with emergency equipment readily available) can be performed to elucidate symptoms. A negative test does not exclude the diagnosis, however, as the presentation is variable.

As with the management of angioedema, anphylaxis treatment should be directed at modifying behaviors and activities. Patients should not exercise alone and should have epinephrine (adrenaline) available at all times. These are usually prescribed as an EpiPen device (a small auto-injector that delivers a single dose of 0.3 mg). Patients must be advised to always have two EpiPen devices with them at all times, so that if they need to use one they will have a back-up device. Patients should be taught to administer the device as an intramuscular injection. They should also be advised not to exercise within 4 to 6 hours after eating and in the case of women it is recommended that they should not exercise in the perimenstrual period. Patients who develop symptoms should stop exercising and administer epinephrine immediately. Antihistamines are also effective in preventing this condition and as with anaphylaxis of any kind may be sufficient to prevent the condition if administered early as an intravenous preparation (IV Piriton 10 mg (UK) or Benadryl 50 mg (USA) are commonly used preparations). In addition, the patient should have 200 mg IV hydrocortisone administered as soon as possible. As with other allergic conditions, sodium cromoglycate (cromolyn sodium), leukotriene antagonists, antihistamines, ranitidine and other H2 antagonists as well as tranexamic acid (an antifibrinolytic agent that is also a potent inhibitor of the complement system) may also play a role in the prevention and treatment of exercise-induced anaphylaxis.

Summary

The respiratory system rarely limits exercise in normal subjects. Some people may, however, present with acute pulmonary conditions of which EIA is the commonest and anaphylaxis the most dangerous. Other common respiratory disorders include coughing and vocal cord dysfunction. Chronic lung diseases such as asthma, COPD, and interstitial lung disease may also impact exercise capacity and endurance; however, these have not been discussed in detail in this chapter. Exercise testing can be useful to distinguish acute and chronic pulmonary causes of shortness of breath during exercise.

Further reading

Harris H. ABC of sports medicine. Pulmonary limitations to performance in sport. *BMJ* 1994; **309**(6947): 113–15.

Helenius I, Lumme A, Haahtela T. Asthma, airway inflammation and treatment in elite athletes. *Sports Med* 2005; **35**(7): 565–74.

Storm WW. Review of exercise-induced asthma. *Med Sci Sports Exerc* 2003; **35**(9):1464–70.

Risk of sudden death in athletes

MF Khan

The frequency of sudden cardiac death (SCD) is estimated to be around 1 in 200,000 young athletes a year and between 1 in 15,000 to 50,000 older athletes a year (see Maron 2001). Although it may appear to be uncommon, the unexpected death of apparently healthy, athletic individuals often receives widespread attention. It is hence important to recognize individuals who may be at a higher risk of SCD by establishing guidelines that document their risk and help to assess each individual's eligibility for competitive exercise.

Aetiology

The distribution of SCD varies geographically, underlying the fact that, especially in those under age 35, the condition is frequently congenital in nature. Also, despite the death being termed "sudden" it most often occurs in individuals in whom there is previously undiagnosed structural heart disease.

In competitive athletes in the US, for example, hypertrophic cardiomyopathy (HCM) is the most common non-ischemic aetiology of SCD (possibly up to 46% of cases in one registry) (see Gibbons *et al.* 1980). However, in a report from Northern Italy, arrhythmogenic right ventricular dysplasia (ARVD) accounted for 22% of SCD in athletes as compared to 2% mortality from HCM (see Maron *et al.* 2003a). The inherited nature of the condition may be also be responsible for the observation that HCM is a more common cause of death in African American athletes as compared to US whites (47% versus 27%) (see Maron *et al.* 2003b).

In all, the prevalence of congenital abnormalities in athletes is estimated at 0.2% (see Maron *et al.* 1996). It is important to note that as a consequence of the much higher prevalence of atherosclerotic heart disease an ischemic etiology is likely the most common cause overall of SCD and is certainly so in subjects over the age of 35.

Table 1 summarizes the causes of SCD.

Table 1 Causes of sudden cardiac death.

Cause of sudden cardiac death	Diagnosis	Recommendations
Hypertrophic Cardiomyopathy	Echo	Low intensity sports in the absence of high risk features
Congenital Coronary Anomalies	MRI	Avoid competitive sport until 6 months after surgery
Arrhythmogenic Right Ventricular Dysplasia	MRI	Avoid all competitive sports
Congenital Long QT Syndrome	ECG and genetic analysis	No competitive sports especially if LQTS 1
Myocarditis	Echo	Avoid competitive sports for 6 months or if cardiac evaluation abnormal
Marfan syndrome	Clinical exam and genetic analysis	Avoid competitive sports if cardiac abnormalities
Mitral Valve Prolapse	Echo	No restriction unless complicated
Atrial Septal Defect	Echo	Avoid sports unless small ASD and no pulmonary hypertension
Coronary Artery Disease	Cardiac stress testing	Low intensity sports if low risk. Avoid if risk higher.

The aetiological factors leading to death in patients with structural heart disease include:

- Syncope
- Tachyarrythmia
- Bradyarrythmia
- Dissection

The less common occurrence of SCD in the absence of structural heart disease can occur due to:

- Commotio cordis – "concussion" to the chest wall.
- Androgen, amphetamine or other illicit drug use – due to the surreptitious nature of its use it is difficult to estimate accurately the prevalence of performance-enhancing or illicit drug use in athletes. A UK survey of 21 gymnasia estimated a 9% use of androgens in men and a 2% use in women (see Korkia and Stimson 1997). It is equally important to note the difficulty in establishing causality in reported cases of SCD in potential drug users.

Athlete's heart

This refers to changes that may occur in a normal heart in response to vigorous training.

Pathology
The changes are benign in nature and do not portend an increased risk of SCD.

Diagnosis
A comparison of these changes with those seen in HCM is summarized in Table 2.

Recommendations
Differentiating these changes from those secondary to a structural abnormality is intrinsic to the process of risk stratification and to making further recommendations for exercise training.

Hypertrophic cardiomyopathy

An autosomal dominant condition leading to myocyte disarray and a phenotypic appearance that varies from normal to asymmetric LV hypertrophy.

Pathology
High-risk features
Features of HCM that portend an increased risk of SCD include:

- Age <45 years
- LVOT gradient >20 mmHg
- Sustained or non-sustained ventricular tachycardia
- Hypotensive blood pressure response to exercise
- Family history of sudden death
- Prior history of syncope

Table 2 Differences between athlete's heart and HCM.

Findings	Athlete's heart	HCM
Family history of HCM	Absent	Present
Echo:		
• LV wall thickness	<16 mm	Often >16 mm
• Septal hypertrophy	Symmetric	Asymmetric
• LV diastolic size	>55 mm	<45 mm
• Diastolic dysfunction	Present	Absent
• LA size	Enlarged	Normal
ECG	LVH	Unusual LVH pattern with deep Q-waves and negative T-waves
Cessation of exercise	LV wall thickness decreases	No change

Adapted from Maron, BJ *et al.* 36th Bethesda Conference on Eligibility Recommendations for Competitive Athletes with Cardiovascular Abnormalities. *J Am Coll Cardiol* 2005; **45**(8): 1325.

The importance of a comprehensive history enquiring specifically about symptoms of presyncope or syncope and of a family history of SCD cannot be overestimated in HCM.

Differential diagnosis

This includes athlete's heart, hypertension, aortic stenosis, storage disorders, e.g. Fabry's disease or infiltrative disorders, e.g. amyloidosis, hemochromotosis. See Table 2 to distinguish HCM from athlete's heart.

Treatment

Beta-blockers and calcium channel blockers are employed to ameliorate symptoms but are not protective against arrhythmias. In patients at high risk of SCD, implantable cardiac defibrillators (ICD) can prophylactically be used to defibrillate arrhythmias. However, ICDs are not a cure and, given the increased risk of SCD associated with vigorous exercise, the recommendations to avoid most competitive sports are not altered by device therapy.

Recommendations

The 36th Bethesda Conference on Eligibility Recommendations for Competitive Athletes with Cardiovascular Abnormalities (see Maron *et al.* 2005) concluded that athletes with a possible diagnosis of HCM should not participate in competitive sports, with the possible exception of low-intensity (low-static/low-dynamic) sports.

See Table 3 for a classification of sports based on static and dynamic components.

Table 3 Classification of sports.

	Dynamic component		
	Low	Moderate	High
Static component			
Low intensity	Cricket Golf Bowling	Table tennis Volleyball	Football Squash Distance running
Moderate intensity	Equestrian Motorcycling	Rugby Sprint running	Basketball Swimming
High intensity	Weightlifting Water skiing	Body building Skiing	Rowing Boxing Cycling

Adapted from Mitchell JH, Haskell W, Snell P, Van Camp, SP. Task Force 8: Classification of sports. *J Am Coll Cardiol* 2005; **45**(8): 1364.

Congenital coronary anomalies

This refers to a congenital abnormality where the coronary arteries arise from an abnormal location.

Pathology

High-risk features

Include an artery that is easily pinched due to angulation and one that follows a course between the pulmonary artery and the aorta.

Diagnosis

Should be considered in athletes under age 30 who present with exertional chest pain, presyncope or syncope. The gold standard for diagnosis used to be cardiac catheterization but is now MRI.

Recommendations

Athletes with uncorrected coronary abnormalities should be excluded from any vigorous exercise. Non-contact sports can be considered 6 months after a correction procedure and only after testing for ischemia to target threshold has been performed.

Arrhythmogenic right ventricular dysplasia (ARVD)

ARVD is an inherited condition that leads to fibro fatty infiltration of the right ventricular myocardium and predisposes to fatal arrhythmia.

Pathology

High-risk features

- Presence of ECG changes
- Significant right ventricular disease on echo
- A family history of SCD

Diagnosis

Changes on an ECG that should alert a provider to the potential of ARVD include:

- Epsilon waves
- Right heart strain
- Incomplete right bundle branch block
- Prolonged S upstroke

Although echocardiography has an acceptable sensitivity and specificity for the diagnosis of ARVD the gold standard for diagnosis is MRI.

Recommendations

The arrhythmia is often exercise induced, likely secondary to right ventricular wall stretch and a catecholamine-sensitive nature. As a consequence, competitive exercise should be avoided.

Congenital long QT syndrome (LQTS)

LQTS is a disorder of myocardial repolarization characterized by a long QT interval on the ECG and associated with an increased risk of SCD.

Pathology

Congenital or acquired (acquired forms are most commonly secondary to medication use and are reversible). Death occurs secondary to malignant arrhythmias, most characteristically torsade de pointes.

High-risk features

Exercise-induced arrhythmic events are particularly associated with congenital LQTS 1. Other features of high risk include palpitations, syncope, seizures and a previous history of SCD.

Recommendations

Athletes with congenital LQTS should avoid all competitive sports.

Myocarditis

An inflammatory disease of the myocardium associated with cardiac dysfunction.

Pathology

Aetiology is varied and can be any of:

- Infectious: viral such as coxsackie or HIV, bacterial such as tuberculosis, protozoal such as tryponosoma (Chagas disease), etc.

- Systemic disease such as sarcoidosis, rheumatoid arthritis or SLE.
- Drug-induced, such as cocaine, penicillins, methyldopa or doxorubicin.
- Others including postpartum myocarditis.

Differential diagnosis includes acute ischemia and pericarditis.

Diagnosis

Suggested by clinical findings of heart failure and characteristic ECG, echo and histological findings. Estimated prevalence in athletes at death is 7% in an autopsy series.

Recommendations

A 6-month period of inactivity is recommended after an acute episode of myocarditis. Any return to vigorous activity should be preceded by a risk assessment including an exercise stress test and Holter monitoring for arrhythmias.

Valvular heart disease

Aortic stenosis (AS) and mitral valve proplase (MVP) are two of the more common valvular diseases that may be encountered in athletes.

Pathology

As the significance of AS increases, cardiac output cannot respond to the increasing demands of exertion. AS is, however, an uncommon cause of SCD likely owing to an early diagnosis from its characteristically loud murmur and subsequent restriction of competitive sports.

MVP is characterized by myxomatous degeneration of the mitral valve leaflets and subvalvular apparatus. The relationship of MVP to arrhythmias and SCD is controversial. The abnormality does, however, predispose to mitral regurgitation (MR), which restricts exercise and increases the risk of SCD.

High-risk features:

- Severe AS (although diagnosis usually precedes this level of severity).
- MVP with moderate to severe MR portends a significantly increased risk of SCD. Isolated MVP, in the absence of MR, does not increase the risk of SCD above the level of the general population.

Recommendations

No restriction on activity if MVP occurs in isolation. If MVP occurs with:

- MR
- prior embolic event
- syncope or documented tachycardia
- family history of SCD

then only low-intensity sports should be considered. Of note, isometric exercise (e.g. weightlifting) should be avoided when associated with MR due to an increased risk of chordal rupture.

Marfan syndrome

This is an inherited connective tissue disorder, characterized by tall stature amongst other features. Marfan syndrome patients may be disproportionately represented in certain sports including basketball, volleyball, etc.

Pathology

Autosomal dominant inheritance. The major cause of mortality is aortic dissection.

Recommendations

Those with Marfan syndrome without evidence of cardiac involvement (primarily aortic root dilation) can participate in medium- to low-intensity sports. All such patients should avoid contact sports (rugby, American football, hurling, etc).

Atrial septal defects (ASD)

ASDs are a communication between the left and right atrial chambers of the heart.

Pathology

The direction of blood flow is determined by the pressure difference between the cardiac chambers and is hence initially left to right. This may eventually reverse (Eisenmenger's syndrome) if right-sided pressures rise above those on the left side of the heart.

ASDs are characterized by location into:

- Ostium premium defects (30% of cases) – involve the ventricular cushion.
- Ostium secondum defects (70% of cases) – do not involve the ventricular cushion.

High-risk features

Cyanotic heart disease (e.g. Eisenmenger's syndrome), significant pulmonary hypertension (HTN), ostium premium defects.

Recommendations

Patients with ostium primum defects should avoid all exercise. In patients with ostium secondum defects if:

- The defect is small with no pulmonary HTN then participation in sports can be considered.
- There is evidence of pulmonary HTN then sports should be avoided until treated.
- There is cyanosis then sports should be avoided all together.

Treatment

Percutaneous closure of ostium secondum defects using "umbrella" or "clam shell" devices is first line therapy. Surgical closure should be considered if percutaneous closure is not possible.

Coronary artery disease (CAD)

CAD is the most frequent cause of exercise-related arrhythmias and SCD, especially in those over the age of 35.

Pathology

Exercise-related death from CAD results directly from myocardial ischemia or from ventricular arrhythmias secondary to the ischemia.

High-risk features

Patients with normal LV function, normal exercise capacity for age and gender and no evidence of ischemia or inducible arrhythmia are considered at low risk. Those with any of these features are considered at increased risk.

Diagnosis

Risk assessment involves a full evaluation of cardiac status including exercise stress testing with echo or radionucleatide imaging and cardiac catheterization if necessary.

Recommendations

The low-risk subset can participate in low-intensity sports and should have an annual evaluation to ensure that their risk status has not changed. Athletes judged to be at very low risk (normal evaluation at a superior workload) could participate in higher intensity activities. Those at higher risk should avoid competitive sports.

Neurocardiogenic syncope

Non-fatal syncope in athletes without structural heart disease is often neurocardiogenic.

Pathology

This cause of syncope is often benign and vasovagally mediated.

Recommendations

No specific restriction on activity is recommended.

Screening

The low prevalence of SCD and the imperfect nature of any evaluation technique make aggressive screening in this population problematic. This is based on the increased likelihood for false positive results with their attendant morbidity and on low-cost effectiveness.

Recommendations are hence initially based more on a careful history and physical exam rather than on non-invasive or invasive cardiac testing. If aspects of an individual's personal or family history or their physical exams leads to a suspicion of a potential underlying cause of SCD then referral to cardiac testing is warranted.

The American Heart Association recommends a history and physical exam by a specialist healthcare worker before participation in organized high school or collegiate sports. ECG, exercise testing and echo are not recommended for younger athletes but can be considered in those over age 40 with moderate to high-risk profiles for CAD.

Further reading

Gibbons LW, Cooper KH, Meyer BM *et al.* The acute cardiac risk of strenuous exercise. *JAMA* 1980; **244**: 1799.

Korkia P, Stimson GV. Indications of prevalence, practice and effects of anabolic steroid use in Great Britain. *Int J Sports Med* 1997; **18**: 557.

Maron BJ. Cardiovascular disease in athletes. In: E Braunwald, DP Zipes, P Libby (Eds) *Heart Disease: A Textbook of Cardiovascular Medicine*, 6th edn. WB Saunders, 2001: Chapter 59, 2052–8.

Maron BJ, Ackerman MJ, Nishimura RA *et al.* 36th Bethesda Conference Eligibility Recommendations for Competitive Athletes with Cardiovascular Abnormalities. Task Force 4: HCM and other cardiomyopathies, mitral valve prolapse, myocarditis, and Marfan syndrome. *J Am Coll Cardiol* 2005; **45**(8): 1340.

Maron BJ, Carney KP, Lever HM *et al.* Relationship of race to sudden cardiac death in competitive athletes with hypertrophic cardiomyopathy. *J Am Coll Cardiol* 2003a; **41**: 974.

Maron BJ, Carney KP, Lever HM *et al.* Relationship of race to sudden cardiac death in competitive athletes with hypertrophic cardiomyopathy. *J Am Coll Cardiol* 2003b; **41**: 974.

Maron BJ, Thompson PD, Puffer JC *et al.* Cardiovascular pre-participation screening of competitive athletes A statement for health professions from the Sudden Death Committee (Clinical Cardiology) and Congenital Defects Committee (Cardiovascular Disease in the Young), American Heart Association. *Circulation* 1996; **94**: 850.

Shin pain

P Thomas

Stress fracture of tibia and fibula

These are more common in runners and dancers of all ages. Symptoms include severe localized pain and the athlete is unable to take part in any sporting activities. Usually they are incomplete fractures. X-rays may be negative in the first 2–3 weeks after the onset of symptoms, but they may demonstrate a radiolucent line, callus formation and soft tissue swelling later on. Techetium 99 bone scan is sensitive after the first 48–72 hours.

Management includes rest into a splint (Aircast brace), protected until the athlete is able to walk without a limp, and also pulsed magnetic field therapy. It takes an average of 6 weeks for recovery (See chapter on Stress fractures in sports).

Medial tibial stress syndrome: MTSS (shin splints)

The deep calf compartment (tibialis posterior, flexor digitorus longus and flexor hallucis longus) is expanded with exercise, producing traction of the fascia at the medial tibial border attachment. Pain and tenderness is present along the medial tibial edge. Techetium 99 bone scan reveals periostitis at the medial tibial edge. Pressure measurements of the compartments are usually normal.

Treatment includes active rest, ice application, anti-inflammatories, physiotherapy massage, stretching and strengthening exercises, gradual increase of work load to adapt the energy needs of an individual sport and conditioning of the muscles to return to sport activities. This treatment programme can take several weeks to months before recovery. Attention to biomechanical correction of the feet such as overpronation will further assist with the recovery. If all these measures fail, then surgery to release the fascia at the medial tibial border attachment may be considered.

Compartment pressure syndromes

See the chapter on Compartment pressure syndromes.

Other causes

- Vascular problems
- Referred pain
- Sciatica from lumbar spine

Further reading

Blue JM *et al.* Leg injuries. *Clin Sports Med* 1997; **16**(3): 467–78.
Hannaford PGH. Shin splints reviewed, medial tibial stress syndrome. *Excel* 1988; **4**: 16–19.

Shoulder – acute dislocation

AA Narvani

The shoulder joint is the most commonly dislocated joint, with its stability being sacrificed for range of movement. Over 95% of shoulder dislocations are reported to be traumatic in nature. The vast majority of the dislocations are anterior (95%), but they may also be posterior (4%) and inferior (1%).

Epidemiology

The incidence of shoulder dislocation is estimated to be 17 per 100,000. It is also very common in athletes with over 70% of all anterior dislocations occurring as a consequence of athletic activity. There appears to be a bimodal distribution with peaks in the second and sixth decades. In the young active population, it is more common in males than in females.

Predisposing factors

Risk factors include:

(1) prior dislocation or subluxation,
(2) increased joint laxity,

(3) involvement in sports that are either violent or force the glenohumeral joint into extreme positions,
(4) excessive retroversion of the humeral head,
(5) neuromuscular conditions such as cerebral palsey.

Pathology

Both static and dynamic factors contribute to shoulder stability. Static factors include:

(1) bony articulation,
(2) labrum,
(3) capsule and its thickenings, which form the various glenohumeral ligaments,
(4) adhesion–cohesion between the intra-articular fluid and joint surfaces,
(5) negative intra-articular pressure producing a vacuum effect.

Dynamic stability is provided by the musculature around the shoulder. This includes the rotator cuff, the deltoid, the long head of the bicep, and the scapula.

As the glenoid only covers around 25% of the humerus, the contribution of the labrum to the stability of the glenohumeral joint is very significant. As well as adding to the depth of the glenoid and increasing the contact area of the glenoid and the humeral head, the labrum also acts as a chock block resisting glenohumeral translation. The labrum also acts as a site for the insertion of the glenohumeral ligaments. In the vast majority of cases with traumatic anterior dislocation, there is disruption of the labrum and the attached inferior glenohumeral ligaments. This is known as "Bankart lesion" and usually occurs as a result of forced external rotation, abduction and extension of the arm forcing the glenohumeral head out of the joint. This detachment of the labrum and the glenohumeral ligaments makes the glenohumeral joint very unstable.

Another common associated injury with traumatic anterior dislocation is a compression fracture at the posterolateral part of the humeral which occurs as a consequence of impaction of the humeral head into the glenoid edge. This is referred to as the "Hills Sach's lesion".

Shoulder dislocation may also be associated with rotator cuff injuries, in particular with the more elderly population.

Clinical features

There is usually a history of trauma. With anterior dislocation, this usually involves an indirect force to the arm in extension, abduction and external rotation, whereas posterior dislocation occurs as a consequence of an axially directed force to an arm that is internally directed and rotated. Commonly, patients complain of severe pain with decreased range of movement.

With anterior dislocation, the arm is held in abduction and external rotation. The arm is retained in adduction and internal rotation with posterior dislocation.

There may be associated neurovascular damage, in particular to the axillary nerve. There may be a history of prior dislocation.

Investigations

Plain radiography involving two views (anteroposterior and axillary or Y view) will demonstrate the dislocation. This may also reveal any associated fractures; however, these may be illustrated with more detail by a CT scan. MRI will demonstrate associated rotator cuff injuries and, when combined with an arthrogram, it will illustrate any damage to the labrum.

Treatment

Acute dislocation will require reduction. Various close reduction techniques are advocated. These include:

(1) Patient lies prone, the affected arm hangs vertically from the table with some weights attached to it. This may take 20 minutes before the shoulder is relocated.
(2) With patient lying supine, while an assistant provides counteraction by pulling a sheet that has been rapped around the chest, the clinician gently pulls and rotates the affected arm to unhinge the dislocated humeral head.
(3) Clinician abducts and externally rotates the affected arm while at the same time disengaging the humeral head with his or her thumb.
(4) Clinician's foot is placed under the athlete's axilla while applying gentle longitudinal traction to the arm (Hippocratic method).
(5) With the elbow flexed to 90°, the arm is externally rotated, elbow brought forward. The arm is adducted next and finally internally rotated. This is known as Kocher's method and is an example of a leveraging technique. With this technique there is a risk of causing fracture and nerve injury.

Reduction of posterior dislocation involves prolonged axial traction on the humerus while manually applying pressure to the humerus head in order to disengage it.

The issue of shoulder immobilization following reduction is controversial. Traditionally, sling immobilization for 3 weeks has been advocated in order to reduce the chances of recurrent dislocation. This concept has been challenged more recently as some studies show even higher rates of recurrent dislocation following immobilization. There are also a number of recent studies that have demonstrated that immobilization in external rotation rather than internal rotation, is better for the healing of an associated labrum tear, and results in fewer recurrent dislocations.

Regardless of whether immobilization is used or not, isometric exercises are initiated as soon as pain subsides. This is followed by range of movement and isotonic exercises. More vigorous exercises including rotator cuff strengthening are initiated once a full passive range of movement is achieved.

The re-dislocation rate is very high in the young athletic population (as high as 90% in some studies). Because of this, some advocate surgical intervention following first dislocation in such athletes. Surgery is in the form of a stabilization procedure and is thought to significantly reduce the re-dislocation rate (as low as 10%). This stabilization procedure may be performed open or arthroscopically.

Return to sport

With both operative and non-operative management, the athlete should only be allowed to return to sport after achieving full strength and range of movement. With non-operative management this may take 2 to 3 months. Following surgery, the average return to sport is between 4 to 6 months, but may be as long as 12 months.

Further reading

Hayes K, Callanan M, Walton J, Paxinos A, Murrell GAC. Shoulder instability: management and rehabilitation. *J Orthopaedics & Sports Physical Therapy* 2002; **32**(10): 1–13.

McCarty EC, Ritchie P, Gill HS, McFarland EG. Shoulder instability: return to play. *Clinics in Sports Medicine* 2004; **23**: 335–51.

Shoulder – instability

AA Narvani

Shoulder instability covers a wide range of pathological conditions that result in an abnormal motion for that joint and may manifest with a variety of clinical features including pain, subluxation or dislocation of the shoulder. It is not the same as joint laxity, which refers to increased-degree glenohumeral translation lying within the physiological range. First reported over 2000 years ago, its management still remains very controversial.

Epidemiology

Shoulder instability is a common problem in athletes. Although primary shoulder dislocation rates are comparable in younger and older patients, recurrent dislocation rate is much more common in the adolescent population. Recurrent dislocation rates following primary dislocation are reported to lie between 70 to 100%, 15 to 65%, and 0 to 20%, in age groups 20 years and under, 20 and 40 years and 40 years or older respectively.

Predisposing factors

Proposed risk factors include:

(i) increased joint laxity
(ii) involvement in sports that are either violent or force the glenohumeral joint into extreme positions
(iii) excessive retroversion of the humeral head
(iv) neuromuscular conditions such as cerebral palsy
(v) young age

Patho-physiology

Both static and dynamic factors contribute to shoulder stability. Static factors include:

(1) *Bony articulation*

(2) *Labrum*

As the glenoid only covers around 25% of the humerus, the contribution of the labrum to the stability of the glenohumeral joint is very significant. As well as adding to the depth of the glenoid and increasing the contact area of the glenoid and the humeral head, the labrum also acts as a chock block resisting glenohumeral translation. The labrum also acts as a site for the insertion of the glenohumeral ligaments.

(3) *Capsule* and its thickenings, which form the various *glenohumeral ligaments*

The superior glenohumeral ligaments' (SGHL) primary function is thought to be limitation of anterior and inferior translation of adducted humerus. The middle glenohumeral ligament (MGHL) resists excessive anterior translation of the humerus when the arm is abducted between 60° and 90°. The inferior glenohumeral ligament (IGHL) is the strongest of the three glenohumeral ligaments, consists of three distinct parts (anterior band, axillary pouch and posterior band), and functions, like a hammock, as the primary restraints against anterior, posterior and inferior translations when the humerus is abducted further than 45°.

(4) *Adhesion-cohesion* between the intra-articular fluid and joint surfaces.

(5) *Negative intra-articular pressure* producing a vacuum effect.

Dynamic stability is provided by the musculature around the shoulder. These muscles include:

(1) *Rotator cuff muscles* (supraspinatus, subscapularis, infraspinatus and teres minor)

These cause compression of the humeral head into the glenoid cavity during motion.

(2) *Scapular rotator muscles* (trapezius, rhomboids, latissimus dorsi, serratus anterior and levator scapulae)

These contribute to posterior and inferior stability of the glenohumeral stability during motion by allowing the glenoid to stay in an anteverted and superior position in order to articulate with a retroverted humeral head.

(3) *Long head of the biceps*

It is thought that biceps contribute to anterior glenohumeral joint stability in external rotation and abduction by resisting the increased external rotation forces that exist in such a position.

The fine balance between static and dynamic stabilizers of the shoulder joint is critical in providing the overall shoulder joint stability. This fine balance may be disturbed in a number of ways.

(I) Labrum lesions

Detachment of the anterior–inferior labrum from the glenoid rim, together with its attached inferior glenohumeral ligament complex, is known as "Bankart's lesion". This can lead to increased anterior translation of humeral head with abduction and external rotation. In addition, there may also be excessive anterior and posterior humeral head translation with flexion, and inferior translation with extension and internal rotation of the shoulder.

"Reverse Bankart's" lesion refers to detachment of the posterior–inferior part of the labrum from the glenoid rim and can lead to increased posterior and inferior humeral head translations.

Superior labral anterior–posterior lesions (SLAP) can also lead to shoulder instability.

(II) *Capsular lesions*
It has been argued that for a complete dislocation to occur as a consequence of capsule lesions, there must exist capsular deformation on the involved side as well as the opposite side of the joint (in order for the humerus to translate excessively, a capsular lesion in one direction must be accompanied by another lesion or capsular laxity in the opposite direction, this is known as the "circle concept"). The capsular lesions may be in the form of tears, redundant capsular pockets or just stretched tissue.

(III) *Glenohumeral ligaments dysfunction*
These can occur either as the result of labrum or capsular lesions (see above).

(IV) *Muscular dysfunction*
This may occur as a result of peripheral and central nervous system lesions, muscular and tendon pathologies.

(V) *Proprioception dysfunction*
It has been shown that ligaments and capsule contain neural structures and mechano-receptors that provide poprioception feedback information which may contribute to stability by mediating muscular reflex stabilization.

(VI) *Altered bony anatomy*
This rarely causes instability on its own. Examples include altered versions of the glenoid or the humerus.

It is important to appreciate that for each patient, more than one of the above factors may play a part in making the shoulder unstable, therefore when managing such athletes all the above factors must be considered.

Clinical features

History

The important features in the patient's history include:

- Presence/absence of *trauma*.
- *Pain* in the shoulder without any history of trauma may be due to shoulder subluxation.
- *Age*.
- *Previous episodes*.
- *Previous treatment* (including type of physical therapy and surgery).
- *Psychosocial* issues.

Examination

This should include:

- Specific tests for *general laxity* (hyperextension of the thumb, fingers, elbows and the knee).

- Specific tests for *shoulder laxity* (anterior/posterior draw tests, Sulcus sign).
- Specific tests for *shoulder instability* (anterior/posterior apprehension tests).
- Detection of *rotator cuff* impingement and assessment of rotator cuff function.
- General shoulder girdle *posture* and detection of any *muscular patterning disorder*.

Investigations

Imaging

Plain radiographs

As well as demonstrating acute dislocations plain films may reveal a Hill Sachs lesion (defect in the humeral head).

CT/CT arthrography

CT allows assessment of bony architecture and, in combination with arthrography, identifies any associated labral tear and ligament laxity.

MRI/MR arthrography

As well as identifying labral pathology, will also illustrate associated rotator cuff pathology. MR arthrography is reported to be more sensitive and specific than MRI alone.

Electromyography (EMG)

This investigation will detect any abnormalities in muscle patterning, and as muscle coordination plays an important part in stability, EMG studies can be of great value in athletes with atraumatic multidirectional instability.

Examination under anaesthesia

Complete examination (see above) under anaesthesia may be of great value in assessment of stability; however, on its own it may not be able to distinguish between laxity and instability.

Arthroscopy

Although an invasive procedure, arthroscopy is the gold standard in identifying structural damages in the shoulder.

Classification

Based on the clinical features and investigations, in order to plan an effective treatment, the instability must be classified. There are many different classifications. One of the most commonly used classification systems is the Thomas and Matsen classification. With this system there are two general types of instability: TUBS and AMBRI.

- TUBS stands for Traumatic Unidirectional Bankart lesion treated by Surgery.
- AMBRI stands for Atraumatic Multidirectional Bilateral usually treated by Rehabilitation but if surgery is required, it should be by Inferior capsular shift.

Although the Thomas and Matsen classification is easy to remember, it has its limitations in that it is very rigid, and does not have a distinct category for patients who suffer from habitual instability with muscle patterning disorder, without any structural damage in their glenohumeral joint.

A less rigid, but more inclusive and practical, system is the Stanmore classification. With this system, the patients are divided into three main polar groups. Type I patients have a good history of trauma with some structural damage to their joint. In type II patients, there is no history of trauma, but structural damage is present. With type III patients there is neither a history of trauma nor any structural damage. The pathology with this type is the muscle patterning problem. In this system each type forms the angle of a triangle. There are also sub-types such as subgroup I(II) (athletes in this sub-group have a history of injury without a subsequent formal reduction). Furthermore, this system is a dynamic classification that allows for a shift in the pattern of instability with time.

Treatment

Management of acute dislocation is discussed in the acute shoulder dislocation chapter (see the chapter on Shoulder – acute dislocation). Management of shoulder instability will be discussed here using the Stanmore classification.

Type I (history of trauma + articular surface damage + Bankart lesion + unilateral laxity + normal muscle patterning)

Treatment of this group is by surgery. This may either be:

- Anatomical repair (such as Bankart's repair). May be performed by open surgery or arthroscopically.
- Non-anatomical repairs (Putti-Plat, Magnuson–Stack, Bristow). These tend to sacrifice range of movement to a greater degree than the anatomical repairs.

Type II (no clear history of trauma, but with a damaged articular surface, dysfunctional capsule and normal muscle patterning).

Those patients who do not have any underlying muscle patterning abnormality, the pure type II, may benefit from surgery intervention.

Surgery is in the form of various capsular shift procedures or laser/radio frequency capsular shrinkage procedures (capsulorraphy).

Those patients who, in addition, have an associated element of muscle patterning disorder (sub-type II(III)), require correction of their muscle patterning abnormality before surgery could be considered. Surgery should only be offered if underlying structural instability remains a problem despite correction of muscle patterning abnormality.

Type III (no clear history of trauma, no articular surface damage, but with abnormal muscle patterning).

Athletes in this group must be treated non-operatively as they require correction of their inappropriate muscle recruitment. These athletes should undergo biofeedback exercises to improve their muscle coordination and position sense with the aim of ultimately improving their scapulothoracic and glenohumeral muscle pattern.

Return to sport

As with other sports injuries, with both operative and non-operative management, the athlete should only be allowed to return to sport after pain relief is achieved, and after regaining a near normal range of movement and strength. Additionally the shoulder must be stable. With non-operative management this may take 2 to 3 months. Following surgery the average return to sport is between 4 to 6 months, but may be as long as 12 months.

Further reading

Backer M, Warren RF. Glenohumeral instabilities. In: JC DeLee, D Drez, MD Miller (Eds) *Orthopaedic Sports Medicine, Principles and Practice*, 2nd edn. Saunders, 2002: 1020–34.

Levine WN, Flatow EL. The pathophysiology of shoulder instability. *Am J Sports Medicine* 2000; **28**(6): 910–17.

Lewis A, Kitamura T, Bayley JIL. The classification of shoulder instability: new light through old windows. *Current Orthopaedics* 2004; **18**: 97–108.

McCarty EC, Ritchie P, Gill HS, McFarland EG. Shoulder instability: return to play. *Clinics in Sports Medicine* 2004; **23**: 335–51.

Shoulder – impingement syndrome/rotator cuff disease

AA Narvani

Recognised more than 150 years ago, this syndrome is one of the most common causes of shoulder pain in athletes. It is particularly common in activities that involve repetitive overhead movements such as swimming, tennis, volleyball, throwing sports and baseball but is seen in many other types of sports as well.

Pathology

The rotator cuff consists of four muscles which include the supraspinatus, infraspinatus, teres minor and the subscapularis. The pathology of rotator cuff disease is complex and multifactorial. Furthermore, it is a spectrum of conditions. An attempt to demonstrate the pathophysiology of the process has been made in Figure 1.

As demonstrated in Figure 1, mechanical impingement of the rotor cuff tendon and tendinopathy of the tendon are interlinked, as impingement of the tendon can lead to its tendinopathy and tendinopathy can cause mechanical impingement by causing swelling of the tendon in the subacromial space. Therefore, the process can develop into a vicious cycle or a positive feedback system, as illustrated by the central square in Figure 1. The percentage contribution of impingement and tendinopathy to the pathological process and symptoms production would be different in each individual athlete. Tendinopathy is characterised by degenerative changes in the tendon.

There are conditions or circumstances that initiate this cycle/positive feedback system or increase the gain of the system. These include the following.

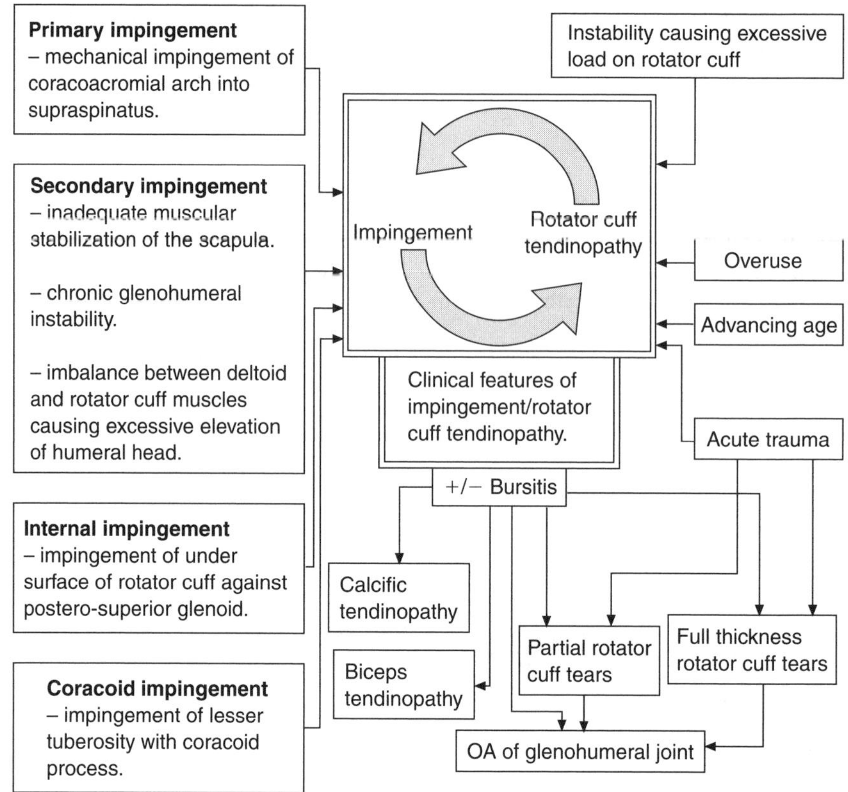

Figure 1 Pathophysiology of rotator cuff tendinopathy/impingement.

Primary impingement

This refers to the direct mechanical impingement of the supraspinatus tendon by structure in the coracoacromial arch (acromion, coracoacromial ligaments and the acromial clavicular joint (ACJ)). Although not the most common cause for impingements in young athletes, it is the most frequent cause overall. As the humerus flexes, abducts and internally rotates, the narrowing of the subcromial space becomes significant and mechanical impingement of the tendon can occur. This position is employed frequently in sports such as swimming, tennis and those that involve overhead throwing. Other factors that contribute to primary impingement include:

(I) curved or hooked acromion
(II) thickening of the coracoacromial ligament
(III) prominent ACJ

Secondary impingement

This is thought to be the most common impingement in young athletes.

The following pathologies can lead to secondary impingement:

(I) A weak serratus anterior may not stabilize the scapula adequately, which can lead to exaggerated angulation of the acromion and therefore mechanical impingement.
(II) In glenohumeral stability, there can be migration of the humeral head anteriorly leading to impingement of the supraspinatus tendon by the coracoacromial arch structures.
(III) If the delicate balance between the rotator cuff muscles and deltoid is disturbed (i.e. weak rotator cuff muscles), deltoid contraction can cause excessive migration of the humeral head, which in turn may lead to impingement.

Internal impingement

This condition is thought to be present in a significant number of athletes who take part in throwing sports and who present with posterior shoulder pain.

In the presence of anterior capsule laxity, the under surface of the rotator cuff can come into contact with the postero–superior aspect of the glenoid as the arm extends, abducts and externally rotates at the same time (as a result of anterior translation of the humeral head). This manoeuvre occurs in the late cocking phase of throwing. This impingement of the under surface of the rotator cuff on the glenoid can become symptomatic.

Coracoid impingement

This is not very common but occurs in athletes with instability, when lesser tuberosity comes into contact with the coracoid process as the arm flexes, internally rotates and adducts.

Overuse

Overuse in athletes who participate in sports that involve overhead and throwing activities, can cause micro-trauma to the tendon. (In throwing athletes, in the follow-through phase of the throwing action, there is eccentric contraction of the rotator cuff as it decelerates the humerus. The large forces generated in the tendon in this can damage the tendon.) This can lead to tendinopathy of the rotator cuff, which is characterized by degenerative histological features. Bad technique and abnormal biomechanics can have the same consequence as overuse.

Advancing age

The incidence of rotator cuff tendinopathy increases with advancing age. This is probably due to the age-related changed in the tendon. As mentioned above the pathological process in tendinopathy appears to be a degenerative one. Degenerative features are commonly observed with advancing age.

Acute trauma

Acute traumatic disruption of the tendon may occur leading to tendinopathy and partial or complete rupture of the rotator cuff. This could occur in the deceleration phase of the throwing motion, as a consequence of direct trauma to the shoulder caused by a fall or contact sport, or with shoulder dislocation.

Tendinopathy as a consequence of instability

The mechanisms for instability causing secondary and corocoid impingements have been discussed above, but they can also lead to rotator cuff tendinopathy directly. In those athletes with shoulder instability, the load on the rotator cuff is greater than in those athletes without instability. This can lead to the tendinopathy of the tendon, particularly if this is present in combination with any of the above conditions.

Clinical features of impingement and tendinopathy

Athletes usually present with gradual onset of shoulder pain, which is made worse by overhead activities. The location of pain is usually over a diffuse area in the proximity of the deltoid.

On examination, inspection may reveal atrophy of rotator cuff muscles. Active abduction is painful. There is usually a painful arc which is between 70° and 120° abduction. The reason for this is that the glenohumeral distance is least in this range and therefore gives the maximum impingement. Neer's sign, which is production of pain with forceful forward elevation of the arm while stabilizing the scapula, is positive. Internal rotation and adduction of the arm while flexing it to 90° in the plane of the scapula is also painful (Hawkin's sign). It is important to test each muscle of the rotator cuff individually to exclude tears (see below); however, because of pain inhibition, there may appear to be rotator cuff weakness in the absence of any tears. This is where Neer's test is helpful. This is positive when there is elimination of pain and therefore restoration of rotator cuff tendon muscles' power, with subacromial local anaesthetic injection.

As already discussed, there are many conditions that could lead to impingement and rotator cuff tendinopathy. Clinical assessment must include attempts at detection of these conditions, as any successful management involves attention and treatment of these underlying causes and predisposing factors.

Investigations

This is a clinical diagnosis; however, the following features may be present on the various imaging modalities.

Plain radiographs may demonstrate;

- Anterior acromial spur (antero-posterior caudal tilt view)
- Subacromial space narrowing (AP view)
- Subchondral sclerosis, cortical fragmentation, cysts of greater tuberosity
- Associated subluxation of humeral head

Ultrasound will demonstrate the tendinopathy, presence of any associated bursa and tears. It is dynamic, non-invasive and cheap, but it is operator dependent.

Magnetic resonance imaging also provides detailed visualization of rotator cuff pathology ranging from mild tendinopathy to full thickness tears.

Treatment

Initially, the athlete is encouraged to discontinue the activity that precipitated the condition. This may involve technique modification by the athlete. A short course of NSAIDs may be prescribed. Some athletes have found other modalities, such as ultrasound, massage and cryotherapy, helpful in controlling the pain. Subacromial cortisone injection can also provide some pain relief and prevent it causing muscular inhibition, therefore allowing adequate physical therapy. Initially, the physical therapy programme should include stretching and range of movement exercises, as contracture of the capsule in athletes can worsen the impingement. Following this, the athlete must progress to strengthening exercises concentrating on all the muscle groups utilized in the athlete's sport, including rotator cuff muscles, scapula stabilizers, even lower limb and trunk muscles.

It is of vital importance to detect and treat any underlying causes that could have led to impingement/tendinopathy. Instability must be addressed and dealt with (see the chapter on shoulder instability). Abnormal scapulohumeral rhythm must be corrected. Any imbalance between deltoid and rotator cuff contraction must be rectified as excessive elevation of the humeral head can lead to, or exaggerate, the impingement/tendinopathy process. Just as important is the amendment of any poor technique and training regime.

Surgery is indicated if there is a complete rotator cuff tear or partial tear greater than 50% (see below) or if there is no symptomatic relief despite about 6 months of non-operative treatment. This would be in the form of either arthroscopic or open procedure. Arthroscopy combined with examination under anaesthesia will reveal other pathologies, such as labral disease, instability and glenohumeral degenerative changes. If it is detected that impingement/tendinopathy is secondary to occult instability, it may be more appropriate to address the instability first with a stabilization procedure. The impingement/tendinopathy itself may be addressed by careful debridement, bursectomy or acriomioplasty.

Prognosis

Two-thirds of patients with impingement/tendinopathy respond to non-operative management. Surgery results in a satisfactory outcome in over 80% of the patients.

Return to sport

As with other sports injuries, return to play is permitted once the athlete is pain free and has regained the majority of his or her muscular strength in order to perform their sport safely. The time this happens is dependent on many factors, including the athlete, sport, underlying cause and type of treatment. The majority of athletes with non-operative management that has been successful return to their sport within a few weeks. With operative management the accepted time for return to sport is between 3 to 6 months postoperatively. Arthroscopic decompression allows earlier return to sport than the open procedure.

Rotator cuff tears

If present in young athletes, rotator cuff tears are usually partial thickness tears, as full thickness tears are uncommon in such a population. They frequently occur on a background of impingement/tendinopathy but occasionally may be as a result of a single traumatic event.

The following test can aid in diagnosis of rotator cuff tears:

(I) "Drop arm test". The athlete is instructed to slowly lower the arm from an abduction position. In presence of a tear, this manoeuvre loses its smoothness.
(II) Test for supraspinatus. A downward force is directed to the arm as the shoulder is abducted 90° and internally rotated. This test will reveal any weaknesses in the supraspinatus by comparing both sides.
(III) Test for infraspinatus. The athlete is asked to externally rotate the shoulder against resistance, with the elbow flexed to 90° at the side.
(IV) "Gerber's lift-off test" for subscapularis. The athlete places their arm behind his or her body with the dorsum aspect of the hand facing the lower back. The clinician then places the palm of his or her hand against the palm of the athlete's hand, and then instructs the athlete to push his or her hand away from the back against resistance.

Ultrasound and MRI are the investigations of choice to confirm the tears. Treatment of partial-thickness tears of less than 50% is similar to that of tendinopathy/impingement. Partial-thickness tears of more than 50% and full-thickness tears require operative intervention in athletes. Surgical repair may be performed by open, mini-open procedures or arthroscopically. It is generally believed that arthroscipic repair leads to quicker recovery, especially when combined with an accurate and adequate rehabilitation programme. Return to sport following surgical repair is also dependent on many other factors, including the patient and the sport. Overall, athletes are expected to participate fully in sports between 8 to 12 months following surgery.

Biceps tendinopathy

The commonest cause of biceps tendinopathy in athletes is rotator cuff impingement/tendinopathy. It also occurs in individuals who undergo a lot of weight training and also in those who suffer from glenohumeral instability. Athletes usually present with anterior shoulder pain, which is made worse by overhead activities. There is localized tenderness over the biceps tendon in the bicipital groove. Passive stretching of biceps would reproduce the pain, as would resisted flexion of the shoulder with an extended elbow and supinated forearm (Speed's test). Resisted supination of the forearm with elbow flexed to 90° leads to localized pain at the long head of the bicep tendon ("Yergason's test"). Ultrasound or MRI will confirm the diagnosis. Management involves NSAIDs, local modalities such as massage and ultrasound. Some athletes may also benefit from steroid injections into the bicipital sheath, which can be performed with image guidance. The underlying cause, such as rotator cuff impingement/tendinopathy and glenohumeral instability must be treated. Surgery is the last option in those who do not respond to non-operative management and the options include debridement, release or tenodesis.

Bicep tendon long head rupture

This may be seen in gymnasts, javelin-throwers, wrestlers, weight lifters and racquet sports. It is more common in older athletes. There may be a history of acute trauma accompanied by sharp pain over the anterior aspect of the shoulder. There is usually a deformity in the anterior aspect of the arm formed by the detached muscle and the accompanying haematoma. Assessment of muscle power will reveal weaknesses. Non-operative treatment involves pain management followed by restoration of mobility and strength. Surgical repair is reserved for young active athletes who are involved in power sports.

Bicep subluxation

This is usually associated with subscapularis disruption as the transverse humeral ligament is damaged, therefore allowing the long head of the bicep to sublux or dislocate. As the arm is internally rotated from external rotation and the abduction position, a painful click may be palpated as the tendon subluxes. Surgery may benefit those with chronic symptoms and those with associated subscapularis tear.

Calcific tendinopathy

The commonest site for this is the supraspinatus tendon. Calcium is deposited on the supraspinatus tendon as a consequence of tendinopathy. Pain is usually intense. There is localized tenderness over the anterior upper part of the shoulder. A plain radiograph will illustrate the calcium deposits. Pain management and mobility are important as stiffness may occur. Cortisone and local anaesthetic injection can improve the pain. In those who do not respond to non-operative management, surgical removal of the calcium deposit is successful in relieving the symptoms.

Further reading

Almekinders LC. Impingement syndrome. *Clinics in Sports Medicine* 2001; **20**(3): 491–503.

Anderson K, Answorth AA. Rotator cuff. *Current Opinion in Orthopaedics* 1999; **10**: 289–93.

Shoulder – acromioclavicular joint injuries

AA Narvani

First recognised by Hippocrates as early as 400 BC, these injuries are extremely common, particularly among athletes. The incidence of acromioclavicular joint (ACJ) dislocation is estimated to be at three or four per 100,000 per annum in the general population. Up to 40% of sports shoulder injuries are due to ACJ disruption. These injuries are more common in males, in particular those in the second or third decades.

Pathology

Since there is very little inherent bony stability of the ACJ itself, the surrounding soft tissue structures play a very important role in providing its stability. These structures include both muscles (deltoid and trapezius, which act as dynamic stabilisers) and ligaments. These ligaments consist of the acromioclavicular (AC) ligament and the coracoclavicular ligaments (compromising the conoid and trapezoid ligaments). It is these two ligament complexes that are damaged in ACJ injuries.

The most practical classification of these injuries is the Rockwood modification of the Allman–Tossy's classification. This modification includes six different types of injury.

More than 90% of the injuries are Types I, II and III, whereas Types IV, V and VI injuries are uncommon (see Table 1).

Mechanism of injury

These injuries may occur as a consequence of direct or indirect force. Direct force, which is thought to be the mechanism of injury in 70% of the patients, occurs when the athlete falls directly on the shoulder with the force pushing the acromion downwards. Indirect force is transmitted through the humeral head to the acromion as the

Table 1 Shoulder – acromioclavicular joint injuries.

Grade	Acromioclavicular lig.	Coracoclavicular lig.	Clavicular displacement
Type I	Sprain	No injury	No displacement
Type II	Complete rupture	Sprain	Mild superior clavicular displacement (less than the diameter of the clavicle)
Type III	Complete rupture	Complete rupture	Clavicle is displaced superiorly with respect to acromion by the diameter of the distal clavicle
Type IV	Complete rupture	Complete rupture	Clavicle goes posteriorly and "button holes" the trapezius muscle
Type V	Complete rupture	Complete rupture	Clavicle is displaced superiorly by twice the diameter of the distal clavicle
Type VI	Complete rupture	Complete rupture	Clavicle displaces inferiorly and becomes stuck beneath the conjoint tendon and coracoid process

athlete falls on his or her outstretched arm. This transmitted force damages the ligament complexes. These injuries are common in contact sports such as rugby, American football and ice hockey but may also occur in sports where falls could occur, such as cycling. Type IV to VI injuries occur with high-energy trauma and therefore may be seen in motor sports.

Clinical features

There may be:

(I) A history of either a fall on the shoulder or onto an outstretched arm.
(II) Pain.
(III) Swelling.
(IV) Localised tenderness.
(V) Deformity at the ACJ.
(VI) Associated injuries such as rotator cuff tear, glenohumeral instability and neurovascular injuries, which must be excluded.

Investigations

Plain radiograph is the investigation of choice. With Type I injuries, X-ray appearance may be normal, but with more severe injuries there is subluxation of the ACJ and there may be widening of the coracoclavicular space. Stress X-rays (not routinely used) may help to distinguish between Type II and III injuries.

Treatment

Treatment is dependent on the type of injury.

Type I Management here is non-operative with NSAIDs, ice packs and sling in the acute phase. Athletes are encouraged to stop wearing the sling after 2–3 weeks. Physical therapy exercises to restore range of movement and strength are started as soon as pain allows.

Type II Same as Type I.

Type III Acute Type III injuries may be managed both non-operatively or operatively. Non-operative measures are the same as those of Type I and II injuries. Surgery may involve acromioclavicular repairs (using wires, pins or hook plates), coracoclavicular repairs (Bosworth screws, cerclage wires, TightRope), dynamic muscle transfers or distal clavicular excisions. Studies suggest that those treated non-operatively have a better range of movement and strength than those treated operatively. In addition, they return to work and sport earlier but the chances that they may be left with a deformity of the lateral end of the clavicle is much higher. Surgery is indicated, however, in those patients who continue to have pain and dysfunction after 3 to 6 months of non-operative measures. In such patients, surgery is in the form of the "Weaver Dunn" procedure, which consists of transferring the coraco-acromion ligament into the intramedullary canal of the clavicle and placing the clavicle into a more anatomical position. Recently arthroscopic reconstruction techniques have also been described.

Type IV There are some recent studies that suggest that these uncommon injuries may be reduced by applying anterior to posterior traction to the acromion of both shoulders; however, the traditional method for treating acute Type IV injuries is by open operative means similar to those suggested for surgical treatments of Type III injuries. Untreated Type IV injuries and those that have presented late are treated with the "Weaver Dunn" procedure. More modern minimal invasive techniques may also be considered, however more research on their effectiveness is required.

Types V and VI The choice with these injuries is operative management (similar surgical techniques to those for acute Type III injuries). Again, untreated ones and those that present late can be treated with the "Weaver Dunn" procedure.

Return to sport

As with other sports injuries, return to sport is permitted once the athlete is pain free, able to achieve a full range of movement and has regained enough strength to perform their sport-specific activities. With non-operative management, as far as Type I and II injuries are concerned, return to sports usually takes 1 to 4 weeks depending on the sport. When Type III injuries are treated non-operatively, return to sport may be slower than Types I and II injuries; surgery is indicated, however, if the athlete has not improved by 3 to 6 months.

Return to sport following operative management usually takes 6 months.

Long-term prognosis

Calcification of the coracoclavicular space appears to be common following both operative and non-operative management of ACJ injuries. This calcification, however, does not usually affect the final clinical or functional outcome.

Degenerative changes in ACJ are seen in about 35% of the patients who have had ACJ injuries. Many with these degenerative changes may, however, not be symptomatic.

Osteolysis of the lateral end of the clavicle can occur after a variable period following these injuries. In most cases, symptoms commonly resolve within 2 years.

Further reading

DeLee JC, Drez D, Miller MD. *Orthopaedic Sports Medicine, Principles and Practice*, 2nd edn. Saunders, 2002: 912–32.

Foy M, Fag P. Medicolegal reporting in orthopaedic trauma, 3rd edn. Churchill Livingstone, 2002: 53–60.

Skin infections in athletes

A Kamvari

Skin infections are very common in athletes due to various forms of trauma related to sports, increased friction and sweating, and occlusive clothing. They can be passed on to other athletes easily due to close contact with each other and with fomites such as weights, mats, pool decks and communal showers.

Skin infections can be divided into three groups depending on the organisms that cause them:

(1) Bacterial skin infections
(2) Viral skin infections
(3) Fungal skin infections

Bacterial skin infections

Impetigo

Impetigo is a contagious infection of the skin caused by staphylococci or streptococci or both. Two forms are recognised:

(1) Vesiculopustular (non-bullous) type with thick golden-crusted lesions.
(2) Bullous type

Aetiology

Non-bullous type is usually caused by group AB haemolytic streptococcus or coagulate-positive staphylococcus aureus.

Bullous type is generally associated with phage group II S. aureus.

Symptoms and signs

Itching is the only symptom. Regional lymphadenopathy may be found.

The bullous form typically begins as multiple fluid-filled vesicles that either coalesce or enlarge forming blister-like lesions. The centre has the classic honey-crusted lesion that, when removed, reveals erythematous plaques draining serous fluid. Non-bullous impetigo starts as small vesicles and pustules with erythematous bases and honey-coloured crusts, which also drain fluid.

There are usually no systemic symptoms but regional lymphadenopathy may be found.

Investigations and treatment

Diagnosis is clinical, or can be confirmed with bacterial cultures. Treatment is with oral antibiotics. In most cases dicloxacillin or erythromycin is effective.

Return to sports

Patients with impetigo should not participate in contact sports such as wrestling, and should be started on oral antibiotic therapy. They may participate in competition after starting antibiotics at least 72 hours previously and have not had new skin lesions for at least 48 hours. The affected area should be protected with a non-permeable bandage that cannot be dislodged during sports.

Folliculitis, furunculosis and carbuncles

Folliculitis is infection of the superficial portion of the hair follicles. Furunculosis (boils) is a deeper infection involving the whole of the hair follicle and the lesions usually contain pus. They typically occur in areas of increased sweating and friction, such as buttocks, the anterior thigh, axilla and the belt line. A carbuncle is several furuncles developing in adjoining hair follicles and coalescing to form a deeply situated mass with multiple drainage points.

Aetiology

Staphylococcus aureus is the causative organism.

Symptoms and signs

Folliculitis is characterised by mildly tender papules or pustules surrounded by erythema. Patients complain of itching and burning in hairy areas.

In furunculosis patients complain about swellings and abscesses that are extremely painful. The pain, fever and malaise are more severe with carbuncles.

Investigations and treatment

Diagnosis is clinical. Treatment for mild foliculitis is topical mupirocin (Bactrobam). More widespread infection may require antistaphylococcal antibiotics (dicloxacillin or cephalexin).

Treatment of furuncles, carbuncles and abscesses include immobilisation of the affected part to avoid over-manipulation of inflamed areas; using moist heat to help localise larger lesions; and incision and debridement after the lesions have matured.

Systemic antibiotics, e.g. erythromycin and cephalexin, may also be needed. Minocycline may be effective against resistant staphylococci.

Return to sports

Athletes engaging in contact sports such as wrestling should not participate in competition until 72 hours after starting antibiotic therapy and have had no new skin lesions for 48 hours. This is not only because of contagiousness to other athletes but also to reduce systemic complications such as bacteraemia and progressive soft-tissue infection.

Cellulitis

Cellulitis is a diffuse spreading infection of the skin affecting deeper tissues, and may be due to several organisms, usually cocci. The lesion is red and hot and has a diffuse border. Cellulitis usually occurs after a break in the skin.

Treatment is systemic antibiotics (penicillin or other broad-spectrum antibiotics). Athletes should not participate in competition until after the symptoms have resolved, to avoid systemic spread.

Otitis externa

See the chapter on Ear, nose, throat conditions in athletes.

Viral skin infections

Herpes simplex

Epidemiology

Approximately 90% of the population acquire herpes simplex (HSV1) infection before the ages of 4 or 5.

Aetiology

Herpes simplex is caused by two closely related viruses, HSV1 and HSV2. Both cause primary and recurrent infections. The virus can remain dormant in the neural ganglia following a primary infection and be reactivated following triggers such as sunlight, fatigue, menstruation and physical or emotional stress.

Signs and symptoms

During the primary infection there may be a prodrome of fever, malaise and lymphadenopathy. After an incubation period of 5 to 10 days, recurrent small grouped vesicles appear, especially around oral or genital areas, which have an erythematous base. The primary symptoms are burning and stinging. The vesicles rupture quickly and crust over within a few days. The crusted lesions may take a couple of weeks to heal completely.

Investigations and treatment

Diagnosis is principally made from clinical history and examination. A Tzanck test may be done to show multinucleated giant cells. Immunofluorescence may detect viral antigens and viral culture may be done but its sensitivity is only 70% to 80%.

Treatment is with oral antiviral medication. Acyclovir, valacyclovir and famcyclovir can all be given.

Return to sports

Vesicular lesions must be dried before the athlete can compete. The dried scabs should be covered with occlusive dressing to provide further protection.

Warts

Warts or verrucae are benign epithelial proliferations due to infection with various forms of human papillomavirus (HPV). They vary widely in shape, size and appearance, and mostly – but not exclusively – occur on the hands and feet. Warts can be periungual, flat, filiform and deep palmoplantar.

Infectivity is low, but can occur from close contact and may occur through fomites such as swimming pool decks, locker room and shower floors, weight lifting and gymnastic equipment. Autoinocculation through scratches, shaving and skin trauma can frequently occur.

Symptoms and signs

There are usually no symptoms. Tenderness on pressure occurs with plantar warts and can impede performance in athletes and should be treated. Occasionally a wart will produce mechanical obstruction (e.g. nostril, ear canal, urethra).

Investigation and treatment

Diagnosis is made by visual inspection. Warts do not have the normal fingerprint lines that calluses and corns retain, and if their surface is scraped using a blade, they show characteristic black pinpoint spots, which are thrombosed capillaries.

Treatment options include:

- Mechanical removal by either surgical excision, electrocautery, freezing with liquid nitrogen, or laser treatment.
- Chemical treatment includes using salicylic acid plasters for plantar warts, or applying preparations of trichloroacetic acid or Verrusol to the warts. Bleomycin injections can be used directly into plantar warts, but must be used with caution.
- Immunologic methods of treatment induce an immune response to suppress warts. These include injecting the wart with agents such as candida or mumps antigens, topical imiquimod and oral cimetidine.

Return to sports
Disqualification from play is not required if athletes start treatment and wear occlusive dressings.

Molluscum contagiosum
Molluscum contagiosum is characterised by single or multiple rounded, dome-shaped waxy papules 2–5 mm in diameter that are umbilicated and contain a caseous plug, caused by a virus in the Poxviridae family. The lesions are skin coloured at first but become pearly grey later on. Typically there are no symptoms, but patients can develop localised eczematous reactions and lesions can become pruritic and may suppurate.

Molluscum contagiosum most commonly develops on the face, hands and forearms, but can be seen on any other surface of skin, including genitalia. They are more common in swimmers, gymnasts and wrestlers. Spread is through skin-to-skin contact and autoinocculation.

Even though the infection is self-limiting, it is advisable for athletes involved in contact sports to be treated.

The treatment of Molluscum contagiosum is exactly the same as for warts.

Return to sports
Contact sports can be resumed 48 hours after resolution of papules.

Fungal skin infections

Tinea pedis
Athlete's foot is a very common fungal skin infection in sports people, mostly due to Tinea rubrum or Tinea mentagrophytes. The hot moist environment in sports footwear is an ideal environment for these fungi to grow and invade the intertriginous web spaces, which is the most common part of the foot for Tinea pedis to occur.

The commonest presenting symptom is itching, which worsens after the removal of socks. There may also be burning or pain from secondary infection with complicating cellulites and lymphangitis. Tinea pedis can present in three forms.

(a) There may be scaly eruption in the intertriginous space, with or without erythema, maceration or fissuring.
(b) Eruption of vesicles and bullae on the mid foot.
(c) Hyperkeratotic scales with minimal erythema on the plantar surface of the foot.

Diagnosis can be reached through clinical history and examination, and confirmed by direct microscopic visualisation of hyphae from skin scrapings.

Treatment is with topical antifungals, either in powder form for mild cases or with creams, such as terbinafine or naftifine or clotrimazole, in moderate cases. Oral antifungals can be used in severe or chronic Tinea pedis. Ketoconazole 200 mg daily for 10 days is usually very effective.

Wet dressings using Burrow's solution applied three times daily can relieve symptoms if maceration or vesicles are present.

There are no specific NCAA guidelines for return to sports with Tinea pedis, but it is advisable to refrain from competition until dissolution of symptoms or to adequately cover the area with non-permeable bandage.

Tinea capitis and Tinea corporis (ringworm)

Tinea capitis is a fungal infection of the head and corporis is of the body. Both are caused by dermatophytes of the genus Trichophyton.

Patients typically present with scaly, erythematous and pruritic ring-shaped plaques. The scalp may have bald patches and, on closer inspection, it can be seen that the hair shafts have been broken.

Scalp and body ringworm is especially common amongst wrestlers and athletes who wear occlusive clothing. Spread is by skin-to-skin contact and there can be Tinea corporis outbreaks amongst wrestlers.

Diagnosis is usually clinical and can be confirmed by visualising hyphae from skin scrapings in 10% potassium hydroxide preparations under a microscope.

Treatment is with topical or oral antifungals. Tinea corporis can be treated by applying terbinafine 1% or clotrimazole 1% twice daily and until 2 weeks after disappearance of the lesions, or orally with ketoconazole, itraconazole, or fluconazole. Tinea capitis should be treated with oral antifungals as above.

Athletes involved in contact sports with extensive Tinea corporis should be disqualified until at least 72 hours after topical treatment has been started, and those with Tinea capitis should have had oral therapy for at least 2 weeks.

Tinea cruris

Tinea cruris is a fungal infection of the groin area and is also known as "jock itch". It is very common amongst athletes and is caused by T. rubrum or T. mentagrophytes. The lesions occur in the crural folds, usually sparing the scrotum, and appear as sharply demarcated, centrally clearing erythematous macular lesions, with or without vesicle formation. Pruritis is a common symptom.

Diagnosis is by demonstrating hyphae microscopically in 10% potassium hydroxide preparations.

Treatment involves drying the affected area and using drying powder 2–3 times daily, and also topical antifungals, e.g. 1% clotrimazole or 1% terbinafine once or twice daily for 2 weeks.

There are no specific NCAA guidelines for return to sports with Tinea cruris.

Tinea versicolor

Tinea versicolor is a mild superficial infection of the skin caused by Pityrosporon orbiculare (Malassezia furfur). It is characterised by pale slightly scaly macules, usually on the trunk that do not tan on exposure to sunlight. There may be slight itching.

Excessive heat and sweating from wearing occlusive and heavy clothes promote the growth and invasion of this yeast in the stratum corneum.

It is diagnosed clinically, but can be confirmed by visualising branching hyphae and spores with direct microscopy.

The condition is not particularly infectious and there are no specific NCAA guidelines for return of athletes to sports.

Treatment is with topical selenium sulfide shampoo once daily for a week, or with 2% ketoconazole cream for 1–2 weeks.

Further reading

Adams BB. Dermatologic disorders of the athlete. *Sport Med* 2002; **32**(5): 309–21.

Sport and exercise at altitude

B Lynn

Aerobic exercise at altitude is limited by the fall in oxygen partial pressure. In mountain terrain it will usually also be cold. This is covered in the chapter on hypothermia (see the next chapter), so this section will deal entirely with the problems of exercise in a hypoxic environment. Note in passing that some of the problems discussed will also be relevant for subjects with low arterial oxygen due to lung disease.

Not a lot happens up to about 1500 m. Above this, the lowered oxygen has several immediate effects, which represent an immediate adaptation. Continued exposure to low oxygen levels causes profound longer term acclimatization. Above 6000 m, if not acclimatized you lose consciousness in minutes.

With acclimatisation, it is possible to survive for some time at altitudes of 6000 m or above, but eventually illness develops (see below). So no human settlements are found above 5000 m.

Immediate adaptation (over a few minutes) consists of an increase in heart rate and pulmonary ventilation, with the latter causing more CO_2 excretion, a lowered $PaCO_2$ and respiratory alkalosis. These adaptations are enough to allow average levels of physical activity. However, maximum aerobic exercise is limited and VO_2max is only 85% of normal. There were no world records in distance events at the Mexico City Olympics! But note that there *were* a lot of records in explosive events, where the reduced air resistance was helpful.

After the initial adaptation, the CO_2 sensitivity of the central chemoreceptor system resets to operate at lower levels suited to the hyperventilation. The resting heart drops back towards pre-altitude values (although the maximum heart rate is reduced). The haemoglobin content of the blood rises by around a third over 2–6 weeks. As discussed in the chapter on blood doping (see the chapter on Drugs in sport – blood doping), many athletes deliberately train at altitude to get this boost in oxygen-carrying capacity. However, although it is an important adaptation for exercise at altitude, the increments in sea-level performance may be small.

There is often substantial weight loss at altitudes above 4500 m. Some loss of appetite clearly occurs, and at higher altitudes there is poor absorption from the GI tract. Maintaining an adequate energy intake therefore requires some attention. It is also important to have plenty of iron to support the haemoglobin synthesis during acclimatization.

Above 4000 m acute mountain sickness (AMS) is common. It has been described as like a really bad hangover! With acclimatization, symptoms usually disappear. The risk is that the condition will progress to HACE or HAPE (see below). If possible, those affected by AMS should descend, then re-ascend more slowly. Certainly they should not ascend further. Acetazolamide is helpful in treating AMS.

High-altitude cerebral oedema (HACE or HACO) is a medical emergency. Cerebral oedema can come on rapidly in hours and can be fatal. It is most common above 5000 m during rapid ascents. Subjects should be moved immediately to a lower altitude. If this is not possible, oxygen can be given if available. Special pressure bags are taken by some high-altitude expeditions, and the subject is placed in a bag that is pumped by foot up to a high pressure. The equivalent of 1500 m descent can be achieved and this can be enough to reduce HACE. Dexamethasone (hydrocortisone)

Table 1 Arterial O_2 saturations and VO_2max at different altitudes.

Altitude, m	Atmospheric pressure, mmHg	Inspired oxygen partial pressure, mmHg	Arterial oxygen saturation, %	Maximum exercise rate, $VO_2max^{\#}$, % sea level value
0 (sea level)	760	160	98	(100)
2300*	580	120	95	85
6500	360	75	70	50
8848^{+}	250	52	–	30

After acclimatization
* Mexico City, 1968 Olympic Games
+ Mount Everest summit

Table 2 Adaptation and acclimatization at different altitudes.

1500–2500 m	Medium altitude	Adaptation sufficient
2500–5000/5500 m	High altitude	Adaptation not sufficient – acclimatization necessary to avoid acute mountain sickness (AMS)
5000/5500–8848 m	Extreme altitude	Acclimatization not possible

is reported to be effective. It is crucial to pick up the early signs of HACE. These include ataxia, exercise intolerance and odd behaviour.

High-altitude pulmonary oedema (HAPE, HAPO) is more common than HACE. It is also a dangerous condition although most people survive. Actions are essentially the same as for HACE, i.e. get to lower altitude or adopt other strategies to raise PaO_2. Nifedipine is reported to help. Again, it is important to spot early signs such as exercise intolerance and a dry cough. The cause of HAPE is raised capillary pressure in the lungs, so it is different from the classical pulmonary oedema from raised pulmonary venous pressure seen in heart failure.

Further reading

Ward MP, Milledge JS, West JB. *High altitude medicine and physiology*, 3rd edn. London: Arnold, 2000.

Sport and exercise in the cold – hypothermia

B Lynn

Exercise in the cold is perfectly safe and enjoyable as long as clothing, equipment and training are suitable – witness the many people who enjoy skiing holidays every year. Basic clothing advice is: plenty of it, in multiple layers. If in doubt put on extra – it is usually possible to remove some or loosen clothing if too hot. A waterproof outer layer is important if it starts raining or snowing. If venturing away from immediate support, then there is a need to learn basic survival skills and carry emergency rations and kit (e.g. survival bags).

Decisions about playing

Definitely cancel at −20°C (ACSM guidance; I think the UK would cancel at a much higher temperature!). At this temperature there is a real risk of frostbite on any exposed areas. Remember to allow for wind chill: light–moderate wind (16 kmph) subtract 8°C; stronger wind, 32 kmph, subtract 13°C.

Note, these are speeds well within the range of running and cycling.

When active in the cold, remember that, during activity, the high metabolic rate is a great protection against hypothermia. Post-activity, or when exhausted, take immediate steps to keep warm.

However, incidents of hypothermia do regularly occur related to sports, notably with water sports and mountain sports. It is essential therefore to understand some of the basics related to hypothermia. Remember that when dealing with likely hypothermia, this will often have occurred because of an accident and that other injuries may be present.

When faced with a hypothermic subject

(1) Try to get rectal or aural temperature
(2) If hypothermia is moderate to severe (see Table 1 for classification), exercise care with moving the subject – it may trigger ventricular fibrillation.

Re-warming

The general rule is to go slowly, no strong surface heating due to the risk of burn injury and the problem of peripheral vasodilatation while the heart is still slow.

From mild hypothermia

Wrap the subject up. Give a hot drink. Space blankets are not practical (too fragile and only help with radiant heat, which is not the main route of loss). Can immerse in a hot bath, but it is advisable to keep legs and arms elevated to maximize venous return.

From moderate/severe hypothermia

Passive re-warming is usually best, leaving the subject to slowly warm up from their own metabolic heat. If in hospital ICU, then internal re-warming from extracorporeal blood shunt or other method can be attempted. For very severe hypothermia, this may be necessary as the metabolism is too low. Remember, however, this practice needs a lot of care. Warming breathed air is thought to help. Total heat gain is small, but some heat may reach vital structures in nearby brainstem. Portable equipment for warmed oxygen is available for use by sea/mountain rescue teams. Once a subject is at 34°C, it is possible to use more active methods. Note that due to immersion diuresis there may be a need to give IV fluids.

General rule: no one is dead until warm and dead!

Cold can cause problems even if core is OK

Cold in the threshold range leads to an increase in accidents in factories, so it probably does in sports activities too. For example, with cold the hands become numb, cannot hold on, or do precise manual tasks.

Table 1 Classification of hypothermia.

Core temperature	Designation	Comments
33–35°C	Mild	Shivering. May become confused.
30–33°C	Moderate	Semi-conscious. No longer able to help themselves.
<30°C	Severe	Loss of consciousness. Stop shivering. Areflexic. Heart very slow.
26–28°C		Onset of ventricular fibrillation, death.

Frostbite

Frozen extremities. Warm up. Only debride after delay to allow area of necrosis to become clearly defined.

Immersion

Hypothermia is a particular danger in water sports. Water has 23× the thermal conductivity of air and a much higher thermal capacity. Remember the *Titanic*: almost all who ended in the water died; almost all who ended in lifeboats survived.

During removal of a subject from the water, if possible *keep horizontal*. Subject can die on the winch to helicopter if upright. The reason is circulatory collapse. Immersion diuresis reduces blood volume, vessels are dilated due to the cold, plus loss of water pressure causes venous pooling in the lower half of the body, venous return then falls catastrophically and the heart fails.

Acute immersion death

Regularly people drown in cold water well before they become hypothermic. The diving reflex on cold immersion can stop the heart! A more common sequence is: tachycardia, vasoconstriction, hypertension, increased cardiac work – a sequence that is a particular risk for anyone with threshold cardiac disease. Another problem is cold-induced hyperventilation, leading to hypocapnia, reduced brain blood flow, disorientation and clouding of consciousness – disastrous in water.

Further reading

Advice on dealing with hypothermic patient. Published on the Internet. Available online at http://www.emedicine.com/emerg/topic279.htm.

Brukner P, Khan K. *Clinical Sports Medicine*, 2nd edn. 2001, Chapter 49. McGraw-Hill.

Edmonds C. *et al.* Diving and subaquatic medicine, 4th edn. London: Arnold, 2002; Chapter 22.

Information on warmed oxygen systems. Published on the Internet. Available online at http://www.hypothermia.org.

Sport and exercise in the heat – thermoregulation and fluid balance

B Lynn

Thermoregulation while exercising under hot conditions

The high metabolic rate during exercise is a major challenge to our thermal homeostasis. The heat generated during exercise of short duration does not increase overall body temperature much. This is because the thermal capacity of the body is large enough to absorb the heat load from short bursts of high activity. The situation for endurance events is quite different.

A marathon runner, weight 70 kg, doing a 3-hour time, will have a metabolic rate of around 900 kcal/hour. Unless it is very cold, simply vasodilating and trusting to passive heat loss is not enough. Fortunately we can sweat at up to 4 litres per hour (man is a very sweaty animal!), evaporation uses 600 kcal/litre, so sweating can dissipate up to 2400 kcal per hour, easily enough to keep our marathon runner cool. But the water and electrolyte lost in sweat has to be replaced. So this is why heat balance on the one hand and fluid and electrolyte balance on the other are so inextricably linked during exercise in the heat.

Two conditions need to be met for sweating to be effective, Firstly, sweat must be able to evaporate easily. This does not happen if the relative humidity is high. If we take our runner and assume a relative humidity of 80% with an ambient temperature of 35°C, then his or her maximal sweating will now dissipate barely 1000 kcal/hour, only just enough to maintain a stable body temperature. The second point is that to continue sweating you need to drink to replace the lost fluid, and you need to drink a lot. Four litres an hour is a lot to drink! How much we need to drink will be considered below.

In practice, body temperature does rise in a controlled manner during exercise. The rise depends mostly on how hard we are exercising and rather little on environmental temperature. During intense exercise the core temperature may rise to 40°C. If core temperature reaches 41°C then heatstroke occurs (see below). So the margin between the temperatures reached normally during intense exercise and temperatures that cause illness is extremely narrow.

How much and what to drink

As pointed out above, thermoregulation during endurance exercise depends on sweating. It is therefore necessary to drink regularly or dehydration occurs. The amount of fluid needed depends on how much we sweat, something that can be assessed by weighing. In games with breaks (e.g. half time in soccer games), this could be done and fluid accurately replaced. In practice we depend on feeling thirsty. Annoyingly, our thirst mechanism is not reliable over short times and most people do not drink enough during endurance sports events. An indication of hydration can be obtained from observing urine colour. If adequately hydrated then urine should not be too dark in colour, and urine should be being passed regularly. Obviously during an event it is not feasible to check urine colour and volume! The best way to find the correct balance is to train under the same conditions as the prospective event and keep careful notes of amounts drunk and whether hydration was adequate. As discussed below, training in the heat will also help with acclimatization.

Sweat contains significant amounts of sodium chloride, so over several hours it is important to replace salt as well as water. The optimal replacement fluid under these circumstances will therefore contain some sodium chloride. Carbohydrate drinks can help performance by delaying muscle glycogen depletion and hence fatigue. So the most popular choice for endurance athletes is a carbohydrate plus electrolyte drink, of which many are available commercially.

Treatment of heat-related problems: exhaustion, heatstroke, hyponatremia

If someone collapses during a sports event on a hot day, heatstroke due to dehydration is the most likely cause. Signs of heatstroke include mental confusion, disorientation, fatigue and nausea. However, there are other possible causes of symptoms and so a rectal temperature should be obtained. Oral temperature can be misleading as the high respiratory volumes during exercise will keep the mouth cool. If heatstroke is confirmed by a rectal temperature of 41°C or above, then immediate steps need to be taken to cool the subject and to give fluid. The sooner this is done, the better, so facilities should ideally be available at the event itself. Cooling can be achieved by immersion in cold water, but may be less effective than expected due to peripheral vasoconstriction. Cold packs over major vessels (neck, groin, axilla) may be useful. If treated promptly, most cases of heatstroke resolve without complications.

Occasionally illness can be due to a fall in blood sodium level due to drinking *too much* water. It is important to distinguish this condition from heatstroke. Clearly, such subjects will not have an extreme rectal temperature, but if they have been exercising hard the rectal temperature may still be elevated. Other signs that can help with diagnosis are dilute urine and tightness of rings, watchstraps, etc. (due to tissue swelling).

Acclimatization

Heat acclimatization is essential if planning to compete in a hot climate. It is surprisingly straightforward to achieve. Exercise sessions of 40–100 min duration in a hot room and at an intensity sufficient to cause lots of sweating will be enough to trigger useful adaptations. Principal changes are: sweating comes on earlier, is at a higher rate, and has a slightly lower electrolyte content. So the key here is getting your sweat glands trained! But note, for this to work you need to drink even more than before. Repeating exercise sessions in the heat daily for 7–14 days is enough to produce good adaptation. Heat acclimatization is lost over weeks rather than days, and significant gains are still present at 3 weeks after the last heat training session.

Prevention of heatstroke

The key matters in prevention have already been mentioned. The first is to drink enough, and to include some electrolyte in the drinks. The second is to prepare for the event by training in the heat enough to get heat acclimatized. There may also be days when endurance events or strenuous training will not be possible outdoors. The ACSM recommendation is that events be cancelled if the wet bulb-globe temperature (WB-GT) is above 28°C. WB-GT determination requires dry bulb, wet bulb and globe thermometers. The wet-bulb thermometer gives an indication of humidity and the globe thermometer measures solar radiant heat load. Finally, hot climates are usually sunny, so care is also needed to avoid sunburn due to UV radiation. Therefore suitable light-coloured clothing, hats and sunscreen are the order of the day.

Further reading

American College of Sports Medicine. ACSM position stand on heat and cold illness during distance running. *Med Sci Sports Exercise* 1996; **28**: 1.

Brukner P, Khan K, Noakes T. Exercise in the heat. In: P Brukner, K Khan (Eds) *Clinical Sports Medicine*, 2nd edn. Sydney: McGraw-Hill, 2001; Chapter 48.

Maughan RJ. Fluid requirements and exercise in the heat. In: RJ Maughan (Ed) *Basic and Applied Sciences for Sports Medicine.* Oxford: Butterworth-Heinemann, Oxford 1999; Chapter 7.

Sport and travelling

P Thomas

The medical team must plan well before traveling, addressing specific factors such as:

- *Region or country to be visited*
- *Climate conditions*

  Variations of temperature and humidity will influence how early before the competition the team should arrive at the location, the choice of clothing, fluid intake, and provision for skin protection factors. Air conditioning must be available and sufficient protection must be taken during training and competition. In locations where the temperature difference between the home country and the visiting area is more than 10°C or the humidity is more than 20% then at least a week's acclimatization is advised. Access to climate chambers for pre-departure training is used by some athletes and teams.
- *Altitude*

  If competition takes place in high altitudes then pre-departure altitude training or a longer period of acclimatization is necessary so the athlete's body will adjust to lower oxygen pressures.
- *Air pollution*

  Air pollution is usually present in many industrial cities and can cause bronchoconstriction and conjunctivitis. Desensitizing nasal sprays and bronchodilators may be required even in athletes who have never experienced symptoms previously.
- *Health hazards*

  (1) Drinking water

  The quality of the local water should always be checked because it can cause gastrointestinal upsets. Bottled or purified water may be required. Ice must not be consumed as it is made from non-purified water and often contains contaminants. The same precautions should be taken when mouth rinsing, tooth brushing or consuming fruits and salads, which have not been peeled or washed by the athlete.

  (2) Food

  The diet available should be of similar quality that the athlete takes back in the home country.

(3) Traveler's diarrhea
This is common due to ingestion of E.coli bacteria which are a different strain from the strain to which the traveler is immune. This is a self-limited condition and treatment consists of 24 to 48 hours' fluid intake and avoidance of solid food and dairy products. Administration of lolepamide could be advised in severe cases.

(4) Accommodation
Accommodation has to be selected close to the training ground, away from noisy traffic and safe with enough room, comfort and entertainment.

- *Medical support and facilities*
  —The access to local medical facilities and the quality of care in the nearby hospital should be examined before departure.
  —A contingency plan should be drawn before departure examining the possibility to stabilize the condition of an injured athlete and then arranging transport to a more specialized centre or even returning home.
  —Substantial traveling medical insurance should be provided for all the traveling members of the team.
  —Physiotherapy items and equipment that are absent at the new location, and considered necessary, should be transported along with the traveling team.
- *Pre-departure assessment and advice*
  An updated assessment for all the traveling members should take place before departure, briefing on hygiene matters and health hazards that may be encountered. Also warnings on banned drugs and medication that may be taken inadvertently by the athletes should be issued.
- *Immunization and disease protection*
  —A list of countries at risk of similar disease, such as hepatitis, malaria, yellow fever and others, must be available to the Medical Officer and appropriate immunizations must take place.
  —Equally, the athlete should be checked if he or she has received an updated booster in tetanus, diphtheria and polio.
- *Equipment and supplies of a range of medicines*
  Range of antibiotics, hypnotics, anti-inflammatories, antacids, laxatives, respiratory preparation, aural drops, ophthalmic preparations, anti-histamines, anti-migraine, ergotamine, contraceptives and topical preparations should all be taken.

The medical team must get advice from the Medical Defense Union or equivalent insurance company on practices in the country of travel and carry sufficient insurance against malpractice.

Further reading

Dirix A, Knuttgen HG. *The Olympic Book in Sports Medicine.* Oxford: Blackwell, 1988; 153–77.
Strauss RH (Ed) *Sports Medicine.* Philadelphia: WB Saunders, 1984; 492–500.

Sports footwear

AA Narvani

Poor footwear can lead to injuries in athletes. In order to aid athletes in selecting footwear, sports clinicians must have a basic understanding of the biomechanics of the foot and different sports as well as the structure and properties of sports shoes. This understanding is vital as many manufacturers are spending tremendous amounts of money and time marketing their products. Clinicians must be able to analyse critically the suitability of many of these products for their athletes.

Function of the foot

As the foot strikes the ground, initially it must be able to accept the vertical impact forces inflicted on it. Following this, early in the stance phase, the foot pronates. This pronation permits force dissipation and absorption of some of the energy from the heel strike. Later on in the stance phase, the foot supinates as it changes from a flexible to a rigid structure. This rigid lever lifts and propels the body during the propulsive stage of the stance phase and therefore prepares for the push off.

Excessive pronation does not permit the formation of the rigid lever required during the toe off. As a result, there may be some instability and internal rotation of the entire lower limb. This internal rotation during weight bearing can in turn lead to excessive forces on many structures such as the medial aspect of the foot, lower leg and the knee, which may result in overuse injuries.

Excessive supination can lead to inadequate shock absorption, which may lead to stress fractures and other overuse injuries.

Function of a sports shoe

A sports shoe must be able to complement and allow the normal function of the foot. It must allow adequate pronation and supination at the required stages. In addition it must provide:

(i) protection of the foot plantar surface,
(ii) traction,
(iii) stability and motion control during activity,
(iv) attenuation of impact forces.

The ideal sports shoe must protect the foot from hot, cold, wet, rough or rocky ground forces. The amount of traction required is very much sports dependent but is determined by the frictional forces between the shoe and the ground surface. Different degrees of stability are required in different sports and different shoe designs must address this. Reduction of the impact forces is brought about by the cushioning properties of the shoe.

Structure of sports shoes

The components of sports shoes are:

(i) Upper and last
(ii) Insert
(iii) Midsole
(iv) Outsole

Upper and last

The upper contains the toe box, tongue, lacing system, mid panels and the heel counter. It holds the midsole and outsole to the bottom of the foot and is also important in providing stability, flexibility and durability. Therefore, it must be constructed from materials that are usually flexible, durable, breathable and light. The toe box guards the toes and the distal part of the forefoot and must be of adequate depth and length so the toes do not rub against it. The tongue and the lacing system determine the fit of the shoe and are also important factors in the stability of the shoes. Padded tongues reduce the risk of superficial injury to the dorsum of the foot by preventing direct contact between the skin and the lacing system. Lacing systems can vary from shoe string to velcro, and even no lacing systems in some modern shoes. In addition to contributing to the fit of the shoe by cupping the heel, the heel counter is also important in providing stability and motion control.

The last of a shoe refers to two different properties. Firstly, it refers to the curvature of the shoe as one looks at the underneath surface. There are three possible designs. Curved-lasted shoes have a forefoot adduction of approximately 25°. Semi-curved shoes have only a 7 to 10° forefoot adduction, whereas straight-lasted ones have no adduction. Last also refers to the attachment technique of the outer to midsole and outsole. The different techniques available influence the flexibility of the sports shoe.

Insert

As well as providing a cushioning effect, the insert dissipates heat and wicks moisture away from the foot. It may also function as an orthotic for structurally abnormal feet.

Midsole

Impact forces may rise to over seven times that of body weight in sports such as basketball. By spreading out the force of impact and preventing full force to be directed at the foot and the leg, the midsole provides most of the cushioning property of the shoe. It is manufactured from a variety of materials including ethyl-vinyl acetate (EVA), polyurethane foams, encapsulated air and gel. It must be appreciated that excessive cushioning may compromise the stability of the shoe leading to exaggerated pronation and supination, which in turn may lead to various injuries. In addition to cushioning and stability, the midsole also influences the flexibility and durability of shoe.

Outsole

The outsole provides the grip of the shoe (traction), which is dependent on the design and material of the outsole and the playing surface. Different sports require varying

Table 1 Properties of different sport shoes.

Type	Example of sports	Properties
Court shoes	Tennis, squash, basketball, volleyball, handball, badminton	• Sports involve repetitive change of direction and sideways shuffling therefore grip is important. • Also important in its stability during sideways shuffle is a low centre of gravity and broad base. • High impact forces are involved in jumping therefore they must also provide adequate cushioning effect.
Running shoes	Running, exercise walking, hiking	• Adequate cushioning required to protect the foot from the high impact forces during heel strike. • Light to reduce energy requirement. • Flexible.
Field sport shoes	Football, rugby, cricket, baseball, American football	• Grip for the surface is vital, therefore these shoes have studs, spikes or cleats. • In kicking sports, these shoes must provide protection for the feet when kicking the ball. Dorsum aspect of the foot has to sustain forces in excess of 1000 N during kicking.
Track and field sports shoes	Track and field sports	Depending on the specific event, different degrees of cushioning, stability, traction and flexibility are required, e.g. sprinting shoes have very basic cushioning properties but are very light in weight.
Winter sports	Skiing, figure skating, ice hockey	Ankle support of vital importance in all.
Specialty sports	Golf, aerobics, cycling, fencing	Properties dependent on each particular sport.
Outdoor sports	Recreational activities such as hunting and fishing	Properties dependent on each particular sport.

degrees of traction, which should be reflected in the design of the shoe. The outsole also plays a role in flexibility and durability of the shoe; however, in most shoes its lifespan exceeds that of the midsole. Materials used in its construction include carbon and/or blown rubber.

The right shoe?

When recommending shoes to athletes, two factors come into play, the specific sport and the athlete's feet.

Sport

Broadly speaking, sports shoes may be divided into seven types. These are presented in Table 1.

Athlete's feet

The most vital requirement for a sports shoe is that it is the correct size and comfortable for the athlete's feet. Incorrect shoe sizes can lead to problems such as blisters, calluses, hallux valgus, metatarsalgia and corns. Three parameters need to be checked before a decision can be made whether a shoe is of correct size. Firstly, the length of the shoe must be correct. As a rough rule, there must be a space equivalent to half to the full width of the thumb between the end of the longest toe and the end of the shoe when pressing the end of the shoe. Secondly, the width of the shoe must be so that one could pinch a small amount of material of the upper across the forefoot. Thirdly, the flexion point of the shoe must be situated where the centre of rotation of the first metatarsal-phalangeal joint lies.

Additionally, particularly in the case of runners, it is also important to assess the gait and the foot arch of the athlete. Those who "underpronate" in the early period of their stance phase, tend to have rigid feet with high arches that do not conform to the ground. These athletes may benefit from "cushioned" shoes that have minimal medial support, maximal flexibility and a curved or semi-curved last. Those who "overpronate" tend to have low arches and may require shoes with maximum medial support with straight lasts in order to restrict and control the motion and the over-pronation during their gait.

Further reading

Asplund CA, Brown DL. The running shoe prescription. *The Physician and Sports Medicine* 2005; **33**(1).

Borom AH, Clanton TO. Sports shoes and orthoses. In: JC DeLee, D Drez, MD Miller (Eds) *Orthopaedic Sports Medicine, Principles and Practice*, 2nd edn. Saunders, 2002: 2275–323.

Stress fractures in sports

M Ramachandran

Briefhaupt originally described stress fractures in military recruits in 1855 (see DeLee *et al.* 2003). They are common in athletes, representing approximately 10% of injuries seen in sports medicine centres. Of these, the lower limb is affected in approximately 95% of those cases. There is no convincing evidence of differences in incidence according to gender, race or geography.

Aetiology

Stress fractures often result from participation in a new activity or from a change in a training programme, such as a change in intensity, duration or frequency of training. Running, especially hurdling and distance running, is thought to be the most common precipitating sport.

General predisposing factors include hard training surfaces, biomechanical causes (e.g. pronated feet, pes cavus, excessive external tibial torsion, limb length inequality, and muscle fatigue), bone density (e.g. osteoporosis, which may be related to amenorrhoea or oligomenorrhoea in female athletes) and previous surgery (e.g. second metatarsal stress fracture following surgery for hallux valgus or rigidus).

Pathophysiology

Stress fractures occur as a result of repetitive loading of bone below its yield strength. When bone is subjected to this increased stress (load) with resultant strain (deformation), remodelling occurs with bone resorption from osteoclasts coupled with bone formation by osteoblasts. If repetitive cyclical loading continues, particularly when relatively greater osteoclastic activity is present or when the reparative capacity of bone is overwhelmed, microdamage occurs and accumulates, resulting in a stress fracture.

The piezoelectric phenomenon underlying Wolff's law, which states that bone remodels itself in direct response to the applied forces, may also be used to explain the pathology of certain stress fractures. Tensile stresses create electropositivity, resulting in bone resorption by osteoclastic activity, while compressive forces create electronegativity, which initiates bone formation by osteoblastic activity. Cyclical tensile forces, therefore, will result in cortical thinning, osteoporosis and the ultimate development of a stress fracture.

Distinction may be made between stress fractures of normal bone that becomes fatigued through abnormal loading (i.e. fatigue fractures) and stress fractures of pathological bone that may fail even under comparatively normal loads (i.e. insufficiency fractures). Both processes are characterised by disrupted bone homeostasis and inadequate repair in the face of repetitive overload.

Sites and sports

The most commonly involved bones are the tibia, distal third of the fibula, shaft or neck of the second or third metatarsals, and base of the fifth metatarsal. Less commonly, the sesamoids, navicular, femur and pelvis may be affected. Stress fractures of the upper limb, ribs, and even the scapula have been described but they are far less common.

Certain sports predispose to specific stress fractures as shown in Table 1.

Clinical features

The typical history is one of pain exacerbated by activity and partially relieved by rest. The pain may begin as diffuse but often becomes localised with time. It may only occur at the end of activity, proceeding to constant pain, including night pain, later on in the disease process. As indicated previously, a recent increase in activity or change in training is often noted. A menstrual history must be taken for female athletes, particularly to exclude the triad of amenorrhoea, disordered eating, and osteoporosis.

On examination, there may be pain on palpation or percussion of the affected area, with localised swelling (which may be due to a local periosteal thickening or callus formation) and occasional erythema. Axially loading the affected bone may reproduce symptoms. The predisposing factors mentioned above should be specifically sought, for example biomechanical factors such as pes cavus.

Differential diagnoses

- Strains and sprains
- Contusions
- Delayed onset muscle soreness
- Shin splints (medial tibial stress syndrome)
- Exertion-related chronic compartment syndrome
- Tumours of bone, especially osteoid osteomas
- Referred pain from the spine
- Morton's neuroma
- Plantar fasciitis
- Metatarsophalangeal joint synovitis

Table 1 Stress fractures encountered in different sports.

Sport	Most common stress fractures
Running	Distal tibia, fibula, metatarsals
Basketball	Navicular, midshaft tibia
Football	Metatarsals, first metatarsophalangeal sesamoids
Dancing	Base of metatarsals, midshaft tibia
Recruits	Distal shaft of metatarsals, calcaneus, proximal tibia

Investigations

Plain X-rays are often unremarkable but may demonstrate periosteal new bone formation, callus and a visible fracture line associated with stress fractures. It may take several weeks before X-ray signs become positive, and sometimes plain films remain negative despite positive bone scans or cross-sectional imaging. The patient's signs and symptoms should therefore guide management.

If X-rays are negative, a triple phase technetium^{99m} bone scan should be considered as the next investigation as it is highly sensitive and may be positive from 48 to 72 hours after injury. The bone scan is diagnostic of a stress fracture if focal isotope uptake is seen in the injured area on the third (delayed) phase of the scan; often all three phases are positive. If the bone scan is negative, a stress fracture is highly unlikely and alternative diagnoses should be considered.

Cross-sectional imaging, such as MRI and CT scanning, can be additional useful diagnostic tools. MRI is being increasingly used as a first-line investigation due to its increased sensitivity for detecting marrow oedema and periosteal reaction in the early stages of the stress fracture process.

Treatment

The five facets of treatment of stress fracture are as follows.

1. Medical treatment

Rest and activity modification are essential components of treatment as they allow for a normal course of bone remodelling, although prolonged rest may result in disuse muscle atrophy. The usual recommended period is 6–12 weeks, although return to sport can be sooner if symptoms resolve. Repeat plain X-rays can be used to confirm progression of healing.

Icing and massage can be used in the early stages, especially when swelling is present. Mild to moderate analgesics, such as non-steroidal anti-inflammatory drugs, are useful to control symptoms.

Casting or bracing is employed to reduce the stresses on the injured area, and surgery is indicated if there is non-union or displacement. Surgery is also indicated in certain fractures that are known to be prone to non-union, e.g. diaphyseal fifth metatarsal stress fractures.

2. Athlete education

It is important that the athlete understands the causes of the injury, including training errors, the intended treatment regime and the methods used to prevent further injury.

3. Cross training

To avoid disuse muscle atrophy and maintain cardiovascular fitness while the stress fracture heals, some form of cross training is recommended, such as cycling, swimming, or the use of rowing machines. As the athlete returns to his or her primary sport, time spent cross training is gradually decreased.

4. Specific exercises

Once past the initial inflammatory stage, specific exercises – such as stretching to maintain range of motion, and muscle strengthening – should be performed, as taught by the physiotherapist, in conjunction with cross training.

5. Programmed return to training

A simple rule of thumb is that, on return to sport, the athlete's volume of training should not increase by more than 10% from one week to the next. Days of stress training should be interspersed with rest or "easy" days.

For example, with running, the athlete should begin with a maximum of 15 minutes of slow running every other day, with 5 minute increases in each session weekly. After he or she can run for 40 minutes without pain, the distance of the longest weekly session may increase by 10%.

Specific fractures

Tibial fractures

This is the most common site for stress fractures, although shin splints and exertional compartment syndromes must be considered in the differential diagnosis. Predisposing factors include rigid cavus feet and excessive subtalar pronation. Treatment is as per the protocol above, but transverse anterior tibial stress fractures must be treated with care as they heal more slowly (average of 6 months) as they are on the tensile aspect of the tibia and are prone to delayed or non-union (persisting as the "dreaded black line"). Pulsed electromagnetic field stimulation is helpful, but internal fixation with bone grafting may be required.

Navicular fractures

These pose a management problem, especially if strict immobilisation and abstinence from weight bearing is not adhered to. Bone grafting should be considered for complete fractures, non-union, cysts and incomplete fractures that do not heal when weight bearing has been avoided.

Metatarsal fractures

In runners, metatarsal fractures occur most commonly in the neck, while in dancers they usually occur in the proximal shaft. The second metatarsal is the most commonly involved. Predisposing factors include flexible pes planus. Treatment includes reduction of activity for 6 to 12 weeks in a cast. When occurring in combination with a cavus foot, plantar fascia release should be considered.

Calcaneus fractures

Most often seen in military recruits, clinical features of this fracture include pain, swelling and exquisite tenderness on both sides of the heel. The differential diagnosis includes plantar fasciitis. Plain X-rays may show the fracture line running perpendicular to the trabecular stress lines, but bone scans are more helpful. Treatment consists of activity modification with or without immobilisation.

Femoral neck fractures

These can occur either on the superior tension (in older patients) or inferior compression (in younger patients) side of the femoral neck. In both populations, patients present with activity-related pain in the groin or anterior thigh. Physical examination may reveal pain with a passive range of motion, particularly internal rotation. Plain X-rays and bone scans are usually sufficient to confirm the diagnosis, although MRI is being used with increasing frequency. For patients diagnosed with early stress reaction or an undisplaced stress fracture of the femoral neck, treatment consists of avoidance of weight bearing on the affected limb until symptoms resolve, with serial X-rays being used as a guide to healing. Next, the individual is permitted to resume partial weight bearing as tolerated, progressing to unprotected weight bearing, walking and then running. If the fracture is displaced or with the more potentially unstable tension fractures, surgical fixation with cannulated screws may be required prior to rehabilitation.

Femoral shaft fractures

This may be confused with a quadriceps contusion as patients often complain of a deep thigh pain. Treatment includes use of crutches for 4 to 8 weeks.

Further reading

DeLee JC, Drez D, Miller MD. *Orthopaedic Sports Medicine, Principles and Practice*, 2nd edn. WB Saunders, 2003.

Miller MD, Cooper DE, Warner JJP. *Review of Sports Medicine and Arthroscopy*, 2nd edn. WB Saunders, 2002.

Sanderlin BW, Raspa RF. Common stress fractures. *American Family Physician* 2003; **68**: 1527–32.

Sterling JC, Edelstein DW, Calvo RD, Webb R. Stress fractures in the athlete. *Sports Medicine* 1992; **14**: 336–46.

Wilder RP, Sethi S. Overuse injuries: tendinopathies, stress fractures, compartment syndrome, and shin splints. *Clinical Sports Medicine* 2004; **23**: 55–81.

Team physician

P Thomas

The duties of the team doctor include:

(1) to recognize common risk factors associated with sport injuries
(2) to know the physical demands of a specific sport
(3) to organize pre-participation assessment and pre-season medical fitness reports
(4) to assess the quality and maintenance of sports equipment and protection guards
(5) to provide on-site medical coverage at events for both the athletes and attendants
(6) to dispense medications
(7) to diagnose injuries and facilitate referrals to other medical specialists

(8) to provide education and information to athletes, coaching staff and parents in a youth academy
(9) to protect confidentiality
(10) to be informed and ensure compliance with the specific Sport Association guidelines
(11) to provide and supervise training for the rest of the medical team, such as physiotherapists, masseurs, etc., in particular the design of emergency policies and procedures
(12) record keeping.
(13) arrange Therapeutic Use Exemptions (TUEs) if it is necessary to prescribe medicines that are on the banned list (see the chapter on Drugs in sport – the administrative framework; doping control procedures).

Pre-season assessment

The team physician is responsible for determining the general health of athletes. Particular attention should be paid to:

- Checking current immunization status and arranging appropriate boosters, etc.;
- Detecting medical conditions that are not healed or may predispose the individual to illness or injury and arranging appropriate medical and rehabilitation treatments;
- Identification of risk behaviours;
- Assessing physical maturity in the young sportsperson;
- Assessing with the coaching staff the fitness level and the recovery from injury/illness to allow an athlete's return to competition.

Medical equipment, the physician's bag

The basic provisions in the medical room and in the match-day bag for "away" competitions include:

(1) Diagnostic equipment: torch, stethoscope, auriscope, ophthalmoscope, sphygmomanometer, thermometer, patella reflex hammer, urine testing strips, eye fluorostrips.
(2) Treatment items: dressings (gauzes, non-adherent dressings), steristrips, eye pads, bandages, slings, splints.
(3) Antiseptic solution, sterile saline, eye washes, syringes, needles, suturing instruments, forceps, air mask and bag, small tracheotomy set.
(4) Drugs: analgesics, local antiseptics, aerosol bronchodilators, anti-emetic agents, anti-diarrhoea agents.

Care must be taken not to use substances that are banned from the Anti Doping Agency. However, an opiate analgesic must be available in cases of severe injury to provide pain relief.

Further reading

Kuland DN. *The Athlete's Physician. The Injured Athlete 1–34.* Philadelphia: B Lippincott, 1988.

Thigh pain (anterior) – quadriceps muscle injuries

AA Narvani and EE Tsiridis

Quadriceps refer to a group of muscles on the anterior aspect of the upper leg formed by rectus femoris, vastus medialis, vastus intermedius and vastus lateralis. The commonest injuries to quadriceps muscles include strains and contusion. This chapter highlights quadriceps strains, as muscle contusions and quadriceps tendon injuries are covered elsewhere.

Quadriceps strain

These injuries occur in athletes who participate in sports that involve eccentric contraction of quadsriceps at high speeds, such as sprinting, track and field, rugby, soccer, American football and other running sports. Most quadriceps strains involve exclusively rectus femoris as it is the only one of the group that crosses both the hip joint and the knee joint.

Predisposing factors

Like other muscular injuries, risk factors could be divided into:

(1) Sports related:
- Participation in sports that involve eccentric contraction of the quadriceps at high speed (see above).

(2) Athlete related:
- Poor posture
- Muscle imbalance
- Limb length inequality
- Previous injury
- Inadequate management and recovery from previous injury.

(3) Training and technique related:
- Poor technique
- Fatigue
- Lack of warm up
- Inadequate flexibility.

Pathology

As mentioned above, rectus femoris is the most vulnerable muscle of the quadriceps for sustaining muscular strain injuries due to the fact that it crosses both the hip and the knee joints. Injuries commonly occur at the musculotendinous junction and are more likely to be distal than proximal, although proximal intramuscular rectus femoris tears have also been described. As with hamstring injuries, the primary mechanism of injury appears to be violent eccentric contraction causing a stretch injury to the musculotendinous junction (due to large force generation with eccentric contractions).

This stretch injury is divided into three main grades:

Grade I This a mild strain as only a few muscle fibres are torn with a small structural integrity disruption at the musculotendinous junction.
Grade II This is a moderate strain with a partial tear, but some of the fibres at the musculotendinous junction do remain intact. There is some strength loss.
Grade IIIA Complete tear/rupture of the muscle (usually at the musculotendinous junction.
Grade IIIB Characterised by bony avulsion at the bone attachment sites.

Clinical features
Clinical features are dependent on the grade of the injury as demonstrated in Table 1.

Investigations
- Plain radiograph may help to exclude femoral stress fracture and myositis ossificans.
- MRI can be of great use by revealing the:
  (i) extent of the injury,
  (ii) grade of the injury,
  (iii) which muscles are involved.

Differential diagnosis
Differential diagnosis includes:

(i) Quadriceps muscle related:
- Quadricep muscular contusions and haematoma
- Myositis ossificans

(ii) Femur related:
- Stress fractures

(iii) Low back pathology:
- Referred pain from low back
- Lumbosacral radiculopathy

(iv) Tumours:
- Soft tissue tumours
- Osteosarcoma of the femur

(v) Others:
- Chronic compartment syndrome
- Apophysitis
- Nerve entrapment
- Sartorius and gracilis strains

Treatment
As with hamstring injuries, the vast majority of athletes with quadriceps muscular sprain injuries are treated non-operatively.

(i) In the acute phase of the injury, efforts should be concentrated on reducing the pain. This may involve using:
- rest
- ice
- compression

Table 1 Grading of the quadriceps muscular injuries.

Grade	Symptoms	Signs
I	• Pain in the anterior thigh. • Presentation may be acute or chronic. • There may be a history of a specific event that started the symptoms (i.e. sprinting), however it is not uncommon for the athlete to continue his or her exercise and present after a good delay, i.e. the following day. • Degree of weakness (may be secondary to pain). • Presence of any of the predisposing factors (see above).	• Small degree of haemorrhage and swelling. • Localised tenderness. • Pain produced by passive stretching of the quadriceps muscle. • Pain produced by resisted active contraction of the quadriceps muscles. • Lack of objective function loss.
II	• Athletes more likely to present with an acute injury. • Athlete may or may not be able to continue with his/her exercise. • More pronounced weakness (actual muscle weakness not just pain related). • Athletes will usually limp but are able to fully bear weight.	• Greater degree of haemorrhage and swelling. • Presence of a painful palpable lesion in the muscle. • Passive stretching causes greater degree by pain. • Smaller degree of resistance felt by clinician before onset of pain during active knee extension against resistance. • True muscle weakness.
III A&B	• Similar to grade II injuries but more severe. • Athlete likely to discontinue his/her exercise and present acutely.	• Similar signs to grade II, but more obvious. • Muscle palpable defect when the muscle contracts, may be felt.

- elevation
- NSAIDs

(ii) Once pain control is achieved, the athlete may progress to the rehabilitation phase. During this phase, attention is focused on

(a) Flexibility

(b) Muscular function

- muscular strength

  isometric
  isotonic (concentric and eccentric)
  isokinetic

- power
- muscular endurance
- muscular coordination

(c) Proprioception
(d) General fitness

(iii) The next stage of non-operative management involves focusing on functional and sport-specific exercises and finally return to sport.
- Walking, running, sprinting, drills
- Sport-specific skills

(iv) Management must also include correction of any of the predisposing factors that could have contributed to the injury in the first place (see above).

Surgery may have a role in those athletes with grade III injuries who demonstrate gross retraction of the quadriceps when they contract. Surgery is by suturing the muscle to the tendon.

Return to sport

As with other sports injuries, return to play is permitted once the athlete is pain free, able to achieve a full range of movement and has regained enough strength to perform their sport-specific activities. Functional testing, which includes assessment of the ability to sprint and to perform specific sporting activities without pain, should also be performed before permitting the athlete to return to play and declaring him or her fit.

The actual time taken for the athlete to return to play depends on the extent of the injury, and can vary from 2 days to 10 weeks; however, the majority of the athletes return to their sports within 4 weeks.

Prognosis

Most quadricep strains usually heal following an appropriate and accurate non-operative regime; however, as with hamstring injuries, an inadequate rehabilitation programme and early return to play can lead to recurrent injury and chronic pain.

In a small number of patients, excessive scar formation may lead to impingement of the femoral nerve (dysfunction of the femoral nerve may also occur secondary to mechanical pressure caused by spasm of the psoas muscle which can be associated with quadriceps injuries).

Further reading

Brown TG, Brunet ME. Adult thigh. In: JC DeLee, D Drez, MD Miller (Eds) *Orthopaedic Sports Medicine, Principles and Practice*, 2nd edn. Saunders, 2002: 1481–504.

Thigh pain (posterior) – hamstring strains

AA Narvani and EE Tsiridis

Hamstrings refer to a group of muscles on the posterior aspect of the upper leg formed by semimembranosus, semitendinosus and bicep femoris. Their injuries are extremely common in athletes and account for significant lost playing time. As they cross both the hip and the knee joints, they have the ability to contribute to both hip extension and knee flexion, but as a consequence can be placed under tremendous forces depending on the positions of the hip and knee joints.

Epidemiology

The most common strain-related injuries faced by sports clinicians, these injuries are common in sports that involve eccentric contraction of the hamstring at high speeds, such as sprinting, track and field, rugby, soccer and other running sports. They are reported to be more common in the 15 to 25 age groups.

Predisposing factors

Risk factors could be divided into:

(1) Sports related:
- Participation in sports that involve eccentric contraction of the hamstrings at high speed (see above).

(2) Athlete related:
- Poor posture
- Muscle imbalance (hamstring to quadriceps ratio of less than 50%)
- Limb length inequality
- Tight hip flexors and anterior hip tilt (may be due to rapid growth in adolescene)
- Previous injury
- Inadequate management and recovery from previous injury.

(3) Training and technique related:
- Poor technique (poor running style; overstriding)
- fatigue
- lack of warm up
- Inadequate flexibility.

Pathology

The primary pathology in hamstring strains appears to be a stretch injury to the musculotendinous junction. As eccentric contractions generate much greater forces than concentric contractions, they are more likely to induce such stretch injuries. Hamstrings span two joints, and are therefore likely to undergo eccentric contractions during various sporting activities.

The initial phase of the injury (first 24 hours) is accompanied with a haemorrhagic response around the injured muscle fibres. This is then followed by necrotic changes of the injured muscle fibres, oedema and an increase in the number of the macrophages in the area (24–48 hours). After 48 hours, as the number of inflammatory cells in the area increases, there is also an intensification of fibroblastic activity.

This stretch injury is divided into three main grades:

Grade I This a mild strain, as only a few muscle fibres are torn with a small structural integrity disruption at the musculotendinous junction.

Grade II This is a moderate strain, with a partial tear but some of the fibres at the musculotendinous junction do remain intact. There is some strength loss.

Grade IIIA Complete tear/rupture of the muscle (usually at the musculotendinous junction).

Grade IIIB Characterised by bony avulsion at the bone attachment sites.

Clinical features

Clinical features are dependent on the grade of the injury as demonstrated in Table 1.

Investigations

- Plain radiograph may reveal the avulsion fractures with type IIIB injuries. It may also demonstrate calcifications in patients with chronic hamstring pain.
- In addition to excluding other injuries, MRI can be of great use by revealing the:
  (i) extent of the injury,
  (ii) grade of the injury,
  (iii) which muscles are involved.

Differential diagnosis

Differential diagnosis includes:

- Hamstring muscular contusions and haematoma
- Referred pain from low back (see back pain chapters)
- Lumbosacral radiculopathy (see the chapter on lumber intervertebral disc herniation)
- Femoral stress fractures (see stress fractures chapter)
- Chronic compartment syndrome
- Apophysitis
- Myositis ossificans
- Nerve entrapment

Treatment

In most cases treatment is non-operative.

(1) In the acute phase of the injury, efforts should be concentrated at reducing the pain. This may involve using:

Table 1 Classification of hamstring injuries.

Grade	Symptoms	Signs
I	• Pain in the posterior thigh. • Presentation may be acute or chronic. • History of a specific event that started the symptoms (i.e. sprinting). • Those with chronic presentation may complain of tightness/pull while participating in sports or some post-exercise pain. • Degree of weakness (may be secondary to pain). • Presence of any of the predisposing factors (see above).	• Small degree of haemorrhage and swelling. • Localised tenderness. • Pain produced by passive extension of knee with hip flexed at 90°. • Pain produced with active knee flexion against resistance. • Lack of objective function loss.
II	• Athletes more likely to present with an acute injury. • Sudden onset of pain in posterior thigh during activity (i.e. sprinting). • More pronounced weakness (actual muscle weakness not just pain related). • Athletes may recall an audible pop at time of the injury.	• Greater degree of haemorrhage and swelling. • Presence of a painful palpable mass in the muscle which will not retract with active contraction of the muscle. • Passive extension of the knee restricted to a greater degree by pain. • Smaller degree of resistance felt by clinician before onset of pain during active knee flexion against resistance. • True muscle weakness.
III A&B	• Similar to grade II injuries but more severe.	• Similar signs to grade II, but more obvious. • Painful mass which retracts with active contraction of the muscle (grade IIIA). • Grade IIIA injuries are generally closer to bone attachment sites than grade II injuries.

- rest
- ice
- compression
- elevation
- NSAIDs

(2) Once pain control is achieved, the athlete may progress to the rehabilitation phase. During this phase efforts are made to restore flexibility, muscular function, proprioception and general fitness.
Flexibility. This is dependent on a range of movements of the joint and soft tissue flexibility. Joint flexibility may be aided by active and passive exercises. Stretching will promote soft tissue flexibility as well as being beneficial in increasing muscular relaxation and preventing formation of excessive adhesions.
Muscular function. Any muscular functioning rehabilitation programme must address muscular strength and power, muscular endurance and finally, but just as important, muscular coordination.
Muscular strengthening involves gradual progression from *isometric* to *isotonic* to *isokinetic* exercises. Progression into the different forms of the muscular-strengthening exercises is dependent on the pain relief achieved with each type of exercise (i.e. once the athlete regains the ability to perform isometric exercises pain free, then isotonic exercises may be started). Isotonic exercises, which involve movement of the joint against a constant resistance, may be concentric or eccentric. As eccentric exercises produce large forces in the muscle, they should only be initiated after the athlete can perform concentric exercises comfortably.
Muscular power training should usually in most cases occur in the later stages of rehabilitation and would involve fast isotonic and isokinetic exercises, progressively faster functional exercises, and activities that are relevant to the athlete's sport, such as hopping and jumping.
Muscular endurance is enhanced by low-force, high-repetitive exercises (load may be increased gradually).
Enhancement of muscular coordination involves athlete and muscular education, and correction of abnormal muscular patterning.
Proprioception. Musculo-skeletal injuries can result in impairment of proprioception due to damaged nerve endings and nerve pathways. If this impairment is not addressed in the rehabilitation programme, further injuries may occur. Correction is performed through a series of progression exercises ranging from standing on one leg to zigzag running and sideway step-ups.
General fitness. During the rehabilitation phase, attempts must be made to maintain the general fitness of the athlete. This may start with water exercises and progress to cycling and running once muscles have been conditioned adequately.

(3) In the next stage of non-operative management, following restoration of flexibility, muscular function, and proprioception, attention is focused on functional and sport-specific exercises and finally return to sport. Functional exercises involve progression from walking to running to sprinting to drills. The athlete should also be taken through sport-specific exercises, which should be followed by return to sport and practice of sport-specific skills.

(4) Management must also include correction of any of the predisposing factors that could have contributed to the injury in the first place (see above).

Surgery should only be considered if there is complete detachment of the musculotendinous complex from the origin or insertion and non-operative management has failed.

Return to sport

As with other sports injuries, return to play is permitted once the athlete is pain free, able to achieve a full range of movement and has regained enough strength to perform their sport-specific activities. The strength of the injured hamstring must reach at least 90% of the strength of the contra-lateral uninjured hamstring. A hamstring–quadriceps ratio of 0.55 must be achieved prior to return to play. Functional testing, which includes assessment of the ability to sprint and to perform specific sporting activities without pain, should also be performed before permitting the athlete to return to play and declaring him or her fit.

The actual time taken for the athlete to return to play depends on the extent of the injury, ranging from a few days for grade I injuries to 6–8 weeks for the more severe grade III injuries.

Prognosis

Most hamstring strains usually heal following an appropriate and accurate non-operative regime; however an inadequate rehabilitation programme and early return to play can lead to recurrent injury and chronic pain.

In a small number of patients, excessive scar formation may lead to impingement of the sciatic nerve (known as hamstring syndrome).

Further reading

Drezner JA. Practical management: hamstring muscle injuries. *Clin J Sport Med* 2003; **13**(1): 48–52.

Hoskins W, Pollard H. The management of hamstring injury – Part 1: issues in diagnosis. *Man Ther* 2005; **10**(2): 96–107.

Thigh – muscular contusions and myositis ossificans

AA Narvani and EE Tsiridis

Muscular contusions refer to injuries that are characterised by escape of blood from disrupted blood vessels, and which usually result from direct force. Myositis ossificans is a benign lesion formed by heterotopic ossification of the muscle calcification, which in most cases occurs as a consequence of severe muscle contusions. As the main mechanism of the injury is direct force, these injuries occur in collision sports such as rugby, soccer, American and Australian football and basketball.

Pathology

The most common site for contusions and myositis ossificans is the anterior region (quadriceps muscles).

Contusion injuries can be divided into three main grades depending on the active range of movement of the knee joint measured at 12 to 24 hours following surgery:

Mild More than 90° of knee flexion possible.
Moderate Knee flexion is less than 90° but more than 45°.
Severe Knee flexion is less than 45°.

Classification of myositis ossificans is based on the radiographic appearance of the periosteal connection of the mass. Three main types have been described:

- broad-based connection
- stalk-shaped connection
- no connection at all

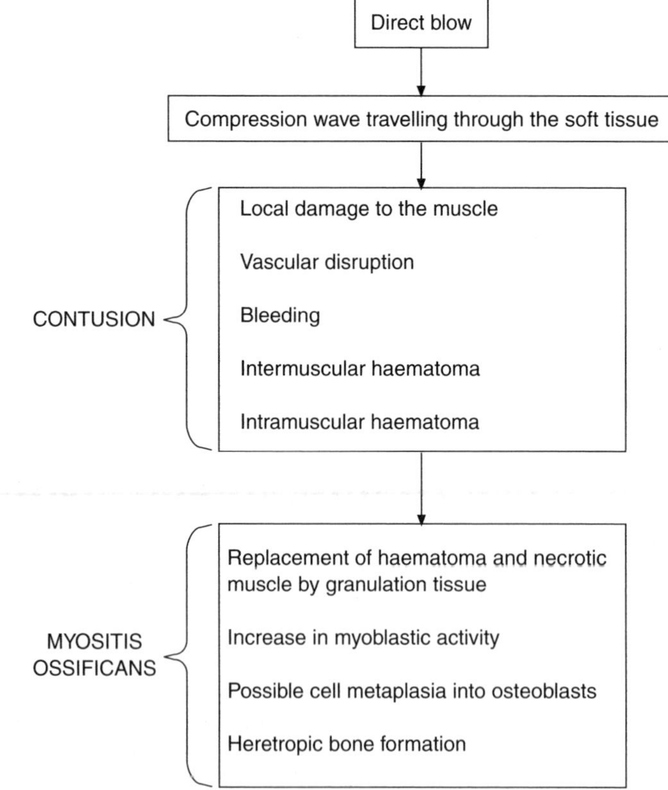

Figure 1 Pathology process of myositis ossificans.

Clinical features

- History of direct blow.
- With severe contusion, the athlete usually has to stop their activity following the blow.
- Localised pain and tenderness.
- Swelling.
- Bruising.
- Knee effusion with more severe injuries.
- Reduced range of knee movement depending on the severity of the injury (see above).
- Palpable mass (with myositis ossificans this may develop up to 4 weeks after the injury).

A possible complication of muscle contusion is development of compartment syndrome. As this is mainly a clinical diagnosis, its features must be looked for by clinicians managing athletes with contusion injuries.

Investigations

- Plain radiograph will also demonstrate the developing myositis ossificans as well as help to exclude other pathologies such as fractures.
- Further imaging such as USS, CT and MRI will aid in distinguishing myositis ossificans from other differential diagnosis (see below). Additionally, biopsy may be indicated to exclude the other conditions.

Differential diagnosis

Appearance of myositis ossificans on the plain radiograph may resemble a series of benign and malignant lesions, these include:

Benign
- Osteochondroma
- Osteomyelitis
- Juxtacortical chondroma

Malignant
- Periosteal osteosarcoma
- Parosteal osteosarcoma
- Synovial sarcoma

Treatment

The vast majority of athletes with contusion and myositis ossificans are treated non-operatively.

(1) In the acute phase of the injury, efforts should be concentrated at limiting the haematoma and reducing pain. This usually involves using:

- rest
- ice
- compression
- elevation
- Immobilisation of the knee in 100 to 120° of flexion started within 12 hours of the injury and sustained for duration of about 24 hours. This is thought to have a tamponade affect, therefore reducing the size of the haematoma.

(2) Athlete may progress to rehabilitation phase once adequate pain control is achieved. During this phase, attention is focused on:
  (a) *Flexibility* (overstretching, however, may result in re-bleeds)
  (b) *Muscular function*
    - muscular strength
      isometric
      isotonic (concentric and eccentric)
      isokinetic
    - power
    - muscular endurance
    - muscular coordination
  (c) *Proprioception*
  (d) *General fitness*

(3) The next stage of non-operative management involves focusing on functional and sport-specific exercises and finally return to sport.
  - Walking, running, sprinting, drills
  - Sport-specific skills

NSAIDs and irradiation may play a part in prevention of further heterotopic bone formation but further research is required to establish this role.

Surgery (excision) has a very limited role in management of athletes with myositis ossificans and should only be considered in those athletes with painful bony mass, persistent loss of motion and function despite adequate non-operative management and in whom at least 6 to 12 months has elapsed since the original injury.

Return to sport

As with other sports injuries, return to play is permitted once the athlete is pain free, able to achieve a full range of movement and has regained enough strength to perform their sport-specific activities. Functional testing, which includes assessment of the ability to sprint and to perform specific sporting activities without pain, should also be performed before permitting the athlete to return to play and declaring him or her fit.

The actual time taken for the athlete to return to play depends on the severity of the injury and may be as much as 10 weeks in athletes with severe contusions. The majority of the athletes, however, are able to return to their sports within 4 weeks.

Further reading

Brown TG, Brunet ME. Adult thigh. In: JC DeLee, D Drez, MD Miller (Eds) *Orthopaedic Sports Medicine, Principles and Practice*, 2nd edn. Saunders, 2002: 1481–505.

Larson CM, Almekinders LC, Karas SG, Garrett WE. Evaluating and managing muscle contusions and myositis ossificans. *The Physician & Sports Medicine* 2002; **30**(2).

Thoracolumbar spine fractures

AA Narvani

Although thoracolumbar spine fractures are more common following road traffic accidents, they are also seen in sports such as skiing, snow boarding, equestrian, parachuting, wrestling, gymnastics, rugby, American football and, of course, automobile racing. It is thought that they account for about 10% of all sporting injuries. These injuries usually occur as a result of major trauma, can be stable or unstable and may or may not be associated with neurological deficits.

Classification

There are a number of classification systems for thoracolumbar spine fractures. The most useful systems subdivide these injuries according to the mechanisms of injury and stability of the injuries as assessed by specific columns involved in the injury (three-column theory of Denis).

Mechanism of injury

With this classification, injuries are differentiated according to the mechanism of injury:

(i) Flexion-compression
(ii) Axial compression
(iii) Flexion-distraction
(iv) Rotational fracture-dislocation mechanism
(v) Other mechanism

Three-column model of Denis

With this model, the thoracolumbar spine is divided into three columns:

(i) *Anterior column*: consists of anterior longitudinal ligament, anterior half of the vertebral body and the anterior portion of the annulus fibrosus.
(ii) *Middle column*: contains the posterior half of the vertebral body, posterior aspect of annulus fibrosus, and the posterior longitudinal ligament.
(iii) *Posterior column*: includes bony and ligamentous structures posterior to the posterior longitudinal structure.

With this classification, one needs at least two intact columns for the fracture to be stable.

Incorporation of the mechanism of the injury and the different columns affected gives the following fracture patterns:

(i) *Wedge compression fractures*
   (a) Caused by flexion compression
   (b) Failure of the anterior column only
(ii) *Burst fractures*
   (a) Usually caused by axial compression
   (b) There is failure of the anterior and the middle columns. In the more severe injuries posterior column may be disrupted as well.
(iii) *Flexion-distraction injuries (Chance fracture)*
   (a) The classical Chance fracture is caused by flexion, the axis of which is anterior to the anterior longitudinal ligament, resulting in a horizontal fracture through the middle and bony elements accompanied by disruption of the supraspinous ligament. In other words the middle and posterior columns fail in tension.
   (b) If the axis of flexion is posterior to the longitudinal ligament, additionally there is also an anterior wedge fracture. This makes the injury very unstable.
(iv) *Fracture-dislocations*
   (a) Usually result from different degrees of shearing, lateral rotation and flexion.
   (b) Involve all three columns and therefore are usually very unstable.
(v) *Others*
   These include isolated fractures of the pars interarticularis, transverse and spinous processes. They are not usually associated with any neurological deficits and are stable; however, they may be accompanied with abdominal and renal injuries as large forces are usually involved.

Clinical features

- There should be strong suspicion of these injuries in athletes involved in major trauma.
- Athletes have back pain with localised tenderness.
- Palpation may also reveal step-offs and spinous process gaps.
- If there is neurological involvement athletes may complain of weakness, numbness, tingling or pins and needles. A thorough neurological examination is required. This should include assessment of the rectal tone and perineal sensation as well as testing for the bulbocavernosus reflex.

Investigations

Plain radiograph

- Should include antero-posterior and lateral views.
- Hairline and undisplaced fractures can be missed.

Computerised tomography

- Will diagnose subtle fractures.
- Gives a more complete detail of the architecture of the bony fracture.
- Provides an indication of the spinal canal occupancy.

Magnetic resonance imaging

- This is the investigation of choice in the presence of any neurological deficits as it is the most sensitive in detecting any compression of the neurological tissue.
- They will also detect ligamentous lesions.

Principles of management

As well as detecting other major associated injuries, the aims of treatment in athletes with thoracolumbar fractures are:

- Prevention and limitation of neurological injury
- Restoration of spinal instability

There are several important basic principles which affect management. These include:

(i) *Adherence to ATLS protocol*
- Spinal immobilisation and log roll in all those with suspected spinal fractures. Initial assessment including airway, breathing and circulation in combination with continued immobilisation. These injuries occur as a consequence of major trauma, therefore they can to be associated with head injuries, abdominal, chest, or limb injuries.

(ii) *Neurological status*
- Despite a number of studies that suggest that surgery may not lead to greater neurological improvement, most clinicians still recommend surgery for athletes with progressive neurological loss or major neurological deficits when there is substantial canal compromise. In such cases, surgery would involve decompression of the neural elements in combination with stabilisation of the injured segment.
- In those athletes for whom surgery is recommended, the timing of surgery is controversial. There does not appear to be clear, conclusive evidence to suggest that early surgical decompression and stabilisation improve neurological recovery. Similarly, there is also a lack of evidence to suggest that neurological recovery is compromised if surgery is delayed by several days.
- The role of steroid use in the acute management of spinal cord injuries also remains controversial. There are some studies that suggest intravenous steroids in acute setting improves neurological deficits; however, there are other studies which have shown no benefits.

(iii) *Stability*
- Stability is defined by White and Punjabi as the "ability of the spine under physiological loads to maintain relationships in such a way that there is neither damage nor subsequent irritation to the spinal cord or nerve roots and, in addition, there is no development of incapacitating deformity and pain". When this ability is lost, the injury is said to be "unstable". How can this

situation be detected clinically? This is when Denis's three-column model can be of great assistance (see above). It is generally thought that if there is damage to two or three columns, then the injury is unstable. Other factors that point towards instability include:
—Progressive neurological deficits
—Greater than 20° of kyphosis
—More than 50% vertebral body height loss
Presence of retropulsed bone fragment in the canal.

- Early surgical stabilisation of unstable fractures can lead to improved fracture reduction, preservation of neurological function and earlier mobilisation. Therefore, surgery is indicated in most athletes with unstable injuries.

(iv) *Deformity*

- This is yet another controversial issue. The relationship between deformity and pain/functional impairment is not clear. Although not universally agreed with, there are those who argue that kyphotic deformity greater than 30° is associated with increased back pain, therefore requires surgical intervention.

(v) *Canal stenosis*

- There are a number of studies that suggest that there is no reliable correlation between the degree of canal stenosis and the severity of neurological deficits. Therefore, non-operative treatment of fractures with canal stenosis of up to 50%, without any neurological deficits, can be successful in selected athletes. Surgery should, however, be offered to those with greater than 50% canal stenosis.

Overall, therefore, there are many controversial issues in management of thoracolumbar fractures. Despite these controversies, non-operative management is clearly indicated for stable fractures that are not associated with any neurological deficits and do not have the potential for progressive deformity. Operative intervention is indicated in athletes with unstable injuries and neurological deficits. Neurologically intact athletes, with greater than 30° kyphosis, 50% loss of vertebral body height and more than 50% stenosis of the canal, should also be considered for surgery.

Management of specific fracture

Wedge compression fractures

As they only involve the anterior column, wedge compression fractures are usually stable injuries and are not associated with any neurological deficit. Those with less than 50% vertebral height loss are treated non-operatively. Depending on the severity of injury, this non-operative management ranges from analgesia and early mobilisation to hyperextension braces or moulded body cast. With greater than 50% vertebral height loss, there is the risk of chronic deformity and pain, and therefore athletes with injuries may be candidates for surgery. Surgery must also be offered to those with progressive deformity, unstable injuries and when there is an associated neurological compromise.

Burst fractures

As these fractures usually involve more than one column, they tend to be more unstable than the wedge compression fractures. The treatment choice can be controversial and may be both non-operative or operative. Burst fractures in athletes with less than 50% height loss, 20° kyphosis and 50% canal stenosis who are neurologically intact, may be treated non-operatively. Athletes with neurological deficits and all those with greater than 50% vertebral height loss, more than 50% stenosis and more than 20° kyphosis are candidates for surgery. Non-operative management involves the use of a well-moulded thoracolumbosacral orthosis, whereas surgery is by decompression and stabilisation.

Fracture-distraction injuries

Sometimes referred to as seat-belt injuries and Chance fractures, these are relatively rare in athletes. Whether treated non-operatively or operatively depends largely on the extent of bony versus soft tissue injury. Those with purely bony injuries are relatively stable and have a good potential for healing, therefore can be treated non-operatively with a thoracolumbosacral orthosis for 3 months. Those with bony injury to the anterior column and soft tissue damage in the middle or posterior column (disc or ligamentous) tend to be more unstable with poorer prognosis for healing, so they can be candidates for surgical stabilisation (particularly if associated with 50% anterior vertebral height loss and 20° kyphosis).

Flexion-dislocation injuries

These are unstable injuries and are usually associated with neurological deficits. They are generally treated with surgical decompression and stabilisation.

Isolated fractures of posterior element structures

Isolated fractures of the pars interarticularis, transverse and spinous processes are usually stable and not associated with any neurological deficits. It is important, however, to exclude other possible associated injuries such as abdominal and renal. Management of the fractures themselves is non-operatively by analgesia and early motion.

Return to sport

Athletes with minor and stable fractures that have been treated non-operatively can return to sport once the fracture has healed provided they have gained pain-free range of movement, and near full muscle strength. Depending on the fracture this can take anything between 8 to 20 weeks. Those who are treated surgically with instrumental stabilisation should generally not be allowed to return to contact sport.

Further reading

Leventhal MR. Fracture, dislocations, and fracture-dislocations of the spine. *Campbell's Operative Orthopaedics*, 10th edn. Mosby, 2003: 1597–690.

Vaccaro AR, Kim DH, Brodke DS, Harris M, Chapman J, Schildhauer T, Routt MLC, Sasso RC. Diagnosis and management of thoracolumbar spine fractures. *The Journal of Bone & Joint Surgery (Am)* 2003; **85A**(12): 2456–70.

Training

B Lynn

Regular physical activity leads to better fitness and better health generally. Inactivity, whether from choice or due to injury leads to reduced fitness – the phenomenon of de-training. So what are the long-term changes that take place in the body in response to regular physical activity?

When beginning a training programme, there will often be rapid increases in performance due to neural changes. One learns better technique with practice and there are also increases in motor unit recruitment and in the ability to tolerate discomfort associated with exercise. In this section, however, the focus will be on the physiological and biochemical changes in muscles and in the cardiovascular and respiratory systems.

The responses to strength training are rather different from those for endurance/aerobic training, so these two topics will be considered separately. However, in both cases four principles will recur: overload, specificity, individuality, reversibility. Overload indicates that to get changes we need to push the system a bit. Not necessarily to the limit, but reasonably close to it. Specificity is sometimes obvious (training for endurance versus strength, for example), sometimes surprising (isokinetic training at a fast velocity producing relatively small effects on strength at lower velocities). And of course, some effects are general (e.g. whatever muscle groups we exercise aerobically, if we do it hard enough and long enough then cardiac performance will improve). But overall the general rule is that all training programmes need to be sport-, activity- or muscle group-specific. Individuality indicates that training programmes need to take account of individual differences. You cannot adopt a "one size fits all" approach. And it is important to understand that the response to training is itself variable from subject to subject. This variation is at least 50% genetically predetermined. Everyone will get some fitness increase from training, but in some subjects the rewards will be greater than in others. Finally, reversibility means, as pointed out above, that if you stop physical activity then fitness immediately starts to decline.

Resistance training, increasing muscle force and power

Resistance training to increase muscle strength and power can be done in several different ways. The traditional method is weight training with free weights. This is still widely used as the equipment is cheap and it is straightforward to progress. But a good technique is required and accidents can happen rather more easily than with other exercise methods. Rather similar exercises can be carried out using fixed gym equipment. A different approach is to use isometric contractions. Repeated strong isometric contractions certainly build up muscle maximum force, but the effects turn out to be quite specific for the muscle length used. So to increase strength and power over the range of movement of a muscle requires making contractions at lengths covering this range. By the time this is done for all the major muscle groups, the training session has become rather long. A relatively new method is to use an isokinetic dynamometer, a machine that sets a constant speed of movement and varies the load. This method is convenient for training at a range of speeds. The machine will also give a performance readout for a range of movements. Finally, we will mention plyometrics. This system involves a series of jumps and so uses gravity to develop dynamic loads.

Optimal training programmes involve sets of 3–12 repeat contractions at close to maximum force (typically 80%), not repeated too often. Using larger numbers of repeated contractions are less effective (in terms of performance improvement per training time).

The effects of all the different exercise systems are broadly the same. Muscle force increases, and does so in proportion to increases in muscle cross-sectional area. Tendons and bones also strengthen. Speed of contraction generally stays the same, or may increase. If we look at the level of individual muscle fibres we find that they get larger, and for strength training the hypertrophy is restricted to fast muscle fibres. There also appears to be some switching of phenotype from FF to FR (e.g. see Harridge *et al.* 1998). This is not perhaps what one might expect as FF are faster and more powerful than FR. However, overall, due to hypertrophy of the fast fibres, there can be an overall increase in speed. Slow (S) fibres do not appear to change to FR or FF, even with specific speed training. Neither do the slow fibres hypertrophy. At the level of the myosin molecule, different versions of the myosin heavy chain (MHC) are found in the three types of fibre, MHC I in S fibres, MHC IIa in FR fibres and MHC IIx in FF fibres. In resistance-trained muscles, there is rather more MHC IIa along with the increase in FR fibres. Interestingly, it has recently been shown in an *in vitro* test that speed of movement of myosins with the MHC IIa heavy chain is increased in samples from resistance-trained muscles (Canepari *et al.* 2005). There may therefore be as yet undefined changes going on in the other parts of the actin or myosin molecules following resistance training that will elevate muscle power.

As pointed out above, training effects on muscles are quite specific. They occur only in the muscles exercised and only for the movements that are trained. For example, isometric training of knee extension at a knee angle of 15° produces useful strength increases when tests are done with this knee angle. When, however, knee extension is tested at 60°, little training effect is seen.

Role of growth factors

The increased muscle fibre size appears to be due to the action of locally synthesised splice variants of insulin-related growth factor 1 (IGF-1). One of these, IGF-1Ec has been designated the mechano growth factor (MGF) as it appears to be preferentially induced by mechanical stresses (Goldspink 2005). Another stimulus for muscle hypertrophy is microtrauma. In all cases hypertrophy involves the satellite cells in muscle. In order for existing fibres to grow they need to assimilate extra nuclei from the satellite cells. It also appears that small numbers of new muscle cells may be generated from satellite cells.

Aerobic training

Muscle

At the muscle level, aerobic, endurance training leads to more S and FR fibres and less FF. There are also striking increases in numbers of mitochondria and in the activity of mitochondrial enzymes. Other metabolic enzymes also increase in activity.

Notable here are enzymes involved in beta-oxidation of fatty acids. Thanks to this, more fatty acid can be metabolised by endurance-trained muscle. This is important as after about 1–2 hours, muscle carbohydrate stores run down. Finally there is a marked growth of capillaries. The main effect of the extra capillaries is probably not to reduce diffusion distances, but rather to ensure that blood flow is not too rapid through any given capillary when muscle blood flow is high. A long enough transit time is required to ensure that there is enough time for gas exchange.

Cardiovascular adaptations

Following aerobic training, ventricular volume increases. There is also an increase in contractility and the functional consequence is that resting and maximal stroke volume are both elevated. The increase in resting stroke volume leads to a balancing reduction in heart rate. The reduced heart rate appears to be caused by increased vagal tone as evidenced by the increased heart rate variability seen in trained athletes under resting conditions. Interestingly, maximum heart rate is unchanged. There is also a useful increase in blood volume, with no change in Hb concentration.

Respiratory system

An important consequence of aerobic training is that the breathing muscles become trained themselves! This helps cope with the greater pulmonary ventilation needed to meet the increased oxygen consumption of trained muscles. There is no change in the pulmonary ventilation/oxygen uptake relationship. Resting tidal volume increases with training and the respiratory rate falls.

Further reading

Astrand P-O, Rodahl K, Dahl HA, Stromme SB. Physical training. In: *Textbook of Work Physiology*, 4th edn. Champagne, Illinois: Human Kinetics Europe Ltd, 2003, Chapter 11.

Canepari M *et al.* Effects of resistance training on myosin function studied by the in vitro motility assay in young and older men. *J Appl Physiol.* 2005; **98**: 2390–5.

Goldspink G. Mechanical signals, IGF-I gene splicing, and muscle adaptation. *Physiology (Bethesda)* 2005; **20**: 232–8.

Harridge SD, Bottinelli R, Canepari M, Pellegrino M, Reggiani C, Esbjornsson M, Balson PD, Saltin B. Sprint training, in vitro and in vivo muscle function and myosin heavy chain expression. *J Appl Physiol* 1998; **84**(2): 442–9.

McArdle WD, Katch FI, Katch VL. Training for anaerobic and aerobic power. In: *Exercise Physiology*, 5th edn. Baltimore: Lippincott, Williams and Wilkins, 2001; Chapter 21.

Unexplained underperformance syndrome

B Lynn

Unexplained underperformance syndrome (UPS) is defined as: persistent unexplained performance deficit (agreed by coach and athlete) despite 2 weeks of relative rest. UPS is rarely seen in sprinters or other athletes in explosive events. However, periods of underperformance, accompanied by excessive fatigue, happen to as many as 20% of endurance athletes involved in heavy training programmes. The link with heavy training led to the older designation of "overtraining syndrome". However, factors other than simply training levels are often involved, notably infective illness and non-sports stresses such as personal problems or exams. Hence the designation "underperformance" is to be preferred.

There is clearly a real difficulty for athletes and coaches in distinguishing between the "healthy" exhaustion felt during periods of intense training and the enervating fatigue of UPS. Athletes and coaches are inevitably pushing the boundaries in attempting to improve fitness and performance. Mostly, it works fine and the heavy training gives improved results. But if adequate rest and recuperation are ignored, then UPS can develop.

Reliable early signs would be helpful. Unfortunately all suggestions so far are non-specific. However, it is clearly worth watching out for fatigue building up, any shift towards more anxious and/or depressed moods, or a slightly elevated resting heart rate. But note, none of these, or the many other signs or symptoms suggested so far in the literature, gives a reliable indication of the onset of UPS. Some coaches have found regularly giving the POMS (profile of mood states) questionnaire useful in heading off problems.

The recommended management is never going to be popular. It is basically a large drop in training levels – perhaps even a period of complete rest – followed by a very gradual rebuilding of training levels. During build up, light levels of training are set and the volume is increased, then intensity is increased later. It typically takes 6–12 weeks to get back to high training loads.

Repeated respiratory tract infections can be a prelude, or accompany, UPS. In some instances it is felt that returning to training too soon after an infection may have triggered UPS. There are reported falls in IgA in saliva and other immune system changes during heavy endurance training. However, not everyone with this pattern develops UPS. Raised levels of the cytokine IL6 have been seen after heavy training. Since IL6 is implicated in some illness syndromes it has been proposed that IL6 plays a part in UPS (Robson 2003).

As mentioned above, UPS can also be associated with psychological stresses, not just overtraining. Clearly attention needs to be paid to these. If UPS is accompanied by mood disturbances, these can be addressed. A frequent problem is UPS accompanied by a depression. In this case antidepressants can be helpful. There is no evidence that antidepressants help in recovery when UPS is not accompanied by depression.

Summary

Unexplained underperformance, despite 2 weeks of rest, defines unexplained underperformance syndrome (UPS).

Commonly due to overtraining, it used to be called overtraining syndrome.

Other stressors may also be involved, not just overtraining.

Management is rest then gradual resumption of training.

Further reading

Angeli A, Minetto M, Dovia A, Paccotti P. The overtraining syndrome in athletes: a stress-related disorder. *J Endocrinol Invest* 2004; **27**(6): 603–12.

Budgett R, Castell LM, Newsholme EA. Overtraining and immunosuppression. In: M Harries (Ed) *Oxford Textbook of Sports Medicine*. Oxford: Oxford University Press, 1998.

Budgett R, Newsholme E, Lehmann M, Sharp C, Jones D, Peto T, Collins D, Nerurkar R, White P. Redefining the overtraining syndrome as the unexplained underperformance syndrome. *Br J Sports Med* 2000; **34**(1): 67–8.

Robson P. Elucidating the unexplained underperformance syndrome in endurance athletes: the interleukin-6 hypothesis. *Sports Med* 2003; **33**(10): 771–81.

Urinary tract injuries

P Thomas

Renal injuries

Haematuria is the symptom present in ruptures or contusions but absent in avulsions where the vascular pedicle is still intact. The pain the athlete experiences is at the renal angle below the twelfth rib. IVP investigation or CT scan will assist diagnosis.

An avulsion that has occurred beyond 12 hours will require a nephrectomy but renal ruptures can be treated with partial or complete kidney salvage. In cases of perinephric tamponade ruptures, then surgery is necessary because of hypovolaemia.

Following renal injury, a persistent hypertension may exist and it will need attention.

Counseling and advice should be provided to the individual athlete with a solitary kidney on the risks, although low, in taking part in contact sports.

Bladder injuries

Such injuries are usually associated with a full bladder during contact sport. A cystogram will assist diagnosis. Intra-peritoneal rupture will require laparotomy and repair. However, with an extra-peritoneal rupture then bladder drainage alone is sufficient in the majority of defects.

Urethral injuries

Usually they occur from a kick to the groin or a fall onto an object such as a bicycle handlebar. The athlete will present with an inability to void or the presence of blood in the urine. A urethrogram is diagnostic. A urine catheter must not be introduced until the diagnosis is made to avoid risk of creating a false urethral passage.

Scrotum injuries

They are common and obvious injuries. They can be classified as contusions, haematoma, torsion or rupture of the testicle. It is important to organise an ultrasound scan to distinguish between a traumatic haematoma and the presence of a tumor, which could be detected in young individuals.

Further reading

Zachazewski JE *et al.* (Eds) *Athletic Injuries and Rehabilitation*. Philadelphia: WB Saunders, 1996.

Index

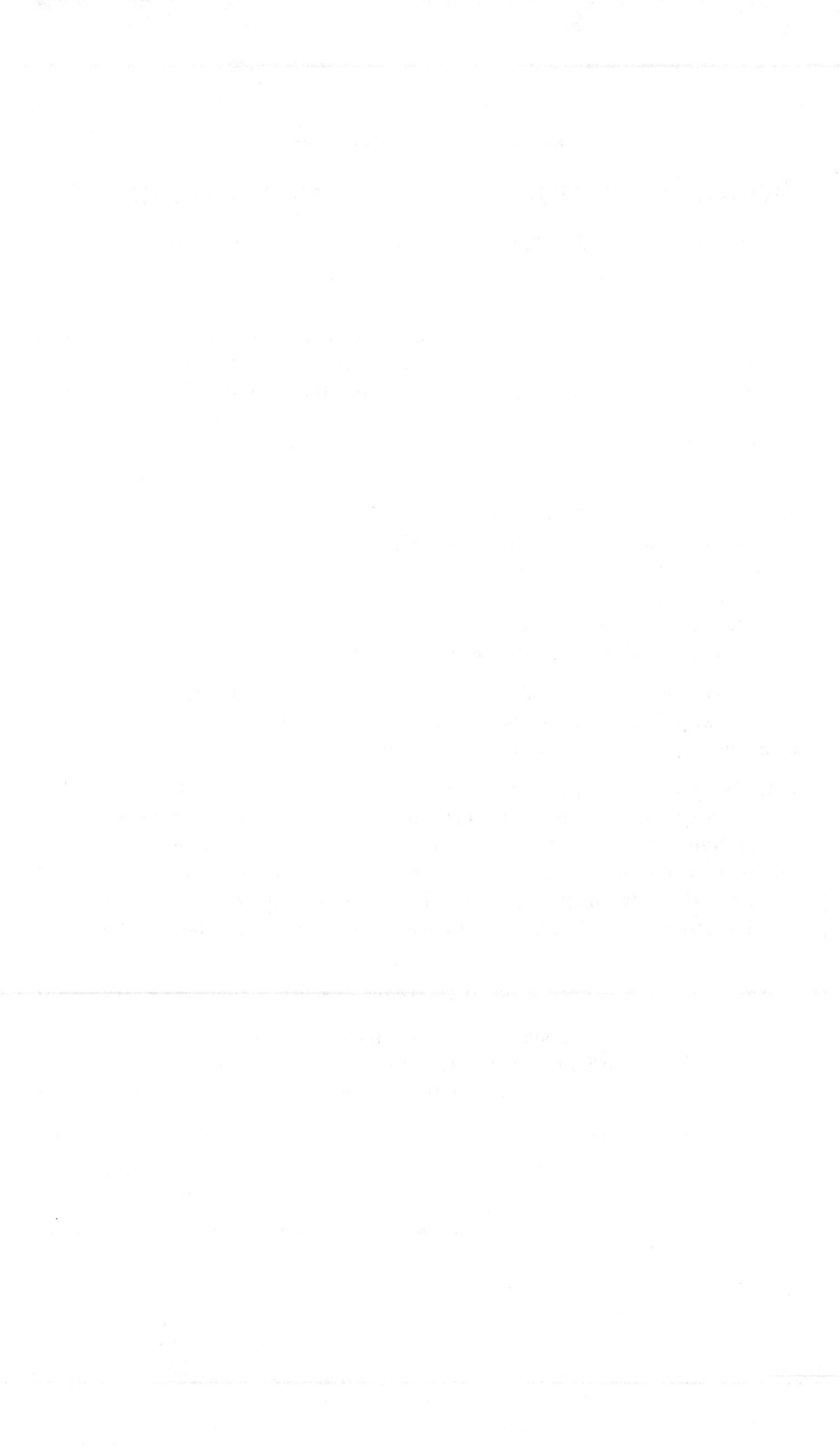

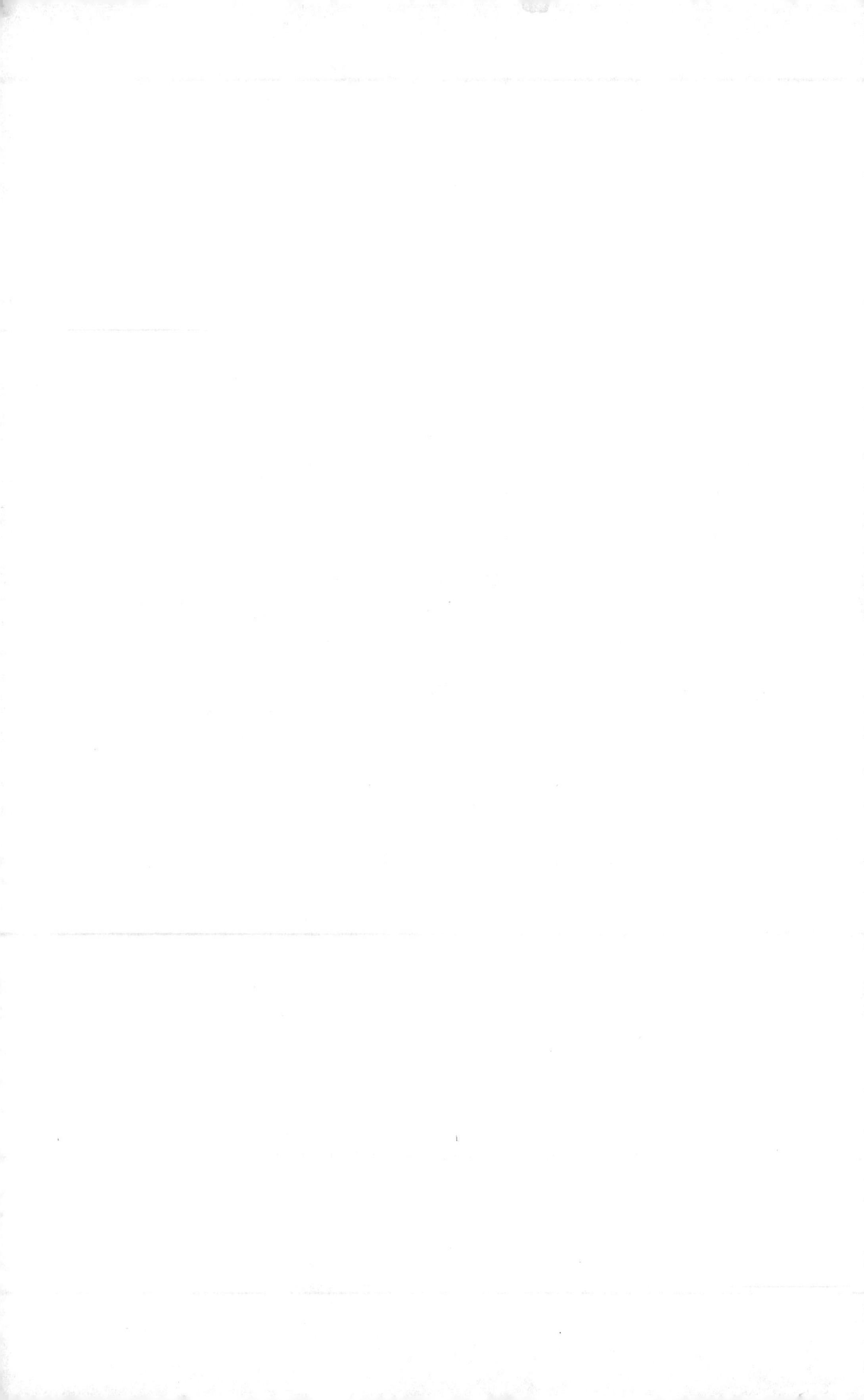